The Handbook:
A Practical Guide for Clinicians

Second Edition

Gary S. Marshall, MD

Professor of Pediatrics
Chief, Division of Pediatric Infectious Diseases
University of Louisville School of Medicine

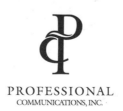

PROFESSIONAL
COMMUNICATIONS, INC.

Professional Communications, Inc.

A Medical Publishing Company

400 Center Bay Drive
West Islip, NY 11795
(t) 631/661-2852
(f) 631/661-2167

PO Box 10
Caddo, OK 74729-0010
(t) 580/367-9838
(f) 580/367-9989

For orders only, please call
1-800-337-9838
or visit our website at
www.pcibooks.com

ISBN: 978-1-932610-37-6

Printed in the United States of America

DISCLAIMER

The opinions expressed in this publication reflect those of the author. However, the author makes no warranty regarding the contents of the publication. The protocols described herein are general and may not apply to a specific patient. Any product mentioned in this publication should be taken in accordance with the prescribing information provided by the manufacturer.

This text is printed on recycled paper.

TABLE OF CONTENTS

TABLES

FIGURES

Preface

In 1982, children in the United States received one shot series (5 DTPs followed by a Td booster), one oral vaccine series (4 or 5 OPVs), and one MMR by 18 years of age…7 injections, a few sugar cubes, and 7 diseases prevented. Today, children and adolescents routinely receive 11 or 12 vaccination series—HepB, rotavirus, DTaP, Hib, PCV7, IPV, yearly influenza vaccine, MMR, varicella, HepA, MCV4, and HPV vaccine (for girls)—as many as 50 injections (47 for boys), 3 oral doses, and 16 dreadful diseases prevented! Unequivocally, vaccination is one of the greatest public health achievements of the 20th century. We enjoy a freedom from contagious diseases that is unprecedented in human history and could not have been imagined by our parents.

As we have gained freedom from disease we have accumulated unforeseen challenges. Providers are faced with dispensing multiple antigens that have catchy trade names and come in various combinations made by different manufacturers, a vaccine alphabet soup that is difficult to keep straight. The business of vaccine practice has become complicated. Parents read on the Internet and hear on television that vaccines are dangerous and that vaccine policy is driven by a conspiracy of unscrupulous profiteers; this leads to vaccination hesitancy that at best prolongs the well child visit, and at worst results in refusal to vaccinate…which leads to outbreaks of disease. Translating the science of vaccinology into layman's terms has become a critical skill as patients bring more in-depth questions into the exam room and demand more sophisticated answers. Adults do not get immunized as they should. There are vaccines for persons with particular risks, and particular risks of vaccines for certain persons. Recurrent shortages, frequent changes in official recommendations, labyrinthine guidances and regulations—these things characterize today's vaccination environment.

The Vaccine Handbook has a simple purpose: to draw authoritative information about vaccines together into a simple, concise, user-friendly, practical resource that can be used in the private office, public health clinic, or on the hospital wards. There are already several excellent books about vaccines. The definitive textbook is *Vaccines*, edited by Stan Plotkin, Walt Orenstein, and Paul Offit (Elsevier; 2008). This book, which is encyclopedic in scope and rich in content, remains the essential reference for specialists and scientists. Books that coherently translate the complex world of vaccinology into terms that lay people can understand include *Vaccines: What You Should Know*, by Paul Offit and Lou Bell (John Wiley & Sons, Inc.; 2003). Two books in particular contain authoritative recommendations: the *Red Book* (*Report of the Committee on Infectious Diseases*), published by the American Academy of Pediatrics (AAP), and the *Pink Book*

(*Epidemiology and Prevention of Vaccine-Preventable Diseases*), published by the Centers for Disease Control and Prevention.

Unlike *Vaccines*, which is geared towards academicians, and unlike books in the popular press, which are geared exclusively towards parents and patients, *The Vaccine Handbook* is geared towards practicing pediatricians, family physicians, internists, obstetrician/gynecologists, nurses, nurse practitioners, physician's assistants, clinic staff, students and residents (some parents might find it useful as well!). Unlike the *Red Book*, which is about infectious diseases, *The Vaccine Handbook* is only about vaccines and the diseases they prevent. It expands on the *Red Book* by including information on the fundamentals of vaccine immunology, development, licensure, policy making, the vaccine safety net and risk-benefit communication. *The Vaccine Handbook* also addresses current public concerns about vaccines, adult vaccination, travel vaccines, billing, legal obligations, and office organization and logistics. It differs from the *Pink Book* as well in the extent to which these topics are covered. Finally, *The Vaccine Handbook* is, well, purple. You can call it *The Purple Book*.

Many things have changed since the first edition was published in 2004. For one, new vaccines have been licensed and recommended for use, including MCV4, LAIV, Tdap, HPV vaccine, zoster vaccine, rotavirus vaccines, and several new combination vaccines. New recommendations have been issued, including yearly influenza immunization for all children, a second dose of varicella vaccine, and universal HepA for children in the second year of life. New concerns about vaccine safety have been raised and addressed in scientific studies. All of these are discussed in the second edition. There also have been some notable additions, including a chapter on the basics of how vaccines work.

The Vaccine Handbook provides enough background for the practitioner to understand the recommendations and explain them to his or her patients. It should be noted that while official recommendations are the foundation of scientific vaccine practice, they have their limitations. They take time to develop and are constrained by precedent, the need for consensus, the big public health picture, and in some cases politics. In addition, not all contingencies and permutations are covered. The language is sometimes definitive (*vaccine X is recommended*), sometimes not definitive (*vaccine X should be considered*), and sometimes vague (*some experts believe vaccine X should be given*). There is even disagreement among sources—the package insert, for example, and the recommendations set forth by the Advisory Committee on Immunization Practices (ACIP) of the Centers for Disease Control and Prevention. Wherever possible, *The Vaccine Handbook* attempts to distill the material down to practical guidances. Where official recommendations do not exist, reasonable suggestions are offered.

One goal we all share is to prevent disease and death without causing harm. Vaccines are a means to this end, and this handbook is intended to provide help along the way.

Gary S. Marshall, MD
Professor of Pediatrics
Chief, Division of Pediatric Infectious Diseases
University of Louisville School of Medicine

Conventions Used in This Book

There is no generally accepted nomenclature for vaccines and no standard for abbreviations. The nomenclature and abbreviations used in this book for disease agents and their respective vaccines are given in **Table 12.1**; they are intended to be intuitive, but the reader may notice some inconsistencies. For example, in some cases, the abbreviation for the agent (eg, "HAV" for "hepatitis A virus") is different from the vaccine (eg, "HepA", which means "hepatitis A vaccine"). In other cases, the abbreviation for the agent (eg, "HPV", which means "human papillomavirus") may be used when referring to the vaccine (eg, "HPV vaccine", which means "human papillomavirus vaccine", or "HPV4", which means "HPV vaccine, 4-valent"). For some vaccines (eg, zoster vaccine), no abbreviation is used. In general, pre-mixed modern combination vaccines are denoted by dashes between the components (eg, "DTaP-HepB-IPV" for a premixed vaccine [Pediarix] containing DTaP, HepB, and IPV); modern combination vaccines that require reconstitution are denoted by a slash mark (eg, "DTaP-IPV/Hib", where the liquid DTaP-IPV is used to reconstitute the lyophilized Hib, creating a combination vaccine [Pentacel]). In general, vaccine trade names use initial capitals only, except where upper and lower case letters are interspersed in the name, as in "TriHIBit". Trademark symbols are not used. Uncommon abbreviations used in the book are defined in the text upon first use; commonly used abbreviations are used in the text without definition.

In general, "age" means that the individual has passed one mark in time but has not yet reached the next relevant mark. For example, "2 months of age" means at or beyond the 2 month birthday but not yet at the 3 month birthday; "4 to 6 years of age" means from the fourth birthday until the day before the seventh birthday. As far as intervals are concerned, "weeks" means 7 days and "months" means 28 days, unless specified as "calendar months". In that case, the interval is to the same date in the appropriate month. For example, for an infant vaccinated on January 6, an interval of 6 calendar months would be on July 6. These definitions are particularly relevant when referring to age indications for vaccines and minimum intervals (eg, **Table 5.1**).

Many organizations provide guidance regarding immunizations. The most generally applicable, authoritative recommendations come from the ACIP, the AAP, and the American Academy of Family Physicians. The recommendations from these organizations are usually very similar, and as such, the ACIP recommendations are referenced in this book. Any differences with other agencies are highlighted.

Each chapter contains a section called "Additional Reading," which includes publications that may be referred to in the text or that provide supplemental information. The list is by no means exhaustive.

Disclaimers

Care has been taken to confirm the accuracy of the information presented herein and to describe generally accepted practices. However, the author, editor, and publisher are not responsible for errors or omissions or for any consequences from application of the information in this book and make no warranty, expressed or implied, with respect to the currency, completeness, or accuracy of the contents of the publication. Application of this information in a particular situation remains the professional responsibility of the practitioner.

The author, editor, and publisher have exerted every effort to ensure that drug selection and dosage set forth in this text are in accordance with current recommendations and practice at the time of publication. However, in view of ongoing research, changes in government regulations, and the constant flow of information relating to drug therapy and drug reactions, the reader is urged to check the package insert and published or posted recommendations for each drug or vaccine discussed, being aware that there may be changes in indications, dosage, or schedule, and that added warnings and precautions may have been issued. This is particularly important when the recommended agent is a new or infrequently employed drug. Some drugs and medical devices presented in this publication have Food and Drug Administration (FDA) clearance for limited use in restricted research settings. It is the responsibility of health care providers to ascertain the FDA status of each drug or device planned for use in their clinical practice.

This book represents a major revision and update of *The Vaccine Handbook: A Practical Guide for Clinicians* (©2004, Lippincott Williams & Wilkins; Philadelphia, PA.). Some of the material from the original work that was contributed by Drs. Penelope H. Dennehy, David P. Greenberg, Paul A. Offit, and Tina Q. Tan is retained here, with the respective authors' express permission. In addition, some of the material in this book was previously published in *The Vaccine Quarterly* (©2007-2008, Wolters Kluwer Health) and is reprinted here with permission.

Acknowledgements

The author is deeply indebted to Drs. Penny Dennehy, Tina Tan, David Greenberg, and Paul Offit for their contributions to the first edition, which have been modified and expanded upon herein with their permission. Appreciation is also extended to the many other people who contributed to this work through conversation and comment, including Dr. Litjen Tan from the American Medical Association and Dr. Bill Atkinson from the Centers for Disease Control and Prevention. Finally, the author would like to thank Dr. Sharon Humiston from the University of Rochester and Dr. Jim Conway from the University of Wisconsin for their superb, comprehensive review of the manuscript and many, many helpful suggestions.

Dedication

For Cherie, Emily and Cullen

Introduction to Vaccinology

Immunization

Immunization is the process of protecting individuals from disease by making them immune. This is most often accomplished *actively* through *vaccination*, the delivery of antigens to the host for purposes of stimulating an immune response. It can also be accomplished *passively* by the administration of antibodies. While not technically correct in all instances, the terms *vaccination* and *immunization* are used interchangeably throughout this book.

■ Active Immunization

Table 1.1 gives one approach to classifying vaccines that have been used in humans. *Live vaccines* replicate in the host and generate immune responses that mimic those induced by natural infection. They are generally *attenuated*, or weakened, in some fashion such that they cause subclinical infection and very little risk of disease. Three approaches to attenuation are represented in our current repertoire of vaccines.

- *Serial passage*—This is the classic method of attenuating viruses, dating back to the 1930s when Thieler passaged yellow fever virus in eggs 200 times in order to weaken it. For viruses, serial passage is now most often accomplished in animal or human cell cultures. The mechanisms of attenuation are not clear but probably involve the accumulation of deletions and mutations that, while adapting the virus to growth in vitro, render the virus less fit (but still capable of replicating) in vivo. The modern prototype live attenuated virus vaccine was developed by Sabin, who passaged the poliovirus serially in monkey cells and demonstrated that oral administration of the attenuated virus protected against polio. Serial passage also was used to attenuate measles, mumps, and rubella viruses for use in vaccines. The virus used to make the varicella vaccine was originally isolated from a child in Japan in the early 1970s. It was serially passaged in human embryonic lung, embryonic guinea pig, and WI-38 (human diploid) cells in order to achieve attenuation, and it is currently produced in MRC-5 (human diploid) cells. The most recent example of the use of serial passage is the human rotavirus vaccine (HRV), which was derived from a strain of rotavirus that circulated in Cincinnati in the late 1980s. That virus was initially passaged 26 times in Vero (African green monkey kidney) cells in order to achieve attenuation.

  Attenuation of bacteria dates back to the mid 1800s, when Pasteur protected animals from anthrax using a form of the bacterium that had been weakened using chemicals. In

TABLE 1.1 — Classification of Vaccines[a]

Live Attenuated			Inactivated				
				Component			
Classic Bacterial	Classic Viral	Engineered Agent	Whole Agent	Toxoid	Purified Subunit(s)	Engineered Subunit(s)	Recombinant
Tuberculosis (BCG)[b]	Adenovirus (oral)[b] Measles Mumps Polio (oral)[b] Rotavirus (human, oral)[b] Rubella Smallpox Varicella Yellow fever Zoster	Cholera (CVD 103-HgR, oral)[b] Influenza (intranasal) Rotavirus (bovine re-assortant, oral) Typhoid (oral)	Cholera: (whole cell)[b] (WC/rBS, oral)[b,c] Hepatitis A Influenza (whole virus)[b] Japanese encephalitis Pertussis (whole cell)[b] Plague[b] Polio (IPV) Rabies Typhoid (whole cell)[b]	Diphtheria Tetanus	Anthrax (cell-free filtrate) Cholera (WC/rBS, oral)[b,c] Hepatitis B (plasma-derived HBsAg)[b] Hib polysaccharide[b] Influenza (split virus) Meningococcal (serogroup B) outer membrane protein vesicle[d] Meningococcal	Hib conjugate Meningococcal conjugate Pneumococcal conjugate	Hepatitis B (HBsAg) Human papillomavirus (L1 protein) Lyme disease (rOspA)[b]

14

polysaccharide
Pertussis (acellular)
Pneumococcal
   polysaccharide
Typhoid (Vi
   polysaccharide)

[a] Listed vaccines are administered parenterally unless otherwise noted.
[b] No longer or never available in the United States.
[c] Contains both whole-inactivated organisms and a recombinant-derived subunit.
[d] Not yet available in the United States.

vitro passage also has been used to attenuate bacteria. For example, Bacille Calmette-Guérin (BCG), a vaccine that protects against disseminated tuberculosis, was a strain of *Mycobacterium bovis* originally isolated from a cow in 1908 and passaged over 200 times in culture (*M bovis* is related to *M tuberculosis*).

• *Heterologous host*—This method dates back to the late 1700s, when Jenner used cowpox to protect humans from smallpox. The modern smallpox vaccine, consisting of a virus called vaccinia, is not the cowpox virus per se but rather a hybrid of cowpox and variola virus (the scientific name for smallpox) that does not exist in nature. Nevertheless, Jenner established the principle that animal viruses can induce immunity to human diseases. Cowpox is not necessarily attenuated for humans—it does cause lesions, as does vaccinia (in fact, if smallpox vaccination does not result in a lesion, it is not considered to have been effective). However, other animal viruses are naturally attenuated for humans. For example, one of the available rotavirus vaccines, PRV, was derived from a bovine strain of rotavirus (WC3) that can replicate in humans but does not cause disease. Unfortunately, it also does not induce sufficient protective antibody to human strains, so it had to be engineered to express immunogenic surface proteins of human rotaviruses. This was accomplished through *reassortment*, whereby the parental strain was cocultured with natural human strains. Bovine viruses that "accidentally" packaged genes for the human G or P proteins (the dominant protective antigens) were selected and propagated. The vaccine strains, then, consist of viruses that in every way are identical to the naturally attenuated bovine virus, except for the fact that each one expresses an immunogenic human protein instead of the corresponding bovine protein.

• *Engineered attenuation*—Today, the attenuated phenotype can be engineered into vaccines. A good example of this is the oral typhoid (Ty21a) vaccine, which was derived from *Salmonella typhi* strain Ty2 after treatment with a mutagenic agent and selection for attenuation. Another example is the live-attenuated influenza vaccine (LAIV). Here, influenza virus was serially passaged in chick embryo cells at successively lower temperatures, selecting for mutants that grow well in the cold (77°F [25°C)]). As it happens, these strains grow poorly at core body temperature. After intranasal inoculation, they replicate well in the relatively cooler nasal passages, thereby generating broad-based systemic and mucosal immune responses. Their attenuation comes in the fact that they cannot replicate in the lower airways and therefore cannot cause pneumonia or more serious influenza syndromes. Each year, a new set of LAIV viruses must be constructed, incorporating genes for the hemagglutinin and neuraminidase (the dominant protective antigens) for the strain anticipated in the next season. This is accomplished through reassortment, as described earlier.

Other approaches to attenuation have been used. For example, the attenuated phenotype can be achieved by something as simple as using an unnatural route of inoculation. The best example of this was the adenovirus vaccine used in the military in the 1970s and 1980s. This consisted of enteric-coated tablets, one containing live (intrinsically unattenuated) adenovirus type 4, and the other, type 7. These viruses are pathogenic in the respiratory tract, but when given in the gastrointestinal tract they replicate without causing disease.

Inactivated vaccines may consist of whole, inactivated microbial agents or specific microbial components that are derived through physical, chemical, or molecular means. Inactivated *whole-agent* vaccines date back to the late 1800s, when Pasteur used killed rabies virus (derived from dried rabbit spinal cords) to protect animals and, eventually, humans against rabies. The modern prototype inactivated whole-virus vaccine was developed by Salk, who grew the poliovirus in cell culture, purified it, inactivated it with formaldehyde, and demonstrated that intramuscular injection of the inactivated virus protected against polio. The hepatitis A, Japanese encephalitis, and modern rabies vaccines are made in much the same way. The modern prototype whole-bacterial vaccine is whole-cell pertussis, which was made from suspensions of cultured *Bordetella pertussis* organisms that were killed and detoxified. Because it contained every antigen from the live organism, this vaccine was both effective and reactogenic.

Component vaccines include toxoids, which are protein toxins that have been chemically modified to reduce pathogenicity but retain immunogenicity. The only current toxoid vaccines are those for diphtheria, tetanus and pertussis. Other component vaccines are made from *purified subunits* of the organism. The original hepatitis B vaccine, for example, consisted of HBsAg that was purified from the blood of persistently infected individuals (these individuals overproduce HBsAg, which is released from the liver into the plasma). Of course, steps were taken to inactivate any live virus that might have also been present. In order to reduce reactogenicity of the whole cell pertussis vaccine, specific immunogenic proteins (inactivated pertussis toxin, filamentous hemagglutinin, pertactin, and fimbrial antigens) were purified from whole organisms and formulated into acellular vaccines. For *Streptococcus pneumoniae, Haemophilus influenzae, Neisseria meningitidis*, and *S typhi*, it was known that the capsular polysaccharide was the immunogenic part of the bacterium. Subunit vaccines were therefore developed using capsular polysaccharide that was stripped from the cell and purified.

Pure polysaccharide vaccines, however, induce only short-term immunity, do not produce immunologic memory, and are not immunogenic in young infants. *Engineered subunits* in the form of protein-polysaccharide conjugates are necessary to overcome these problems (see below). Subunits can also be produced through *recombinant DNA* technology. The prototype here is the recombinant-derived hepatitis B vaccine, in which the gene for HBsAg was inserted into yeast cells, which then produced large quantities of the protein for purification. A similar method was used to produce the quadrivalent HPV vaccine. In this case, the gene for the L1 protein was expressed in yeast cells. The nice thing about L1 is that it spontaneously aggregates into virus-like particles, which in every way look like viruses on the outside but which carry no genetic material and are, therefore, incapable of replicating.

Table 1.2 lists general characteristics of live and inactivated vaccines. These properties have very real consequences in practice, affecting storage conditions, scheduling, expected efficacy, contraindications, and the potential for adverse reactions. Some implications of these characteristics, as well as exceptions to the generalizations, are given in the footnotes, and the following section on vaccine immunology provides explanations for some of these characteristics.

■ Passive Immunization

Passive immunization is the process by which short-term protection from disease is conferred through the administration of antibodies. This process occurs naturally during the last 2 months of pregnancy, when large quantities of IgG are transferred across the placenta to the fetus, and it explains the relative protection that newborns enjoy against invasive pneumococcal and *Haemophilus influenzae* type b infections, among others. Passive immunization is necessary for patients with humoral immune defects who cannot synthesize their own antibody; in these cases, *polyclonal immune globulin* is used. For example, patients with agammaglobulinemia receive monthly infusions of IGIV to prevent a broad range of infections. Polyclonal immune globulin is also used to prevent certain specific infections, such as measles and hepatitis A, because the titer of antibody to these agents is sufficiently high in the general population from whom the immune globulin is derived.

Passive immunization also is useful for individuals at risk for particular infections; in such cases, *hyperimmune globulins*, derived from donors with high antibody levels to the pathogen, are used. One example is varicella zoster immune globulin (VariZIG), which is used for prevention of chickenpox in exposed immunocompromised individuals. Another example is hepatitis B immune globulin (HBIG), which is used in neonates born to mothers who are chronic hepatitis B carriers and also in other susceptible individuals who are exposed to the virus. It should be understood that hyperimmune globulins also contain antibodies to pathogens besides the one they target; this is true because the individuals from whom they are derived, while selected for their

18

high antibody titers to specific pathogens, also have antibodies to other agents. Although immune globulin products are made from blood, current donor screening and processing of the antibodies make the risk of transmission of blood-borne pathogens negligible. Antibodies can be *engineered* for prevention of specific diseases, as in the case of RSVmAB (Synagis), a monoclonal antibody that has the effector (constant) region of human IgG but the combining (antigen recognition) region of a mouse monoclonal antibody specific for the RSV F protein (which mediates fusion of the viral envelope to the host cell membrane—blocking this prevents infection). *Antitoxins*, also known as heterologous hyperimmune sera, are also used for passive immunization. These are produced in animals like horses and target toxins such as diphtheria, botulism, and tetanus.

Whether passive immunization occurs *intentionally*, as when IGIM is administered for prevention of hepatitis A, or *unintentionally*, as when antibodies accompany blood products transfused for other reasons (eg, IGIV for Kawasaki disease), passively acquired polyclonal antibodies can inactivate live-attenuated viral vaccines, such as measles and varicella. RSVmAB, which is specific for RSV alone, does not inactivate live vaccines. Yellow fever vaccine (which is also live-attenuated) does not appear to be inactivated by commercially available polyclonal immune globulin products in the United States, probably because the titer of yellow fever antibody in the donors from whom these products are derived is low. **Table 5.2** gives the recommended intervals between receipt of antibody-containing blood products and live vaccines.

Basic Vaccine Immunology

Entire textbooks have been written about the immune response, and many of the details have been worked out at the molecular level. Despite the complexity, only a few basic concepts are necessary in order to understand how vaccines mediate protection against disease. These concepts shed light on the differences between various types of vaccines, the duration of protection, dosing schedules, and other aspects of vaccine practice that are delineated elsewhere in this book.

Vaccines are designed to generate pathogen-specific antibodies and T cells by stimulating the *adaptive immune system*, which recognizes and remembers specific pathogens and learns to respond to them more strongly after each exposure. What follows is a simplified version of the immune mechanisms that underpin vaccination—in essence, what you need to know to understand how vaccines work.

■ Antibodies
Antibodies are proteins that bind to 3-dimensional patterns, or *epitopes*, that are present on *antigens* (substances on the microbe that are foreign to the host and engender immune responses).

TABLE 1.2 — Generalizations About Live and Inactivated Vaccines

Characteristic	Live Vaccines	Inactivated Vaccines
Immune response	Humoral and cell-mediated	Mostly humoral[a]
Dosing	1 dose usually sufficient[b]	Multiple-dose primary series and booster doses usually required[c]
Adjuvant[d]	Not neceessary	May be necessary[e]
Route of administration	SC, PO, or intranasal	SC or IM
Duration of immunity	Potentially lifelong	Booster doses usually required[f]
Person-to-person transmission	Possible[g]	Not possible
Inactivation by passively acquired antibodies	Possible[h]	Less likely[i]
Use in immunocompromised hosts	May cause disease	Cannot cause disease
Use in pregnancy[j]	Fetal infection theoretically possible[k]	Fetal damage theoretically unlikely
Storage requirements	Reflect need to maintain viability	Reflect need to maintain chemical and physical stability
Simultaneous adminstration at separate sites	Acceptable	Acceptable
Interval between doses of the *same* vaccine given in sequence	Minimum intervals apply	Minimum intervals apply
Interval between doses of *different* vaccines given in sequence	Minimum intervals apply	No minimum intervals[l]

a Some inactivated vaccines stimulate limited humoral responses. For example, polysaccharide vaccines (eg, the original Hib vaccine, MPSV4, and PPSV23) induce short-lived IgM responses and do not result in immunologic memory. Engineering can overcome these limitations, as in the conjugation of polysaccharides to protein carriers. Protein vaccines can induce memory responses that are T-helper cell dependent.

b Although 1 dose of MMR or varicella vaccine may be sufficient to induce long-lasting immunity, second doses are given before school entry to ensure that children who did not seroconvert to the first dose have another chance to do so (the second dose is therefore not a booster in the classic sense). Live oral vaccines such as OPV, PRV, HRV, and typhoid Ty21a are given in multiple-dose series.

c Some inactivated vaccines, such as PPSV23 for older adults, are given as a single dose. In this case, individuals have probably been previously primed by natural exposure to *Streptococcus pneumoniae*. At the present time, MCV4 is given as a single dose to adolescents; ongoing studies could indicate that reimmunization is necessary.

d Adjuvants are substances that enhance immune responses by slowing the release of antigen or by enhancing delivery to, increasing uptake by, and inducing maturation of antigen-presenting cells. The most common adjuvant used in vaccines is alum, a generic term for a variety of aluminum salts.

e One Hib vaccine, TIV, MCV4, MPSV4, PPSV23, IPV, JE vaccine, and rabies vaccine do not contain adjuvants.

f Long-term protection has been demonstrated for some inactivated vaccines, such as HepA and HepB, in the absence of booster doses.

g This phenomenon has been relevant for OPV, where horizontal transmission probably contributed to immunity at the population level but also on rare occasion from smallpox vaccinees represents a real risk to susceptible close contacts. Transmission of vaccinia from smallpox vaccinees represents a real risk to susceptible close contacts. Transmission of MMR, Ty21a, PRV, HRV, and YF vaccine has not been documented but is extremely rare. Transmission of varicella vaccine and LAIV has been documented but is extremely rare.

h This phenomenon is most relevant for MMR and varicella vaccine and is the reason why these vaccines are not given in the first year of life, when passively acquired maternal antibodies can interfere with take. Receipt of antibody-containing products does not affect the take of Ty21a, LAIV, or the YF vaccine. Although deferral of rotavirus vaccine is indicated for 42 days after receipt of an antibody-containing product (unless this will preclude giving the first dose at the recommended age), the risk of decreased take is largely theoretical. See **Table 5.2** for recommended intervals between antibody-containing products and live vaccines.

i Passively acquired maternal antibodies may interfere with the take of HepA; vaccination is therefore recommended in the second year of life. To avoid antigen-antibody interactions, antibody-containing products are not administered at the same site as inactivated vaccines.

j Most vaccines are classified as Pregnancy Category C (see Chapter 7, *Vaccination in Special Circumstances*).

Continued

TABLE 1.2 — *Continued*

k This possibility leads to the general recommendation that live vaccines are contraindicated in pregnancy, although there are some exceptions (see *Chapter 7*).

l The AAP suggests a minimum interval of 1 month between Tdap and MCV4 if the vaccines are not given on the same day (the concern here is that both vaccines contain diphtheria toxoid [it is used as the carrier protein in MCV4]—too many doses of diphtheria toxoid in sequence can cause increased reactogenicity). However, the ACIP does not recommend a minimum interval.

Antibodies constitute the humoral, or soluble, arm of the adaptive immune system, and are produced as several different immunoglobulin *isotypes* (IgG, IgA, IgM, IgE, IgD) that differ in function. A given antibody with a given antigenic specificity can be produced as one of several different isotypes. Antibody binding is *specific* in that each antibody molecule binds best to one particular epitope; any given antigen may have many different epitopes, and any given microbe may have hundreds of different antigens. Binding of antibodies to viruses or toxins can lead to *neutralization*, ie, the blocking of ligands or receptors that are critical for infectivity or toxicity. Binding of antibodies to bacteria can lead to *opsonization* (coating of the organism) so that it can be pulled out of circulation by cells of the reticuloendothelial system or so that it can be killed by *complement-mediated lysis* (fixing of complement proteins on the surface, forming a *membrane attack complex* that kills the organism). Binding of antibodies to virus-infected cells can lead to *antibody-dependent cell-mediated cytotoxicity*, whereby the infected cell is flagged for destruction by natural killer cells, monocytes, and eosinophils.

Antibodies are the only element of the adaptive immune system that can *prevent* viral infection because they can neutralize the virus before it has a chance to replicate in cells. They are also the mainstay of protection against bacterial invasion since they facilitate destruction of the inoculating organism before it has a chance to reproduce. The battle between antibodies and pathogens takes place at different sites. At mucosal surfaces, where most pathogens try to gain entry, secretory IgA and serum IgG antibodies that leak across from the vascular space are important. Live vaccines that replicate at the mucosal surface (eg, LAIV) have the advantage of inducing strong local IgA responses that can neutralize pathogens before invasion. Vaccines given intramuscularly or subcutaneously are not as good at generating secretory IgA at mucosal surfaces, although this does happen. A vaccine that induces high levels of serum IgG not only can protect against bloodstream invasion or infection in extravascular spaces, but also can block infection at mucosal sites before the organism gains a foothold.

Antibodies are produced by plasma cells, which are derived from B lymphocytes or B cells. B cells have immunoglobulins on their surface (mostly IgM) that express one and only one antibody specificity. During ontogeny, genetic rearrangements lead to a diversity of B-cell clones, each with its own unique antibody specificity (those B cells that emerge from this process with surface immunoglobulins that recognize self antigens are deleted). People are, therefore, walking around with millions of B cells, each precommitted to recognizing one and only one epitope. When a given B cell binds to its antigenic match, it becomes activated and proliferates (this is known as *clonal expansion*); the daughter cells eventually differentiate into plasma cells, the factories that secrete large amounts of antibody.

There are two basic pathways through which antibody production occurs, and the differences between them are important to understanding how vaccines work.

■ The Extrafollicular Reaction

The extrafollicular reaction, one of the pathways for antibody production, is best exemplified by the immune response to polysaccharides (**Figure 1.1**). A precommitted B cell encounters its polysaccharide match (at the site of inoculation with a vaccine or perhaps in a lymph node to which the vaccine antigen was transported), leading to activation, proliferation, and rapid differentiation into plasma cells, which migrate to the red pulp of the spleen and intramedullary areas of lymph nodes. There the plasma cells begin to produce antibodies. It is important to understand that these are *germline* antibodies, ie, antibodies transcribed from genes that were present in the B cell to begin with. Germline antibodies have low affinity for their corresponding antigens because the genes from which they are transcribed, the sequence of amino acids, the shape of their combining site, and thus their ability to bind to the antigen was determined by a random process way back when the person was a fetus. These B cells (and their genes) were selected during ontogeny because they recognized nonself antigens, not because they would someday bind especially tightly

FIGURE 1.1 — Polysaccharide Antigens and the Extrafollicular Reaction

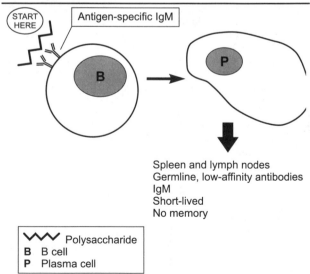

See *The Extrafollicular Reaction* section within the text for a complete explanation.

to those particular antigens. Furthermore, most of the antibodies produced in the extrafollicular reaction are of the same isotype that was present on the B-cell surface, namely IgM, which does not offer the functional benefits of other isotypes such as IgG. Finally, the plasma cells produced through the extrafollicular reaction ultimately die out—no more antibodies produced, no more protection, no ability to remember the encounter and respond more quickly or decisively the next time.

This is called the *extrafollicular reaction* because it takes place outside of the germinal centers of lymph nodes. Antigens that elicit this response are called *T-independent* because the responding B cells differentiate without much T-cell interaction. The characteristics of T-independent responses—rapid production (days to weeks) of short-lived, low-affinity, predominantly IgM antibodies without induction of memory—are hallmark features of the response to pure polysaccharide antigens, such as those in the original *H influenzae* vaccine, PPSV23, and MPSV4. To compound the problem with polysaccharides, children <2 years of age do not mount robust T-independent responses, making these vaccines poor immunogens in that age group.

It is important to point out that there is some crossover between the immunologic pathways. For example, some degree of T-cell help (see below) may be available to extrafollicular B cells, such that some isotype switching occurs and some memory may be generated.

■ The Germinal Center Reaction

Underpinning the adaptive immune system is the much more primitive *innate immune system*, capable of initiating the battle against an invading microorganism in a nonspecific fashion. Cells of the innate immune system—most notably dendritic cells and monocytes—carry receptors that recognize conserved patterns among pathogens (*pathogen-specific molecular patterns*) that are not found in self tissues. Among the most important of these are *Toll-like receptors* (TLRs), each of which recognizes a different pattern. TLR3, for example, recognizes double-stranded viral RNA; TLR2 binds lipopolysaccharide, and TLR6 binds bacterial flagellins. Engagement of pattern-recognition receptors activates the cell, which then secretes *cytokines* (intercellular communication molecules) that activate and recruit other cells, setting up an inflammatory reaction. The end result might be destruction of the invader through processes such as phagocytosis. Importantly, this is a one-time occurrence—once the pathogen is destroyed, there is no memory of the encounter that might facilitate a response the next time around.

Why do vaccinologists care about innate immunity if it provides no memory? The answer lies in the fact that activation of the innate immune system can trigger an adaptive immune response. The key link is provided by *antigen-presenting cells* (APCs), the most important of which are dendritic cells (**Figure**

1.2). Immature APCs circulate through the body or reside in tissues (immature dendritic cells in the dermis are called *Langerhans cells*). When a pathogen-specific molecular pattern is encountered—in the form, for example, of an injected vaccine antigen—the APC cells begin to mature, express new receptors on their surface, and migrate through lymphatic vessels to regional lymph nodes. Some of them also engulf the antigen, degrade the proteins into small peptides, load the peptides into the groove of *major histocompatibility complex (*MHC*) class II molecules* (MHC-II), and express those molecules on their surface.

The mature APC is now activated (secreting proinflammatory cytokines and expressing costimulatory molecules on its surface), flagged (by the surface expression of antigen-derived peptides in the context of MHC-II), and has migrated to the follicular region of the lymph node. At this stage the APC is ready to engage immature *helper T lymphocytes* (Th cells) by interacting with the *T-cell receptor* (TCR) and the *CD4 coreceptor* (both are on the Th cell). Each Th cell is predetermined to recognize a particular peptide/MHC-II flag by virtue of its TCR and CD4 coreceptor (like the surface immunoglobulin of B cells, the TCR has a unique antigenic specificity; the diversity of TCRs is generated during fetal development by a random process, much like the generation of germline antibodies, and those T cells that emerge from this process with receptors that recognize self antigens are deleted or inactivated). Through soluble cytokines and costimulatory receptor-ligand interactions, contact with the right APC results in activation and maturation of the Th cell into one of two antigen-specific subtypes: Th1 or Th2 cells. Th2 cells have some direct antimicrobial functions, particularly against parasites. More importantly, though, Th2 cells seek out their unique B-cell matches in order to help them make antibody (to the antigen from which the peptide in the MHC groove was originally derived). B cells are primed to be helped by engulfing some of the bound antigen, digesting the proteins, and presenting the peptides on their surface in the context of MHC-II, much like dendritic cells do.

Th1 cells also have direct antimicrobial functions, particularly against viruses. More importantly, though, Th1 cells seek out *cytotoxic T cells* (Tc cells) and macrophages, coaxing them into performing cytotoxic functions (see below). Several factors determine whether a Th cell differentiates into a Th1 or Th2 cell during immunization; among these are the dose of antigen, route of administration, and the effect of *adjuvants*, substances that potentiate the innate immune response. These factors, therefore, also determine whether humoral or cellular responses will predominate.

The interaction between B cells and Th cells takes place in the germinal centers of lymph nodes, hence the name of the reaction. The signals provided by Th2 cells, as well as the persistence of antigen shuttled there by APCs, drive B cells to undergo massive clonal proliferation—producing millions of daughter cells capable

FIGURE 1.2 — Antigen-Presenting Cells and the Germinal Center Reaction

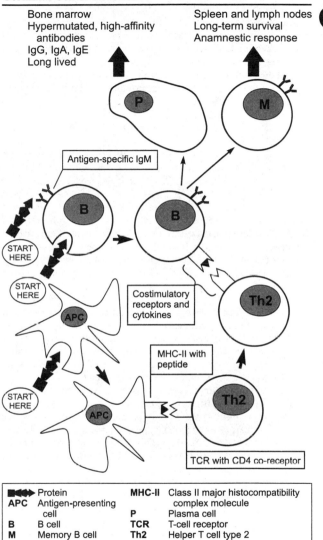

See *The Germinal Center Reaction* section within the text for a complete explanation.

of making the same antibodies. As they proliferate under these conditions, the B cells undergo a process of somatic hypermutation, whereby the genes encoding the immunoglobulin combining region mutate at exceptional rates, randomly producing a spectrum of antibodies with varying affinities for the antigen. Those B cells expressing high-affinity antibodies are selected for and clonally expanded. The end result is a set of dominant B-cell clones that produce high-affinity antibodies, ones that bind the antigen better than the germline antibodies produced in the extrafollicular reaction. The only problem is that this process takes a week or two to get rolling.

Two other things happen in the germinal center. First, signals from Th2 cells drive *isotype switching* as B cells transform into plasma cells. The end result is large numbers of plasma cells that migrate to the bone marrow and produce high-affinity IgG (as well as other isotypes). Second, Th2 cells drive the parallel evolution of *memory B cells*, which migrate to the spleen and lymph nodes and wait there—sometimes for decades—until they again encounter the antigen, at which time they rapidly proliferate and differentiate into plasma cells that produce antibody. This is called the *anamnestic response*. It should be mentioned that memory Th cells are also generated, but their numbers wane with time.

The germinal center reaction has many implications for vaccination.

- *Stimulating innate immunity*—The more innate immunity is stimulated, the more robust the adaptive immune response will be. For example, intradermal vaccination generally stimulates more robust responses than intramuscular injection, probably because there are more immature dendritic cells lying in wait in the dermis. As another example, we know that live viral vaccines are more immunogenic than inactivated ones. One reason is that live viruses can disseminate and encounter dendritic cells at multiple sites, ultimately establishing multiple foci of germinal center reactions. Another reason is that live vaccines carry more recognizable pathogen-specific molecular patterns that are capable of activating innate immune cells. Inactivated vaccines may need help in this regard from adjuvants. The most widely used adjuvant today is alum, an amorphous mixture of aluminum salts that adsorbs antigen, promotes inflammation, and facilitates uptake by APCs.

- *Priming and boosting*—Ultimately, the magnitude and duration of the antibody response to inactivated vaccines depends on the immunologic set point following primary immunization. In other words, the more germinal centers that are formed, the more long-lived plasma cells and memory B cells there will be. In addition to optimizing antigen dose and using adjuvants, *primary immunization* is enhanced by multiple doses of the vaccine given in succession, classically separated by 1 or 2 months (as in the 2-, 4-, and 6-month schedule for primary DTaP immunization). These doses are given too soon to exploit memory responses, but they do drive the process of affinity maturation in the germinal centers. Following priming, vaccine schedules take advantage of anamnestic responses, which boost the level of high-quality antibody (**Figure 1.3**). The need to wait until the germinal center reaction is complete explains the longer interval between the primary series of a vaccine and the booster doses (as in the 15- to 18-month dose of DTaP). The response to booster doses of vaccine mimics what happens when the natural pathogen is encountered.

• *Specificity*—Hypermutated, high-affinity antibodies specifically target single epitopes. For this reason, most inactivated vaccines are very specific in the protection they afford. For

FIGURE 1.3 — Time Course of Antibody Responses

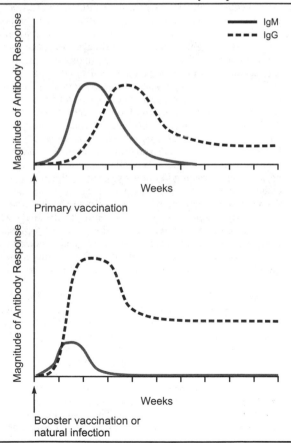

example, IPV contains formalin-inactivated, disrupted viral particles from three different serotypes of poliovirus because the antigens from any given serotype do not induce antibodies that will neutralize the other serotypes. Germinal center reactions by and large generate *homotypic* responses, ones directed against the antigen used as the vaccine. *Heterotypic*, or *cross-protective*, responses occur only if there is sufficient similarity between the antigens of different strains, or if there is a common antigen between them. Tc cells offer much more potential for cross-strain protection (see below).

• *Persistence of antibody*—The germinal center reaction peaks in several weeks, after which it is terminated. The mechanisms by which serum antibodies persist for long periods of time—something so critical to maintaining protection—are not yet worked out. Some models suggest that there is more or less constitutive differentiation of memory B cells into plasma cells, stimulated by persistent antigen, reinfection, or exposure to cross-reactive antigens. Other models propose there is nonspecific, or so-called "bystander", activation of memory B cells, although recent data suggest this mechanism is less important. These models have important implications for vaccine programs. For example, early studies of the varicella vaccine showed persistent if not *rising* titers of antibody over time. But these studies were done at a time when the wild-type virus was still circulating; therefore, immunized individuals might have experienced repeated subclinical reinfections with natural virus, coaxing memory B cells to differentiate into plasma cells and boosting antibody production. As transmission of natural varicella decreased, some studies began to show waning immunity over time (this observation made it less likely that antibody persisted because of boosting from periodic reactivation of latent vaccine virus). Although technically intended to immunize those individuals who failed to seroconvert after the first dose (so-called *primary vaccine failures*), the second dose of varicella vaccine that is now recommended also serves to boost immunity in those individuals whose antibody levels have fallen low enough to allow *take*, or replication of the vaccine virus.

Other models suggest that plasma cells derived from the germinal center reaction can live for a very long time. Either way, for some vaccines, it is necessary to periodically conjure up the anamnestic response through booster vaccination. One thing is clear—to prevent infections with a short incubation period (*N meningitidis* is a good example), one must have a sufficient amount of circulating antibody at the time of encounter with the pathogen. Anamnestic responses, while brisk, are not fast enough to be of much help when dealing with rapidly replicating bacteria. They may be sufficient, however, for pathogens with longer incubation periods. Thus, for example, although antibodies to HBV, and along with them protection from *infection*, may wane with time, protection against *disease* does not wane—there is plenty of time for memory responses to kick in before the virus can do damage.

1

- *Making better immunogens*—As mentioned above, polysaccharides are poor immunogens. Vaccinologists have learned, however, to harness the power of the germinal center reaction to enhance their immunogenicity (**Figure 1.4**). The polysaccharides are chemically attached to protein carriers—among the variety of carriers used are an outer-membrane protein from *N meningitidis* (as in PRP-OMPC or PedvaxHIB), a mutant diphtheria toxin called CRM_{197} (PCV7 or Prevnar), tetanus toxoid (PRP-T or ActHIB), and diphtheria toxoid (MCV4 or Menactra). B cells that are precommitted to producing anti-*polysaccharide* antibody are stimulated by their encounter with the antigen. They also engulf the bound antigen, digest it, and present peptides from the *protein* portion of the vaccine on their surface in the context of MHC-II (polysaccharides cannot be presented in this context). So what you have is a B cell committed to making anti-*polysaccharide* antibodies that is displaying a *peptide* flag on its surface. All it takes now is for APCs to display the same peptides and stimulate Th2 cells, which then find their B-cell matches and help them make antibody through the germinal center reaction. In essence, the Th2 cells "think" they are helping B cells make antibodies to the protein antigen from which the peptides were derived, but in fact the flagged B cells make polysaccharide antibody. By converting a *T-independent* response to a *T-dependent* one, the shortcomings of polysaccharides as antigens are overcome. **Table 1.3** summarizes the advantages of protein-polysaccharide conjugate vaccines.

- *Genetic determinants of antibody responses*—Germinal center reactions depend on the interplay of various cells that engage each other through MHC molecules loaded with peptides derived from the pathogen (or vaccine). The genes encoding MHC molecules demonstrate a large degree of diversity, such that one person's MHC molecules might be better able to present a given peptide than another person's. This is one way that genetic background influences vaccine responses.

■ **Cytotoxic T Cells**

Tc cells are the main effectors of the adaptive cellular immune response. Like Th cells, they express the TCR on their surface, which has a unique antigenic specificity encoded in the germline. Unlike Th cells, which express CD4, Tc cells express the CD8 coreceptor, which directs engagement with *MHC class I molecules* (MHC-I). Like MHC-II, MHC-I loads pathogen-derived peptides into its groove and presents those peptides on the cell surface. However, instead of coming from the digestion of exogenous proteins that were engulfed by the cell, the peptides loaded into

FIGURE 1.4 — Response to Protein-Polysaccharide Vaccines

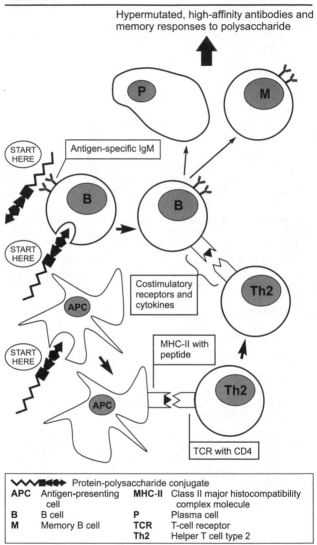

See *The Germinal Center Reaction* section within the text for a complete explanation.

TABLE 1.3 — Advantages of Protein-Polysaccharide Conjugate Vaccines

Property	Type of Vaccine	
	Polysaccharide	Protein-Polysaccharide Conjugate
B-cell response	T-cell independent	T-cell dependent
Pathway	Extrafollicular	Germinal center
Antibody generation in young infants	No	Yes
Induction of immune memory	No	Yes
Anamnestic or booster responses	No	Yes
Long-term protection	No	Yes
Reduced carriage of the organism at mucosal surfaces	No	Yes[a]
Herd immunity	No	Yes[b]

[a] Robust serum IgG levels allow for leakage onto mucosal surfaces, where colonizing bacteria are killed.
[b] Fewer colonized people means less transmission of the pathogen from person to person, indirectly protecting people who are not vaccinated.

MHC-I are actually made inside the cell—by infecting viruses or other intracellular pathogens.

MHC-I is expressed on APCs as well as on all nucleated host cells. Naïve Tc cells, predetermined to recognize a particular peptide/MHC-I flag, engage infected APCs that express those particular peptides in the context of MHC-I (**Figure 1.5**). While this leads to activation of the Tc cell, the Tc cell does not become a killer until it receives additional signals—those coming in the form of cytokines from Th1 cells, which in turn have been activated by engagement of APCs expressing pathogen-derived

FIGURE 1.5 — Cytotoxic T-Cell Response

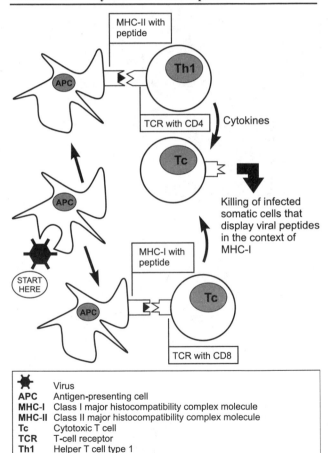

✹	Virus
APC	Antigen-presenting cell
MHC-I	Class I major histocompatibility complex molecule
MHC-II	Class II major histocompatibility complex molecule
Tc	Cytotoxic T cell
TCR	T-cell receptor
Th1	Helper T cell type 1

See the *Cytotoxic T Cells* section within the text for a complete explanation.

peptides in the context of MHC-II (Th1 cells have other functions as well, such as activation of macrophages). The respective, critical role of the two different types of Th cells is obvious—Th2 cells help B cells produce high-quality antibodies and memory cells, and Th1 cells help Tc cells become killers (and memory cells as well).

What does a Tc cell kill? Remember that Tc cells recognize peptides in the context of MHC-I, and all cells express MHC-I. Therefore, Tc cells find and destroy infected cells that express pathogen-derived peptides on their surface in the context of MHC-I. How does a Tc cell kill? One mechanism is through the release of *cytotoxins* that create holes in the cell membrane. In addition, Tc cells can induce *apoptosis*, or programmed cell death, through the release of certain enzymes and through cell-surface receptor-ligand interactions.

It is important to point out that there is some crossover between the immune mechanisms delineated above. For example, some exogenous peptides can be presented to a limited extent in the context of MHC-I; therefore, some inactivated vaccines can induce Tc responses.

The unique characteristics of Tc cells and their generation have several implications for vaccination:

- *Viruses versus bacteria*—Tc cells are much more important in controlling viral infections than in controlling bacterial infections. The reason is simple—most bacteria are fully capable of replicating independently outside of cells, and therefore do not generate APCs or somatic cells flagged with peptide/MHC-I ("somatic cells" refers to all cells on the body except gametes, or sex cells) . Viruses, on the other hand, are obligate intracellular pathogens—they can only replicate by usurping the host cell machinery for protein synthesis. Therefore, infected APCs and somatic cells are routinely flagged with peptide/MHC-I—unless the virus has evolved a mechanism to cloak the infected cell in anonymity by preventing the surface expression of peptide/MHC-I (cytomegalovirus and adenovirus, for example, evade the immune response in this fashion).

  Vaccines against bacterial pathogens are designed to maximize high-quality antibody production (some part of this involves the generation of large pools of Th2 cells). The ideal vaccine for a viral infection would maximize high-quality antibody production as well as lead to the generation of Tc cells.

- *Preventing versus limiting infection*—Tc cells operate *after* infection has taken place; they limit but do not prevent infecion. Unlike antibody, a Tc cell cannot kill a free virion that lands on a mucosal surface or enters the bloodstream. It must first wait until a cell is infected and expressing viral peptides. The (live-attenuated) varicella vaccine induces both antibody and Tc cells directed against VZV. If a vaccinated person is exposed to the virus, the first line of defense is the antibody that resides at the site of inoculation or in the immediate local environment. That antibody could neutralize the virus, thus preventing *infection*. If it does not, and the virus gains entry into cells and begins to replicate, memory Tc cells are called into action to destroy those cells, thus preventing *disease* (in this case, chickenpox). Antibody may also play a role in the destruction of infected cells through antibody-dependent cell-mediated cytotoxicity.

Differences between the varicella vaccine and the zoster (shingles) vaccine (which is the same live-attenuated virus given in a higher dose) are instructive. First, the main goal of the zoster vaccine is to expand the pool of Tc memory cells. By definition, people who get herpes zoster (shingles) are already infected with VZV (herpes zoster is the reactivation of endogenous, natural VZV that has been latent in the person since he or she had chickenpox). Early in the process of reactivation, infected cells begin to express viral peptides on their surface, and the idea is to have Tc cells ready to pounce on those cells before the disease can manifest. Second, in order for the vaccine itself to stimulate Tc cells, it must first infect host cells so that its peptides can be expressed in the context of MHC-I. The reason the zoster vaccine has so much more virus in it (14 times the amount) than the varicella vaccine is precisely the fact that it must avoid neutralization by any naturally occurring antibody in order to gain entry into host cells.

- *Live versus inactivated vaccines*—Because they replicate within cells, live viral vaccines are much better at inducing Tc cells than are inactivated vaccines. This is in addition to other factors that have already been mentioned, such as their enhanced ability to stimulate innate immune responses and their ability to amplify and disseminate antigens.
- *Cross-protection*—B cells recognize epitopes that are conformational in nature, in essence 3-dimensional structures that are represented on antigens on the pathogen surface. A good example of such an antigen is the hemagglutinin (HA) molecule of influenza virus, a glycoprotein that protrudes from the viral envelope and mediates attachment to cells. The trivalent inactivated influenza vaccine (TIV) is very good at eliciting antibodies to HA that can block infectivity—but those antibodies are specific to the strain of influenza virus that was used to make the vaccine. If antigenic drift occurs during a given season—that is, if the HA of the prevailing virus has a slightly different sequence and conformation—the vaccine will not be as effective.

Tc cells, on the other hand, recognize peptides that are derived from any protein made by the pathogen, some of which are more conserved between strains than are surface molecules. Just like TIV, LAIV elicits strain-specific antibodies directed at HA. However, it can also induce Tc cells that recognize peptides derived from the nucleocapsid of the virus. The advantage here is that nucleocapsid proteins are well conserved from one strain to another. Thus LAIV can induce Tc-cell responses capable of limiting infection due to strains whose HA has drifted from the vaccine strain.

Additional Concepts

A few additional basic concepts are necessary to fully understand the world of vaccinology.

■ Correlates of Protection

Ideally, vaccines are shown to be effective in randomized, blinded, placebo-controlled trials, where one group of subjects gets the vaccine, another gets the placebo, and the measured outcome is *efficacy*, or ability to prevent the disease (or infection). This works if the disease is prevalent, such that the number of subjects needed in a clinical trial is within reach. For diseases that are relatively rare, demonstrating efficacy may not be feasible. In such situations, *immunogenicity*, or the ability to generate an immune response, is relied upon as a *surrogate* of efficacy. As will be seen, however, the connection between immunogenicity and efficacy is not that straightforward.

Surrogates of protection against a disease are useful for other reasons as well. For example, it may not be possible to study vaccine efficacy in every population that will ultimately be targeted for immunization. How can we be sure that a vaccine demonstrated to be effective in one age group will be effective in another? Or, for that matter, in individuals of different ethnic groups, those with underlying medical conditions, or those living in different geographic areas? If we knew which immunologic tests predicted protection, we could be reassured that if the immunologic criteria were met, protection would likely ensue. Immune correlates or surrogates also drive preclinical development, in the sense that scientists choose antigens, delivery systems, and dosing schedules that maximize immune responses thought to be important in protecting people from disease. Surrogates also are critical to quality assurance—each new production lot of vaccine cannot be studied for efficacy, but it *can* be studied for immunogenicity and, in particular, for its ability to generate responses that are relevant in some way to protection. Likewise, there are many vaccination scenarios that must be studied in practice. For example, a new vaccine might be effective in clinical trials, but in real life it needs to be given concomitantly with other vaccines. It would be very difficult to study efficacy under every permutation of concomitant use; instead, investigators rely on surrogates to determine if concomitant use is likely or unlikely to compromise protection. For new combination vaccines, noninferiority (with respect to a relevant immune response) to concomitant administration of the separate vaccines must be demonstrated (see Chapter 2, *Vaccine Infrastructure in the United States*).

For some diseases, there are generally accepted, albeit imperfect, surrogates of protection. For example, studies in the prevaccine era showed that children who had naturally occurring anticapsular polysaccharide (polyribosylribitol phosphate [PRP]) antibody levels ≥0.15 mcg/mL were protected from invasive *H influenzae* disease; those with levels <0.15 mcg/mL were not. One would interpret this to mean that circulating levels of anti-PRP antibody ≥0.15 mcg/mL are enough to kill *H influenzae* that happens to gain entry into the bloodstream. Studies utilizing the unconjugated PRP vaccine showed that antibody levels ≥1.0 mcg/mL immediately following vaccination correlated with protection against disease. Are we to assume, then, that children with postvaccination levels ≥1.0 mcg/mL ultimately wind up with steady-state levels ≥0.15 mcg/mL, the presumed protective level? Or is it that the antibody induced by vaccination with PRP is of poorer quality, such that more of it is needed to provide protection?

The situation becomes even more complex. Protection may be mediated before the organism enters the bloodstream, at the site of mucosal colonization. Little is known, however, about mucosal surrogates of protection. How much secretory IgA or extravascular IgG is enough to prevent colonization? What role does prevention of colonization play in prevention of disease? How about the role of inoculum size (assuming there is a correlate of protection necessarily assumes there is an average inoculum)? In addition, the *H influenzae* surrogates were derived from studies of natural infection and vaccination with PRP. We know, however, as discussed, that the kinetics of the immune response to protein-polysaccharide conjugate vaccines and the quality of antibody differ markedly from unconjugated polysaccharide vaccine. Is, therefore, a surrogate of protection derived from studies of natural infection and PRP vaccine relevant to the use of conjugate vaccines?

Another example of the problem with interpreting surrogates of protection comes from observations made with HepB. Studies suggest that circulating levels of HBsAb ≥10 mIU/mL at the time of exposure to HBV perfectly predict protection from infection. In this sense, then, HBsAb ≥10 mIU/mL is a surrogate of protection. However, studies also show that antibody wanes with time—often to levels <10 mIU/mL—even though protection does not. Therefore, there must be another (unmeasured) surrogate of long-term protection.

One also needs to ask how antibodies are being measured. Clearly, quantitation of high-avidity antibodies that kill or opsonize *H influenzae* would correlate more closely with protection than measurement of antibodies that bind to PRP in an enzyme-linked immunosorbent assay. Similarly, quantitation of antibodies that neutralize viruses in vitro might be more relevant than measurement of antibodies that bind to viral proteins—unless one knows exactly which proteins are involved in generating neutralizing antibody. Even then, there is no guarantee that a protein-binding assay will measure antibodies that bind to the neutralizing epitopes, and that binding to those epitopes actually correlates with neutralization in a functional assay. For some infections (eg, tetanus), antibodies to the *organism itself* are not relevant, but antibodies to *toxins produced by the organism* are. The situation becomes even more complex when one considers that for some diseases, protection may be mediated as much by Th and Tc cells as by antibody. In as much as Th cells help B cells make antibodies, antibody levels may be an indirect measure of cellular immunity.

Fortunately, vaccine development does not depend on establishing immunologic correlates of protection. For example, there is no consensus on correlates of protection against rotavirus (candidates include mucosal IgA and T cells), even though highly effective vaccines have been developed. Likewise, debate continues about the correlates of protection against pertussis. Most agree that antibody to pertussis toxin is necessary; some say it is sufficient, but some say immunity is incrementally enhanced by antibodies to filamentous hemagglutinin, pertactin, and fimbrial antigens. No one really agrees on the actual levels of antibody that are necessary. Yet whole-cell pertussis vaccines have been in use since the 1940s and acellular vaccines since the 1990s—each licensed based on the demonstration of efficacy against disease in clinical trials.

In the last few years, however, acellular pertussis booster vaccines for adolescents and adults were licensed without proof of efficacy—and despite the fact that there are no agreed-upon correlates of protection. The basis for licensure was the demonstration of levels of antibodies to pertussis antigens that were similar to the levels found in infants who had received DTaP, a vaccine already proved to be effective against disease. Similarly, MCV4 was licensed because the levels of antibody following vaccination were equivalent to those achieved after immunization with MPSV4, which was also known to be protective.

■ Herd Immunity

Vaccines protect people in two ways. First, they stimulate adaptive immunity in vaccinated individuals. The level of protection depends on the quality, magnitude, and duration of the individual's response. Since no vaccine is 100% effective, even vaccinated individuals can become infected—*if* they are exposed to the disease. Exposure, in turn, depends on transmission of the pathogen from person-to-person (an exception is tetanus, which is acquired from the environment, not other people). What if transmission were interrupted because there were enough immune individuals in the population? Then everyone—susceptible vaccinated and unvaccinated individuals alike—would be indirectly protected.

The term *herd immunity* was coined in 1923 by Topley and Wilson in drawing a distinction between (but acknowledging the relatedness of) the immunity of individuals and protection of the community in which the individuals live. It refers to the fact that susceptible members of "the herd" are protected by the presence and proximity of immune members who prevent propagation of the infection. For every disease that is transmitted from person to person, there is probably a *herd-immunity threshold*—a critical proportion of the population that must be immune in order for transmission to be squelched. Although simple in concept, the herd-immunity threshold depends on a complex interplay of many factors, including contagiousness of the pathogen, mode of transmission (eg, fecal-oral vs respiratory droplet), and whether the disease is endemic or comes in epidemic waves. Ideally, one would want to know what proportion of a population needs to be vaccinated in order to protect the entire population. This will depend on the above factors, as well as on the efficacy of the vaccine and the reality that neither vaccination nor exposure is evenly distributed within a population. For example, there may be pockets of susceptible individuals (eg, undervaccinated inner-city residents) or foci of close contact (eg, college dormitories).

In addition, the microbial ecology of the pathogen must be taken into account. For measles virus, there is no carrier state and there is no reservoir of infection other than humans. Thus a vaccine that prevents individual infection will prevent transmission and amplify the protective effect on individuals through herd immunity. For *H influenzae*, in contrast, there *is* a reservoir of infection—the nasopharynx of young children. A vaccine that prevents invasive infection but not nasopharyngeal colonization arguably would not result in herd immunity, since transmission could still occur from vaccinated children who remain colonized. Fortunately, protein-polysaccharide conjugate vaccines are very effective at reducing colonization.

Figures 1.6 and **1**.7 give modern-day examples of herd immunity in action. In the early 1990s, the incidence of hepatitis A in Butte County was six times higher than in California as a whole. Beginning in 1995, children 2 through 17 years of age were routinely immunized with HepA. Within 5 years, the incidence of hepatitis A had fallen dramatically among children, as one might expect (**Figure 1**.6). However, the incidence also had fallen in all other age groups—groups that were not targeted for immunization. Preventing hepatitis A infection in children was enough to prevent transmission to, and infection among, adults. Economic models suggest that herd immunity effects more than double the cost savings from universal HepA immunization of young children.

Similarly, **Figure 1**.7 illustrates the impact that routine childhood PCV7 immunization has had on invasive pneumococcal disease in unimmunized older individuals. In this case, herd immunity was mediated by decreases in nasopharyngeal colonization among vaccinated children. However, there is a cautionary tale to tell here. Vaccination only affects colonization with vaccine

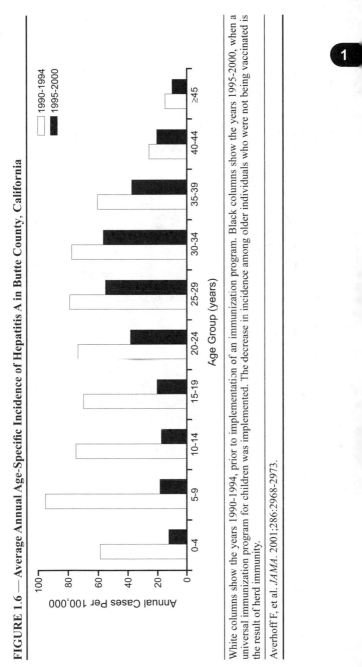

FIGURE 1.6 — Average Annual Age-Specific Incidence of Hepatitis A in Butte County, California

White columns show the years 1990-1994, prior to implementation of an immunization program. Black columns show the years 1995-2000, when a universal immunization program for children was implemented. The decrease in incidence among older individuals who were not being vaccinated is the result of herd immunity.

Averhoff F, et al. *JAMA*. 2001;286:2968-2973.

FIGURE 1.7 — Annual Projected Cases of Invasive Pneumococcal Disease Due to PCV7 Serotypes (4, 6B, 9V, 14, 18C, 19F, and 23F) in the United States

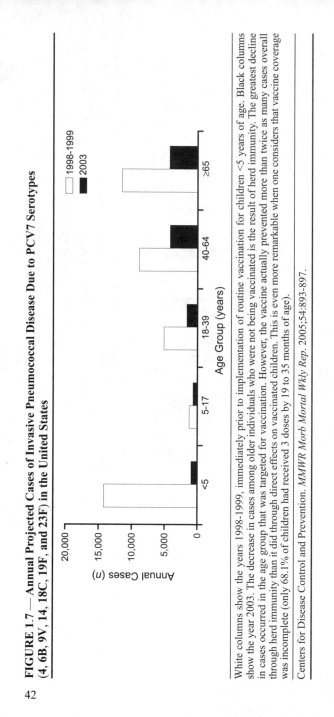

White columns show the years 1998-1999, immediately prior to implementation of routine vaccination for children <5 years of age. Black columns show the year 2003. The decrease in cases among older individuals who were not being vaccinated is the result of herd immunity. The greatest decline in cases occurred in the age group that was targeted for vaccination. However, the vaccine actually prevented more than twice as many cases overall through herd immunity than it did through direct effects on vaccinated children. This is even more remarkable when one considers that vaccine coverage was incomplete (only 68.1% of children had received 3 doses by 19 to 35 months of age).

Centers for Disease Control and Prevention. *MMWR Morb Mortal Wkly Rep.* 2005;54:893-897.

serotypes. When these serotypes disappear from the nasopharynx, other serotypes take over, something called *serotype replacement*. Some of those serotypes—19A, for example, in the case of *S pneumoniae*—are themselves capable of causing invasive disease. In fact, invasive disease due to nonvaccine serotypes has *increased* in the PCV7 era, although the overall rate of invasive disease (all serotypes included) has dramatically declined. The challenge is to stay one step ahead of the organism by developing vaccines that include the emerging serotypes.

■ Goals of Immunization Programs

Some historians believe that smallpox has killed more people since civilization began than all other infectious diseases combined. Although global eradication through vaccination was conceived by Jenner as early as 1801, it did not become a real possibility until 1967, when the following factors converged: 1) the World Health Assembly resolved to eradicate the disease and increased funding was secured; 2) large amounts of stable, lyophilized vaccine became available and reference testing centers were established; 3) a highly effective bifurcated needle was adopted for administration; and 4) the strategy of ring vaccination was developed, wherein active cases were hunted down and their contacts vaccinated. As a result, the last natural case of smallpox on the planet occurred in 1977 (the last case in the United States was in 1949), and on December 9, 1979, the WHO certified that smallpox had been eradicated. It was remarked that smallpox eradication was one of the few things that needed to be done only once in the history of the world.

In many ways, *eradication* represents the Holy Grail of vaccination programs, the end result of progressive *control* and *elimination* as defined in **Table 1.4**. Because there is no reservoir of variola virus in nature and there is no human carrier state, the elimination of natural disease was felt to be definitive. In the United States, routine vaccination of civilians ceased in 1972, health care workers in 1976, and military personnel in 1990. Until 2001, the only individuals in the United States who continued to be vaccinated were laboratory and animal care workers with potential exposures to orthopox viruses, and health care personnel conducting clinical trials with recombinant vaccinia virus vaccines. Between 1984 and 2001, no country routinely immunized civilians.

The terrorist attacks of September 11, 2001, raised the concern that the end-game for smallpox should not have been eradication but rather *extinction*. After eradication, worldwide stocks of variola virus were consolidated at the CDC and the Institute of Virus Preparations in Moscow (now the Russian State Centre for Research on Virology and Biotechnology, Koltsovo, Novosibirsk Region, Russian Federation). It is now known that the Soviet Union had an active program to weaponize variola virus, and with the political unrest and economic hardship that ensued in Russia during the 1990s, it remained possible that the virus and the

TABLE 1.4 — 1997 Dahlem Conference Definitions of Vaccine Program Goals

Term	Definition
Control	Reduction of disease incidence, prevalence, morbidity, or mortality to a locally acceptable level as a result of deliberate efforts; continued intervention measures are required to maintain the reduction
Elimination of disease	Reduction to zero of the incidence of a specified disease in a defined geographic area as a result of deliberate efforts; continued intervention measures are required
Elimination of infection	Reduction to zero of the incidence of infection caused by a specific agent in a defined geographic area as a result of deliberate efforts; continued measures to prevent re-establishment of transmission are required
Eradication	Permanent reduction to zero of the worldwide incidence of infection caused by a specific agent as a result of deliberate efforts; intervention measures no longer needed
Extinction	The specific infectious agent no longer exists in nature or the laboratory

Hinman A. *Ann Rev Pub Health*. 1999;20:211-229.

technology to deliver it may have fallen into the hands of terrorists or rogue nations. Even a single case of smallpox anywhere in the world would strongly imply an intentional release and would be considered an international medical and strategic emergency. The destruction of remaining lots of variola virus was debated in the 1990s, but on December 20, 2001, the WHO recommended against this—the virus was spared execution in order to facilitate continued research into molecular diagnosis, genetic analysis, serologic assays, animal models, antiviral drugs, and vaccines.

Many diseases have been *controlled* through vaccination. Beyond smallpox, three diseases—polio, measles, and rubella—have been *eliminated* from the United States, meaning that indigenous cases no longer occur. Because infection can still be imported from outside the country, as was demonstrated by the measles outbreaks in Arizona, California, Wisconsin, and elsewhere in 2008, elimination should be viewed as a step along the way to the ultimate goal of global eradication. Worldwide efforts to eliminate and ultimately eradicate hepatitis B, measles, rubella, and polio are under way. One could argue, though, that in the post-9/11 era, the ultimate goal should be *extinction*, where the virus no longer exists in nature or laboratories. Even that, however, may not be enough—the genome of polio virus is known, and live virus could theoretically be reconstructed from the raw genetic materials.

What does it take to eliminate or eradicate a vaccine-preventable disease? First, it takes favorable disease characteristics, including a readily recognizable clinical syndrome, easy diagnosis, few subclinical infections, a short period of contagion, absence of persistence and nonhuman reservoirs, little strain variability, and lifelong immunity after natural infection. Then it takes a safe, effective, stable, easily stored and transported, cheap vaccine. Then it takes political will and the collaboration of governments, organizations, and many individuals. Finally, eradication takes money. While eradication requires intensive effort and expense over a short period of time, it can be viewed as very cost-effective when one considers that once achieved, vaccination may no longer be necessary.

Public Health Impact of Vaccination

It is difficult to summarize the tremendous impact that vaccines have had on our general well-being. Vaccination ranks among the top ten great achievements in public health during the 20th century and is partially responsible for the dramatic increase in life expectancy that was seen during that period of time. **Table 1.5** shows the impact on specific diseases by comparing the peak number of cases and deaths in the prevaccine era to the most recent numbers. The decline in cases for almost all of these diseases has been nothing short of spectacular, although a few things are worth pointing out. Pertussis, for example, declined to historic lows in the 1970s but has resurged since then. Some part of this is more awareness, active surveillance, and better diagnostic tools, such that more cases are being detected. Part of it is also the fact that immunity induced by childhood vaccination does not last long, and that until recently there have been no vaccines available to boost pertussis immunity in adolescents and adults. **Table 1.5** also reflects the abrupt resurgence of mumps that occurred in the Midwest in 2006, which was probably due to a virus imported from Europe. That outbreak, which disproportionately affected young adults, was driven by waning vaccine-induced immunity and the close-contact living situation of college students.

New strategies have been adopted for diseases that have stubbornly persisted. For example, immunization against hepatitis A targeted at high-risk individuals and communities could only bring us so far; the adoption of a universal childhood immuniza-

TABLE 1.5 — Historical Morbidity and Mortality From Vaccine-Preventable Diseases

Disease	Historical Peak		Most Recent	
	Cases	Deaths	Cases[a]	Deaths[a]
Vaccine Programs Initiated Before 1980				
Diphtheria	30,508	3065	0	0
Measles	763,094	552	55	0
Mumps	212,932	50	6584	0
Pertussis	265,269	7518	15,632	27
Poliomyelitis (acute)	42,033	2720	0	0
Poliomyelitis (paralytic)	21,269	3145	0	0
Rubella	488,796	24	11	0
Congenital rubella syndrome	20,000	2160	1	0
Smallpox	110,672	2510	0	0
Tetanus	601	511	41	4
Vaccine Programs Initated After 1980				
Hepatitis A	254,518	298	15,298	18
Hepatitis B	74,361	267	13,169	47
Invasive:				
Haemophilus influenzae type b	>20,000	>1000	<50	<5
Streptococcus pneumoniae	64,400	7300	41,550	4850
Varicella	5,358,595	138	612,768	19

[a] Reported cases are given for programs initiated before 1980; estimates are provided for programs initiated after 1980.

Roush SW, et al. *JAMA*. 2007;298:2155-2163.

tion program in 2006 should bring the number of cases down much further. Similarly, the one-dose varicella program initiated in 1995 was very successful, but because of breakthrough disease in vaccinees (primary vaccine failure) could only bring us so far; the adoption of a routine 2-dose childhood schedule and catch-up immunization for everyone else should close the deal. The issue for invasive *S pneumoniae* disease is more complicated. We will need vaccines that cover more serotypes, especially the ones that have become more prevalent since PCV7 was introduced in 2000.

Studies have shown that the *clinically preventable burden*, which is the proportion of disease aborted by a preventive service in usual practice, is higher for the routine childhood immunization schedule than for virtually every other routine public health intervention, including things such as colorectal and breast cancer screening.

Vaccines also make economic sense—a study of the 2001 US birth cohort showed that for every $1 spent on routine childhood immunizations (which at the time did not include rotavirus vaccine, HepA, PCV7, influenza vaccine, MCV4, or HPV vaccine), $5 was saved in direct costs and an additional $11 was saved in societal costs. **Table 1.6** shows the data from that study and gives you a hint of what the world would be like without vaccines.

ADDITIONAL READING

Vaccine Immunology

Amanna IJ, Carlson NE, Slifka MK. Duration of humoral immunity to common viral and vaccine antigens. *N Engl J Med.* 2007;357:1903-1915.

Huang AYC, Rigby MR. The immune response: generation, regulation, and maintenance. In: Stiehm ER, Ochs HD, Winkelstein JA, eds. *Immunologic Disorders in Infants & Children. 5th ed.* St Louis, MO: Elsevier; 2004.

Plotkin SA. Immunologic correlates of protection induced by vaccination. *Pediatr Infect Dis J.* 2001;20:63-75.

Qin L, Gilbert PB, Corey L, McElrath MJ, Self SG. A framework for assessing immunological correlates of protection in vaccine trials. *J Infect Dis.* 2007;196:1304-1312.

Siegrist CA. Vaccine immunology. In: Plotkin SA, Orenstein WA, Offit PA, et al, eds. *Vaccines. 5th ed.* St Louis, MO: Elsevier; 2008.

Additional Concepts

Armstrong GL, Billah K, Rein DB, Hicks KA, Wirth KE, Bell BP. The economics of routine childhood hepatitis A immunization in the United States: the impact of herd immunity. *Pediatrics.* 2007;119:e22-e29.

Fine PE. Herd immunity: history, theory, practice. *Epidemiol Rev.* 1993;15:265-302.

Hinman A. Eradication of vaccine-preventable diseases. *Annu Rev Pub Health.* 1999;20:211-229.

Public Health Impact

Centers for Disease Control and Prevention (CDC). Impact of vaccines universally recommended for children—United States, 1900-1998. *MMWR Morb Mortal Wkly Rep.* 1999;48:243-248.

Coffield AB, Maciosek MV, McGinnis M, et al. Priorities among recommended clinical preventive services. *Am J Prev Med.* 2001;21:1-9.

TABLE 1.6 — Effect of Routine Childhood Vaccines on the 2001 US Birth Cohort[a]

Scenario	Cases of Disease	Vaccine-Preventable Deaths	Total Costs (Direct and Indirect)
Without routine childhood vaccines	14,330,376	33,564	$46,557,000,000
With routine childhood vaccines[b]	708,372	463	$482,000,000

[a] $N = 3,803,295$.
[b] Analysis does not include rotavirus vaccine, HepA, PCV7, influenza vaccine, MCV4, or HPV vaccine.

Zhou F, et al. *Arch Pediatr Adolesc Med.* 2005;159:1136-1144.

2

Vaccine Infrastructure in the United States

Vaccine Development and Licensure

A tremendous amount of effort is involved in developing vaccine candidates. The biology of the infectious agent and pathogenesis of the disease must be elucidated. Correlates of immunity, and the laboratory tools to measure them, must be developed. Animal models of vaccine efficacy need to be investigated. Issues such as immunopotentiation, formulation, and delivery need to be worked out, and consistent test lots must be produced. These steps in preclinical development may take place in academia, industry, or governmental research institutions, or through collaborations between these groups. **Figure 2.1** illustrates the process of vaccine development and licensure in the United States.

Once candidate vaccines are ready for testing in humans, the process is rigorously overseen by the Food and Drug Administration (FDA), an operating division of the Department of Health and Human Services (HHS). In general, the financial risk of clinical development is borne by industry. The investment, which typically runs into the hundreds of millions of dollars, may or may not pay off in terms of a marketable product. Either way, it is important to understand that no vaccines reach the public without industry, since pharmaceutical companies — not academic medical centers or governmental agencies—manufacture and distribute the final products.

The FDA group that sets standards for purity and consistency is the Center for Biologics Evaluation and Research, commonly referred to as CBER, which acts under the authority of Section 351 of the Public Health Service Act and sections of the Federal Food, Drug, and Cosmetic Act. The World Health Organization (WHO) provides guidance for products that are used internationally. Laboratory testing for vaccine purity and consistency is required before and after licensure. An intensive search is performed for known viral, bacterial, and fungal agents that may contaminate vaccines, and potency tests are applied. Manufacturers are required to conform to Good Manufacturing Practices (GMPs), a vast collection of rules and guidances that cover everything from raw-materials quality assurance to record keeping, cleanliness standards, personnel qualifications, inhouse testing, process controls, warehousing, and distribution. They must also adhere to Good Laboratory Practices (GLPs), an analogous set of guidances for the laboratory. Several large lots of vaccine (each containing tens of thousands of doses) with identical potencies must be produced in a manner that is consistent

FIGURE 2.1 — Schematic of the Process of Vaccine Development and Licensure in the United States

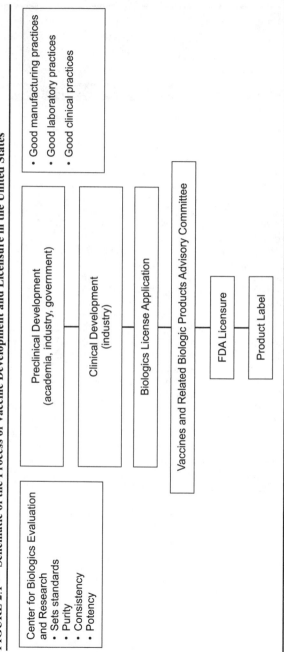

Center for Biologics Evaluation and Research
• Sets standards
  • Purity
  • Consistency
  • Potency

Preclinical Development (academia, industry, government)

Clinical Development (industry)

Biologics License Application

Vaccines and Related Biologic Products Advisory Committee

FDA Licensure

Product Label

• Good manufacturing practices
• Good laboratory practices
• Good clinical practices

and reliable. In addition, manufacturers are required to provide information regarding appropriate storage and handling. Fulfilling the requirements of CBER often takes between 5 and 10 years.

After a candidate vaccine is approved as an investigational new drug for use in clinical trials, studies for safety, immunogenicity, and efficacy are performed. A set of guidances called Good Clinical Practices (GCPs), analogous to GMPs and GLPs, sets the standard for the conduct of clinical trials. Some trials are conducted by the Division of Microbiology and Infectious Diseases of the National Institutes of Health (NIH) through Vaccine and Treatment Evaluation Units; as of November 2007, there were eight such funded units, most of them at academic medical centers. Other studies, generally involving candidate vaccines that are further along in development, are conducted at academic medical centers or private offices by pharmaceutical companies (or clinical research organizations contracted by the pharmaceutical companies) using local principal investigators who are overseen by institutional review boards or human studies committees. Either way, strict federal guidelines apply regarding the protection of human subjects and the management of potential conflicts of interest.

Prelicensure trials proceed in three phases, followed by a postmarketing phase (**Figure 2.2**):

- *Phase 1*—These trials usually involve <100 volunteers and are intended to provide basic information on safety and tolerability. Because of their small size, they can detect only extremely common adverse events. Subjects are often not drawn from the intended vaccine target population. For example, pediatric vaccine candidates might undergo initial testing in adults until basic safety is assured.
- *Phase 2*—These trials enroll hundreds of subjects and provide information about the vaccine's immunogenicity, dose, and common side effects. Studies are performed in the proposed target group and may also provide some information on efficacy.
- *Phase 3*—These studies enroll thousands to tens of thousands of subjects, using sample sizes large enough to ensure that questions about safety and efficacy will be answered (they are often referred to as pivotal studies). Subjects are carefully followed for adverse events in the immediate postvaccination period, usually for as long as 42 days. Longer periods of observation allow for assessment of protection from disease and longevity of immune responses. Large trials also evaluate the consistency of responses and look at concomitant use with other vaccines. This phase of development includes the transfer of manufacturing to full-scale facilities, which must operate under GMPs and are subject to rigorous inspections (the plant itself must be licensed).

Phase 3 trials of new vaccines, that is vaccines for diseases that previously were not vaccine-preventable, include

FIGURE 2.2 — Sequential Stages in the Testing of Vaccines in Humans

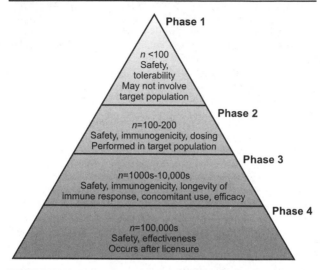

placebo recipients; therefore, efficacy against disease can be determined and adverse events related to the vaccine can be pinpointed. Phase 3 trials of new versions of existing vaccines generally pit the new vaccine against the existing one. Here, prevention of disease may not be a feasible end point, since the disease itself may be unusual. The end point, therefore, may by necessity be immunogenicity, with the inference being that if the new vaccine is as immunogenic as the existing one (which is known to be protective), it should provide equal protection; these are often called immunogenicity bridge studies. Noninferiority is statistically defined for each study and is usually agreed upon before the trial is conducted. Pressure to make sure that vaccines are as safe as possible before licensure has driven the size of phase 3 trials upward—the studies that went into the licensure of PRV and HRV, for example, each involved >70,000 children, more than any other prelicensure studies since the Salk vaccine trials of the early 1950s.

- *Phase 4*—Prelicensure trials cannot detect very rare side effects, adverse events with delayed onset, or potential reactions in culturally or ethnically diverse populations. Formal postmarketing studies, which may involve large cohorts of vaccinated children followed prospectively, are designed to detect such rare events. These studies are supplemented by the surveillance systems described below. Postmarketing studies also may look at *effectiveness*, or how a vaccine performs in real life, outside the context of a controlled clinical trial.

After phases 1 through 3 studies are completed, the manufacturer submits a Biologics License Application (BLA) to the FDA. The BLA contains all of the data necessary to determine if a license should be granted. It is important to point out that the file is not submitted blindly—rather, its content is determined in a dynamic process of evaluation and negotiation between the FDA and the manufacturer. Around the time of the BLA submission, the manufacturing facilities are inspected and all aspects of vaccine production are evaluated. Once the BLA is accepted, the formal evaluation process begins—a process that generally takes a year or two, depending on whether supplemental information or additional studies are requested by the FDA. In 1992, the Prescription Drug User Fee Act (PDUFA) went into effect, authorizing the FDA to collect fees from manufacturers submitting a file. The continued reauthorization of PDUFA has allowed FDA to expand its staff and shorten the time to approval—the current goal is to act on 90% of standard new BLAs within 10 months.

Eventually, the manufacturer may be invited to present the entire case for licensure to the Vaccines and Related Biological Products Advisory Committee (VRBPAC), especially if the vaccine is the first in a class or if there are questions about safety or efficacy. VRBPAC consists of 12 core voting members appointed by the FDA Commissioner. Although most members have recognized expertise in fields related to vaccinology, one member who is identified with consumer interests may be appointed. In addition, a nonvoting representative of the pharmaceutical industry may be invited; this ensures that all interested parties have input into vaccine licensure decisions. VRBPAC makes recommendations to the FDA Commissioner regarding whether to license the product, what the indications should be, and whether any additional data are needed.

In general, the FDA Commissioner follows the VRBPAC recommendations, and licensure is usually granted within a few months. The FDA also approves a package insert (PI), synonymously referred to as the product information or label. The PI contains official indications, statements about efficacy, contraindications, warnings, precautions, and adverse events. When people refer to labeled indications, they are referring to the specifics contained in the PI.

There are several things to bear in mind regarding the PI:
- The labeled indications are based on the data in the BLA. So, for example, if the studies in the file only included individuals in a certain age group, the label will specify approved use only in that age group. That will not change, even if new studies are published, unless the manufacturer submits a supplemental BLA that is subsequently approved.
- Official recommendations are sometimes at odds with the PI. For example, Comvax (HepB-Hib) is labeled for use only in infants of HBsAg-negative mothers, but use in infants

of HBsAg-positive mothers is considered acceptable by the Advisory Committee on Immunization Practices (ACIP). Thus there is a difference between the labeled *indications*—which are derived strictly from the PI, and therefore from the FDA—and the *recommendations*, which are derived from authoritative professional bodies (see below). One question to consider is which of the two—the PI or the recommendations—sets the authoritative reference standard in malpractice litigation. Most people would agree that the recommendations supersede the PI in this respect because they are based on a more comprehensive dataset and they represent the opinion of medical peers.

- The PI does not provide guidance for all situations. For example, the Boostrix (Tdap) PI (June 2007) states that there are no immunogenicity or safety data for the concomitant administration of Boostrix with other vaccines. The next sentence reads, "When concomitant administration of other vaccines is required, they should be given with separate syringes and at different injection sites." While this would seem self-evident, one is still left to wonder if other vaccines—MCV4 and HPV vaccine in particular—can be given at the same time. Fortunately, ACIP recommendations usually answer these questions; in this case, concomitant administration of Tdap, MCV4, and HPV vaccine is recommended.
- Taking a conservative approach, the PI often mentions adverse events that have been reported but not proved to be caused by the vaccine. Thus, for example, the RotaTeq (PRV) PI mentions Kawasaki disease as an adverse event that has been reported postmarketing. While this is true at face value—namely, that Kawasaki disease has been reported to the Vaccine Adverse Events Reporting System (VAERS) following RotaTeq administration—the number of cases reported does not exceed what one would expect as background, and data from postmarketing studies do not support a causal relationship. Nevertheless, the mere fact that Kawasaki disease was added to the PI has led to unnecessary concern on the part of parents and providers.
- The PI determines how a vaccine can be advertised and marketed. Company field representatives must restrict their claims about the product to the information contained in the PI. Likewise, promotional programs must remain within the label, and it must be specified during continuing medical education programs when off-label uses of a product are mentioned.

With the above caveats, the PI does contain valuable information. The provider should be familiar with its contents, especially the specifics regarding proper storage and handling.

Figure 2.3 gives an overview of the various agencies and committees involved in making and executing vaccine policy in the United States. The Centers for Disease Control and Prevention (CDC), an operating division of HHS, includes the National Center for Immunization and Respiratory Diseases (NCIRD), an interdisciplinary program that merges vaccine-preventable disease science and research with immunization program activities. NCIRD, formerly known as the National Immunization Program, provides leadership in the planning, coordination, and conduct of immunization activities throughout the country. It assists health departments in implementing immunization programs, supports establishment of vaccine supply contracts for state and local programs through the Vaccines For Children (VFC) Program, assists in the development of information-management systems, administers research and operational programs, provides clinician educational programs, and supports surveillance for vaccine-preventable diseases.

The ACIP is the principal body that makes recommendations for use after a vaccine is licensed. The ACIP provides advice and guidance to the Secretary of Health and Human Services, the Assistant Secretary, and the Director of the CDC regarding the most appropriate application of vaccines to control communicable diseases in the civilian population. It is the only entity in the federal government to function in this capacity. There are 15 members who are all appointed by the Secretary (none of them are federal government employees); persons who are knowledgeable about consumer perspectives and/or social and community aspects of immunization programs are included, as are infectious diseases specialists. In addition, there are eight nonvoting members representing a variety of other governmental agencies involved in vaccine policy, distribution, and financing, as well as liaison members from professional organizations. Members with financial conflicts of interest concerning particular vaccines cannot vote on recommendations that pertain to those products. This includes members who receive research funding from the manufacturer.

The committee meets three times each year and makes recommendations regarding target populations and indications; on occasion, recommendations regarding things such as contraindications and precautions are made that deviate from the PI. In making its recommendations, the ACIP considers a product's labeled indications and dosing schedule, disease burden, safety data, feasibility, cost-benefit and risk-benefit analyses, and input from other stakeholder groups. Oftentimes, data that are not included in the BLA are considered, which explains why the recommendations may differ from the label. The process usually involves the formation of working groups on specific topics; these groups are chaired by

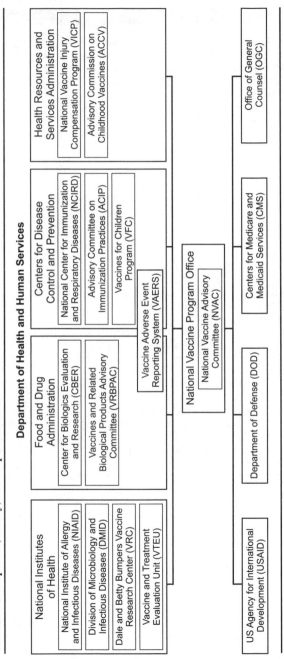

FIGURE 2.3 — Governmental Agencies and Advisory Committees Involved in Vaccine Development, Policy, and Implementation

ACIP members but often include outside experts. There are four permanent working groups:

- *Childhood/Adolescent Immunization Schedules*—This group recommends changes to the routine childhood and adolescent schedules, which are published every January. Since 1995, the ACIP schedule has been harmonized in its characteristic graphic layout with the recommendations of the American Academy of Pediatrics (AAP) and the American Academy of Family Physicians (AAFP).
- *Adult Immunization Schedule*—This group recommends changes to the routine adult schedule, which are published every October.
- *Influenza Vaccine*—This group makes recommendations regarding influenza immunization, which are published annually for the upcoming influenza season.
- *General Recommendations*—Every 3 to 5 years, the ACIP publishes a document entitled *General Recommendations on Immunization*, commonly referred to as the "General Recs," which provides background and technical guidance regarding vaccination. Specific topics include timing and spacing of doses, contraindications and precautions, administration technique, storage and handling, special situations, record keeping, and adverse-event reporting, among others. These topics are elaborated upon elsewhere in this book, and Chapter 5, *General Recommendations*, gives a useful distillation of general rules for immunization.

Supplemental recommendations pertaining to newly licensed vaccines, programmatic issues, changes in previous recommendations, and informational items ("Notice to Readers") are published periodically in the *Morbidity and Mortality Weekly Report* and on the Internet (http://www.cdc.gov/vaccines/pubs/ACIP-list.htm. Accessed August 15, 2008). Provisional recommendations are also posted on the Internet (http://www.cdc.gov/vaccines/recs/provisional/default.htm. Accessed August 15, 2008), oftentimes many months before the recommendations are published in the *MMWR*. A comprehensive summary of ACIP recommendations is released every 1 to 2 years in a book entitled *Epidemiology and Prevention of Vaccine-Preventable Diseases*, commonly known as the "Pink Book."

The AAP Committee on Infectious Diseases also develops policy recommendations on the use of vaccines. While these are developed independently, every attempt is made to achieve congruity with the ACIP recommendations. From time to time, however, there are subtle but important differences. AAP recommendations on vaccination are included the *Report of the Committee on Infectious Diseases*, a comprehensive summary of infectious diseases that is published every 3 years and is commonly called the "Red Book." The AAP also partners with the

CDC in the Childhood Immunization Support Program (http://www.cispimmunize.org. Accessed August 15, 2008), with goals to promote quality improvement and best immunization practices, improve delivery, and enable effective communication.

The ACIP has one other important function: it determines which vaccines should be added to the VFC program. In general, a specific resolution is passed for each vaccine that is routinely recommended.

The National Vaccine Program Office (NVPO) was created in 1986 to coordinate the activities of all federal agencies in developing and implementing the National Vaccine Plan (available at http://www.hhs.gov/nvpo/vacc_plan. Accessed August 15, 2008), which calls for "optimal prevention of human infectious diseases through immunization and ... optimal prevention of adverse reactions to vaccines." The NVPO strives to improve collaboration with the commercial vaccine industry, global organizations, consumer groups, and academic institutions. The National Vaccine Advisory Committee (NVAC) makes recommendations to the NVPO regarding the supply of safe and effective vaccines, research priorities, areas of cooperation, and ways to achieve optimal prevention of infectious diseases through vaccine development while minimizing adverse reactions. The 17 members include physicians, researchers, and individuals involved in manufacturing and public health, and representatives from parent organizations.

Monitoring Delivery

Once vaccines are licensed and recommended for use, delivery to the appropriate individuals needs to be monitored. *Coverage* refers to the proportion of eligible individuals who receive a recommended vaccine. *Timeliness* assesses whether vaccinated individuals receive the recommended doses of a vaccine within the recommended age range; it can be measured as the proportion of individuals who receive the vaccine on time or as the cumulative number of days a given vaccine or vaccine series is delayed. Both coverage and timeliness are important measures of the quality of immunization care. Through effective monitoring, racial and ethnic disparities can be discovered, underserved groups can be identified, the effectiveness of intervention programs can be assessed, uptake of new vaccines and the effect of shortages can be tracked, and correlates of quality can be determined. Some of the mechanisms by which these ends are achieved in the United States are listed.

■ National Immunization Survey (NIS)

Conducted annually since 1994, the NIS is a random digit-dialing telephone survey of households in the United States. Historically focused on vaccine coverage among children 19 to 35 months of age, it was expanded in 2006 to include adolescents

13 to 17 years of age. Respondents provide information about vaccinations as well as sociodemographic information. For those children whose parents give permission, validating data are obtained from their providers. The survey includes all 50 states and selected urban and county areas; the 2006 report included data from 21,044 provider-reported vaccination records. **Figure 2.4** shows the results of the NIS over the past decade. The good news is that in general, coverage rates for individual vaccines have improved. The bad news is that coverage for the primary child-hood series (4 doses of DTaP; 3 doses of IPV; 1 dose of MMR; 3 doses of Hib; 3 doses of HepB; 1 dose of varicella vaccine, referred to as "4:3:1:3:3:1") lags behind. The 2006 survey demonstrated increases in coverage for PCV7 and varicella vaccine, although the rates for these vaccines, as well as for DTaP, still fell below the *Healthy People 2010* target of 90% (see Chapter 3, *Standards, Principles, and Regulations*). Disparities continued to exist between states—4:3:1:3:3:1 coverage ranged from 83.6% in Massachusetts to 59.5% in Nevada. Rates varied by race and ethnicity, with the differences largely due to socioeconomic factors—children living below the poverty level were less likely to be vaccinated.

FIGURE 2.4 — Immunization Coverage Rates Among Young Children

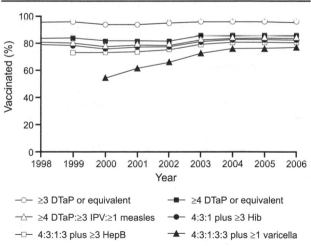

The graph shows the percentage of children 19 to 35 months of age who received the indicated vaccines.

Centers for Disease Control and Prevention. *MMWR*. 2007;56(RR-4): 880-885; Centers for Disease Control and Prevention. *MMWR*. 2003;52 (RR-4):728-732.

The 2006 survey also shed light on adolescent immunization. Coverage for 1 dose of Tdap, which was recommended in 2005, was only 10.8%. Coverage was 81.3% for 3 doses of HepB and 86.9% for 2 doses of MMR. Only 11.7% of adolescents had received MCV4. None of the *Healthy People 2010* targets for adolescents 13 through 15 years of age were met. This made it clear that we have a long way to go to in promoting immunization of adolescents.

NIS data have been instrumental in uncovering poor timeliness as an issue in vaccine delivery, one that is masked by good coverage rates. A study using 2003 NIS data and involving 14,810 children showed that during the first 2 years of life, children spent a median of 172 days underimmunized; 37% of underimmunized children had cumulative delays of >6 months. Eighteen percent of children who were considered fully covered by 24 months of age were actually undervaccinated for >6 months. In some states, <5% of children had received the 4:3:1:3:3 (4 DTaP, 3 IPV, 1 MMR, 3 Hib, 3 HepB) series exactly as recommended. Poor timeliness could leave children vulnerable to disease.

■ National Health Interview Survey (NHIS)

This survey covering a broad range of health issues has been conducted by the CDC's National Center for Health Statistics since 1957. The current sample size target is 35,000 households containing about 87,500 persons. The NHIS is an important source of information about adult vaccine coverage.

■ Behavioral Risk Factor Surveillance System (BRFSS)

This state-level, random digit-dialing telephone survey of noninstitutionalized civilians 18 years of age and older has been conducted by the CDC since 1984. More than 350,000 adults are surveyed every year, making the BRFSS the largest ongoing health survey in the world. The data obtained are very useful for issues such as influenza and pneumococcal vaccine coverage (**Figure 2.5**). The BRFSS showed that influenza vaccine coverage for high-risk individuals 18 to 49 years of age during the 2005-2006 season was only 30.5%. Coverage among individuals 50-64 years of age was 36.6%. Only 69.3% of individuals ≥65 years of age received a flu shot in the 2005-2006 season. We clearly have a long way to go in encouraging immunization of adults as well as adolescents.

■ School Surveys

Retrospective school entry surveys are the most common form of state and local level surveillance. Coverage data are collected from the health records of randomly selected schools, and an assessment is made of vaccine coverage. Audits are performed to validate school entry data. The data necessarily lag several years behind current performance because children are 5 or 6 when they enter school. In addition, no information on the timing of immunizations is obtained. A recent study looked at coverage

FIGURE 2.5 — Immunization Coverage Rates Among Adults

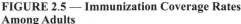

The graph shows the percentage of adults ≥65 years of age who received an influenza vaccine in the past year and the percentage who ever received pneumococcal vaccination.

Behavioral Risk Factor Surveillance System. Centers for Disease Control and Prevention Web site. http://apps.nccd.cdc.gov/brfss. Accessed August 15, 2008.

rates for kindergarten students during the 2006-2007 school year. Approximately 75% of states had reached the *Healthy People 2010* objective of ≥95% coverage for all vaccines among kindergarten attendees (this goal is higher than the general goal of 90% because settlings such as kindergarten represent a higher risk of spread of vaccine-preventable disease). These data highlighted the success of school mandates in ensuring that children are fully immunized.

■ **Special Area and Population Surveys**

These studies involve small geographic units such as counties or census tracts or specific populations in a local area, such as Medicaid participants. Largely supported by federal grants, special surveys can target needy groups and ensure accountability within the public and private health care sectors. The National Nursing Home Survey, which is conducted on an episodic basis, is an example of a targeted survey.

■ **Healthcare Effectiveness Data and Information Set (HEDIS)**

The National Committee for Quality Assurance, an independent nonprofit organization, monitors the performance of managed health care plans through HEDIS, a set of standardized measures. Immunization rates on preschoolers, children, adolescents, and adults are captured through administrative claims, encounter data, and chart review.

Monitoring Effectiveness

Vaccine-preventable disease activity must be monitored in order to assess the effectiveness of immunization programs. A variety of mechanisms are in place to accomplish this at the population level. Efforts are coordinated by the CDC's Epidemiology Program Office and the NCIRD, in collaboration with groups such as the Council of State and Territorial Epidemiologists. Over 60 diseases are now reportable through the National Notifiable Disease Surveillance System (NNDSS). Disease reporting by the states is voluntary, and reporting of diseases within states is mandated through legislation or regulation; for these reasons, the list of notifiable diseases varies from state to state. Reporting to the CDC occurs weekly through the National Electronic Telecommunications System for Surveillance; the CDC analyzes the data and launches investigations when appropriate. Active surveillance systems are in place for certain diseases such as measles, mumps, rubella, congenital rubella syndrome, diphtheria, tetanus, pertussis, poliomyelitis, and varicella. Laboratory-based surveillance programs, such as that for influenza, supplement these programs. Additional surveillance for invasive bacterial infections, such as those due to *S pneumoniae*, *H influenzae*, and *N meningitidis*, is done through the Active Bacterial Core, which is part of the CDC's Emerging Infections Program Network. This system stores demographic information on cases and collects bacterial isolates for further laboratory testing.

The New Vaccine Surveillance Network (NVSN) was established in 1999 in order to evaluate the impact of new vaccines and new recommendations. The network currently consists of three sentinel sites at academic medical centers: the University of Rochester in Rochester, NY, Vanderbilt University in Nashville, TN, and the Cincinnati Children's Hospital Medical Center in Cincinnati, OH. These sites conduct inpatient and outpatient surveillance for vaccine-preventable diseases, including seasonal surveillance for acute respiratory illness and acute gastroenteritis. Special targeted studies look at vaccine effectiveness.

The Vaccine Safety Net

No medical intervention is 100% safe. For therapeutic interventions—antibiotics, for example, in patients with pneumonia—there is an inherent tolerance for risk, because without therapy, the illness will intensify. Preventive interventions such as vaccines, in contrast, are usually given to people who are perfectly healthy; as a consequence, the tolerance for adverse events is much lower. Moreover, everyone gets vaccines but only selected people get medicines. Therefore, the consequences of even rare adverse events are significant at the population level. It has been said that when a medicine is given, disease is treated, but when vaccines are given, nothing happens. The truth is, of course, that disease prevention through vaccination is just as active a phenomenon as treating pneumonia with antibiotics. The difference is that with antibiotics, it is about what you see happen (the pneumonia improves), whereas with vaccines, it is about what you do not see happen (disease does not occur).

Major components of the vaccine safety net in the United States are listed in **Table 2.1**. Monitoring for safety begins as soon as a candidate vaccine is proposed for testing. Prelicensure evaluation is described earlier in this chapter. Aspects of postlicensure safety monitoring are described below.

■ **Vaccine Adverse Event Reporting System (VAERS)**

VAERS is a postmarketing surveillance system created by the National Childhood Vaccine Injury Act of 1986 (Public Law 99-660) and coadministered by the FDA and the CDC. Anyone can submit a report about any event that they feel is related to vaccination, and the reporting of certain events is mandated by law (provider responsibilities with respect to VAERS reporting are described in *Chapter 3*). Information from VAERS reports is entered into a database, and selected serious events and deaths are compiled and analyzed. Between 1991 and 2001, a total of 128,717 reports were received, representing approximately 11.4 reports per 100,000 net doses distributed. The most common adverse events reported were fever (25.8%), injection site hyper-

TABLE 2.1 — The Vaccine Safety Net in the United States

- FDA Center for Biologics Evaluation and Research (CBER)
- Good Manufacturing Practices (GMP)
- Good Laboratory Practices (GLP)
- Good Clinical Practices (GCP)
- Phase 1, 2, and 3 prelicensure trials
- Review and licensure by the FDA
- Review and recommendation by authoritative bodies such as the Advisory Committee on Immunization Practices (ACIP), the American Academy of Pediatrics (AAP), and the American Association of Family Physicians (AAFP)
- Phase 4 (postlicensure) studies
- Industry pharmacovigilance programs
- Vaccine Adverse Event Reporting System (VAERS)
- Vaccine Safety DataLink (VSD)
- Clinical Immunization Safety Assessment (CISA) Network
- Brighton Collaboration
- Ad-hoc groups such as the Task Force on Safer Childhood Vaccines (TFSCV) and the Immunization Safety Review Committee (ISRC) of the Institute of Medicine (IOM)

sensitivity (15.8%), rash (11.0%), injection site edema (10.8%), and vasodilatation (10.8%). Approximately 14% of reports described serious adverse events. Most reports were from vaccine manufacturers (36.2%), health departments (27.6%), and providers (20.0%). The proportion reported by providers increased from 11.4% in 1991 to 35.3% in 2001. Overall, only 4.2% of reports were filed by parents or patients.

A significant limitation of VAERS is that it only receives information regarding vaccinated persons in whom an adverse event occurs. Because it does not receive information about the number of vaccine doses administered or the occurrence of adverse events in unvaccinated persons, causal relationships between vaccines and particular adverse events cannot be established. In addition, underreporting, poor data quality, incomplete reports, differences between public and private sector reporting rates, lack of consistent diagnostic criteria for disease, and simultaneous administration of multiple vaccines limit the information that can be derived from VAERS. Moreover, significant reporting biases exist. For example, increased reporting is seen immediately after licensure and when particular vaccines are "in the news." As another example, many of the reports of autism following administration of thimerosal-containing vaccines have been filed by attorneys. For all of the above reasons, VAERS is vital for hypothesis *generation*, but not useful for hypothesis *testing*.

Despite these limitations, VAERS is the only surveillance system that covers the entire US population, and it includes the largest number of case reports temporally associated with vaccination. It serves to generate the signal that triggers further investigation, and can provide early warning of potential problems, including new, rare, or unusual adverse events. A good example of the utility of VAERS data was in prompting investigation of the relationship between the rhesus rotavirus vaccine and intussusception. Unfortunately, VAERS data have also been misunderstood by the media and misused by antivaccine activists, who have made the erroneous supposition that temporal association means causation.

■ The Vaccine Safety DataLink (VSD)

The VSD is an active surveillance system created by the CDC in 1990 and operated by the CDC's Immunization Safety Office. Information regarding vaccination, medical outcomes, birth history, and census is collected through large, linked, computerized databases from eight health maintenance organizations in Seattle, WA, Portland, OR, Oakland, CA, and Los Angeles, CA, Denver, CO, Minneapolis, MN, Marshfield, WI, and Boston, MA. Approximately 6 million people of all ages are studied through this process, amounting to 2% of the entire US population. Given these numbers, relatively rare adverse events can be detected. Strengths of the VSD include improved reporting, reduced recall bias, and the ability to study unvaccinated control subjects. For these reasons, the VSD is an excellent way to test hypotheses and determine if the relationship between a vaccine and an adverse event is causal or coincidental. A recent priority has been to develop mechanisms for rapid-cycle analysis to reduce the lag time between the occurrence of adverse events and assessment of risk factors. This methodology will be particularly useful for monitoring the safety of newly licensed vaccines.

■ Clinical Immunization Safety Assessment (CISA) Network

Before the creation of the first CISA centers in 2001, there was no coordinated effort to evaluate and treat vaccine adverse events in individual patients. The CISA network is a partnership between academic medical institutions and the CDC that systematically evaluates patients who experience adverse events after immunization. Major goals include studying the pathophysiologic basis of adverse events, understanding risk factors (including host genetics), and providing evidence-based guidelines for vaccination, revaccination, and evaluation of adverse events following vaccination. CISA centers as of 2008 are located at Johns Hopkins University (Baltimore, MD), Northern California Kaiser Permanente (San Francisco, CA), Vanderbilt University (Nashville, TN), Boston University (Boston, MA), Stanford University (Palo Alto, CA), and Columbia Presbyterian Hospital (New York, NY). Recent research priorities have included investigations of Guillain-Barré syndrome temporally associated with vaccination, hypersensitivity reactions, use of live vaccines in patients with DiGeorge syndrome, encephalitis following MMR, illness following yellow fever vaccine, and myopericarditis following smallpox immunization.

■ The Brighton Collaboration

The Brighton Collaboration, launched in 2000, is an international organization that aims to facilitate the development, evaluation, and dissemination of high-quality information about the safety of vaccines. Participants are volunteers from patient care, public health, pharmaceutical, regulatory, scientific, and professional organizations. The primary objective is to develop standardized definitions of adverse events following immunization, which should enhance comparability of data. In addition, Brighton aims to establish guidelines for collection, analysis, and presentation of safety data.

■ Ad-Hoc Committees and Task Forces

From time to time, ad-hoc committees and task forces are constituted to address particular issues. The National Childhood Vaccine Injury Act of 1986, for example, mandated the establishment of the TFSCV, comprising representatives of several PHS agencies. The charge was to make recommendations promoting the development of safer vaccines and assuring improvement in licensing, manufacturing, processing, testing, labeling, warning, use instructions, distribution, storage, administration, field surveillance, adverse reaction reporting, recall of reactogenic lots, and research. The task force report, released in 1998, emphasized the need to assess and address public concerns about the risks and benefits of vaccines, conduct research on the biological basis for vaccine reactions, foster partnership between stakeholders, enhance the ability to detect adverse events, and improve coordination of effort between agencies.

A good example of an ad-hoc committee is the Immunization Safety Review Committee (ISRC), convened in 2001 by the Institute of Medicine (IOM), a private, nonprofit, nongovernmental organization of distinguished scholars. The ISRC consisted of 15 members with expertise in pediatrics, internal medicine, infectious diseases, immunology, epidemiology and biostatistics, public health, nursing, ethics, and risk communication, among other disciplines. Committee members were subject to strict selection criteria in order to avoid real or perceived conflicts of interest. The committee was charged with reviewing nine different vaccine-safety hypotheses selected by an interagency vaccine group representing the NVPO, NIP (now the NCIRD), NIH, Department of Defense, the FDA, National Vaccine Injury Compensation Program, Health Care Financing Administration, and the Agency for International Development. Each review assessed scientific plausibility based on epidemiologic and clinical evidence of causality and experimental evidence for biologic mechanisms, as well as the significance of the issue in a broader societal context. Before release, the committee's reports were reviewed and critiqued by an independent panel of experts overseen by the National Research Council's Report Review Committee. **Table 2.2** summarizes the findings of the ISRC.

■ The Safety Net in Action

The release of rhesus-human reassortant rotavirus vaccine-tetravalent (RRV-TV; RotaShield) in the United States and its rapid withdrawal illustrate how well the safety net works. The vaccine was licensed based on demonstrated safety and efficacy in clinical trials wherein nearly 11,000 children received the vaccine in its final formulation. With universal use, the vaccine was expected to prevent 55,000 hospitalizations and 25 deaths each year. Before licensure, an ACIP Working Group, the NIH, and the AAP considered the possibility of an association between the vaccine and intussusception but rejected a causal relationship based on statistical analyses of the few cases that did occur. Nevertheless, the package insert listed intussusception as possible adverse reaction and postlicensure surveillance was mandated. The vaccine was licensed in August 1998. By July 1999 there were 15 reports of intussusception in the VAERS database, and several population-based investigations suggested a causal relationship. The CDC recommended suspension of vaccination, and by October 1999 the product was withdrawn from the market.

It is estimated that intussusception attributable to RRV-TV occurred once for every 11,000 children vaccinated, although some argue that the risk was actually much less. In any event, the risk was so small that it could not have been detected in the prelicensure trials, given the number of children enrolled. However, the vaccine safety net performed remarkably well, such that in a very short period of time the potential danger signal was detected, studies were conducted, and use of the vaccine was suspended. As a result of this experience, new-generation rotavirus vaccines have been tested in tens of thousands of children before licensure in order to detect even a weak association with intussusception. Even these massive trials, however, cannot detect extremely small associations. Therefore, rigorous postmarketing studies will need to be done. Ultimately, the decision to use any new vaccine will necessarily need to balance the known risks, however small, with the known complications of disease, and society will need to answer the question as to where the threshold for risk tolerance should be set.

Financing

Table 2.3 illustrates a simple truth: for any given individual in the United States, the total cost for all routinely recommended vaccines has skyrocketed, driven by the increased number of vaccines that are recommended for universal use and the increased cost of newer vaccines. Layered on top of the purchase price for vaccines are the costs associated with administration, from personnel time, storage, and equipment to wastage and insurance.

The system for financing immunization in the United States rests on a unique partnership between the public and private sectors—more than half of the purchase cost is borne by public entities, but most of the vaccinating is done in private settings. As seen in **Figure 2.6**, only 46% of the purchase cost of routine childhood vaccines is borne by the private sector; most of this is reimbursed through private insurance, but some comes directly out-of-pocket. Many states have laws requiring insurers to cover childhood immunizations, at least to some degree. Some mandate coverage in accord with the recommended childhood immunization schedule, while others make reference to appropriate pediatric vaccines. Some states prohibit deductibles and coinsurance, and while self-insured employers may be exempt from such regulation, federal statutes prohibit employers providing vaccine coverage as of May 1, 1993, from reducing that coverage. Insurance plans vary in terms of which vaccines they cover for both children and adults and to what extent they reimburse for vaccine administration. In general, managed care plans are more likely than indemnity plans to cover vaccines and to promote their use. Delays in covering new vaccines are common—some

TABLE 2.2 — Immunization Safety Review Committee Findings

Report Date	Topic	Findings
April 2001	*Measles-Mumps-Rubella Vaccine and Autism*	Reject causal relationship at the population level
		Cannot exclude possibility that MMR contributes to autism in a small number of children
October 2001	*Thimerosal-Containing Vaccines and Neurodevelopmental Disorders*	Hypothesis is biologically plausible
		Evidence is inadequate to accept or reject a causal relationship
February 2002	*Multiple Immunizations and Immune Dysfunction*	Reject causal relationship for increased risk of heterologous infections and type 1 diabetes
		Evidence is inadequate to accept or reject a causal relationship for allergic diseases
		Evidence for proposed mechanisms of allergy and autoimmunity is weak or theoretical
May 2002	*Hepatitis B Vaccine and Demyelinating Neurological Disorders*	Reject causal relationship for incident multiple sclerosis and multiple sclerosis relapse
		Evidence is inadequate to accept or reject a causal relationship for other demyelinating diseases
		Evidence for proposed mechanisms is weak
October 2002	*SV40 Contamination of Polio Vaccine and Cancer*	Evidence is inadequate to accept or reject a causal relationship for cancer
		Evidence is moderate that SV40 exposure could lead to human cancer

March 2003	*Vaccinations and Sudden Unexpected Death in Infancy*	Reject causal relationship for DTwP and for multiple simultaneous vaccinations
		Evidence is inadequate to accept or reject a causal relationship for DTaP, Hib, HepB, OPV, and IPV
		Evidence for proposed mechanisms is theoretical
October 2003	*Influenza Vaccines and Neurological Complications*	Accept causal relationship between 1976 swine influenza vaccine and Guillain-Barré syndrome
		Evidence is inadequate to accept or reject a causal relationship for other influenza vaccines
		Reject causal relationship for relapse of multiple sclerosis
		Evidence is inadequate to accept or reject a causal relationship for incident multiple sclerosis, optic neuritis, and other demyelinating disorders
		Evidence for proposed mechanisms is weak or theoretical
May 2004	*Vaccines and Autism*	Reject causal relationship between MMR and thimerosal-containing vaccines and autism
		Evidence for proposed mechanisms is theoretical

Immunization Safety Review. Institute of Medicine of the National Academies Web site. http://www.iom.edu/?ID=4705. Accessed August 15, 2008.

TABLE 2.3 — Cost of Vaccines (US$) in the Routine Childhood Schedule[a]

Sector	1987	2003	2007[b]	
			Boys	Girls
Public	34	437	924	1214
Private	116	705	1338	1700

[a] The total cost of all vaccines recommended in the routine childhood schedule is given. Public sector cost is based on the VFC contract price. Private sector cost is estimated from catalog prices. The cost of the least expensive products was used in the calculations.

[b] The difference between boys and girls in 2007 is due to the HPV vaccine, which is only recommended for girls.

Hinman AR, et al. *Clin Infect Dis*. 2004;38:1440-1446; and CDC Vaccine Price List. Centers for Disease Control and Prevention Web site. http://www.cdc.gov/vaccines/programs/vfc/cdc-vac-price-list.htm. Accessed August 15, 2008.

insurers wait until official recommendations are published before they will provide reimbursement.

Medicare, an entirely federal insurance program, is an important source of funding for adults 65 years of age and older. Part B, which requires a monthly premium, covers influenza vaccine and PPSV23 without deductibles or coinsurance. HepB is also covered for individuals of any age with end-stage renal disease or other high-risk conditions. Part D, a prescription drug plan that also requires a monthly premium, covers the zoster vaccine. Future vaccines for older adults should also be covered under Part D but may be subject to prior authorization requirements to determine medical necessity. Medicare reimbursement includes the cost of administration.

Medicaid is another source of vaccine funding for adults, but coverage and reimbursement rates vary widely from state to state.

Public sector funds for vaccination include the following sources:

• *The Vaccines for Children (VFC) Program*—Created in 1993 by the Omnibus Budget Reconciliation Act, VFC is a federal program that guarantees immunization services for children 18 and younger who are 1) Medicaid-eligible; 2) uninsured; 3) underinsured and receiving immunizations at federally-qualified health centers (FQHCs) or rural health clinics (RHCs); or 4) American Indian or Alaska Native.

Through this program, vaccines are purchased by the CDC at reduced rates and provided to participating private practices and public clinics free of charge. Providers are prohibited from charging the patient for the vaccine. Whereas they *can* charge patients administration fees, within limits established by the Centers for Medicare and Medicaid Services, they cannot

FIGURE 2.6 — Childhood Vaccines According to Funding Source, 2005

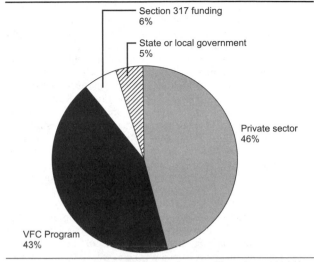

Section 317 funding
6%

State or local government
5%

Private sector
46%

VFC Program
43%

Data from Vaccine Manufacturers Biologics Surveillance Data, 2005 (does not include influenza vaccine) as cited in Rodewald LE.

Rodewald LE. Implementing new vaccines and vaccine recommendations. Paper presented at: National Vaccine Advisory Committee; September 26, 2006; Washington, DC. http://hhs.gov/nvpo/nvac/sep06 .html. Accessed August 15, 2008.

deny vaccination if the patients cannot pay the fee (claims for these fees can still be submitted to Medicaid for those children who are enrolled). There are no regulations regarding charges for the office visit itself or nonvaccination services.

Any private provider who sees eligible children can participate in the program; this has resulted in a shift toward private sector delivery of vaccines, establishing an anchor point for the medical home for many children. Vaccines that are routinely recommended by the ACIP are included in the VFC program through separate ACIP resolutions. However, significant delays in securing a federal contract may occur. During such delays, state Medicaid programs are bound to cover ACIP-recommended vaccines.

It is important to remember that VFC is an *entitlement* program, which means that Congress is obliged to appropriate the funds necessary to purchase the covered vaccines, no matter how much they cost. At the same time, there are an increasing number of children who are falling out of the system, namely those who qualify for VFC because their private insurance does not cover all routinely recommended vaccines (the underinsured) but who must receive their VFC vaccines at FQHCs or RHCs. The simple fact is that many of these children do not make it to these sites, and the fall-back position—namely, to receive the uncovered vaccines at the local health department—is less of an option as the other public funding sources listed below become more inadequate.

There is no VFC-equivalent program for adults.

• *Section 317 Funds*—States, territories, protectorates, and several designated cities may purchase vaccines through block grants under Section 317 of the Public Health Service Act. The majority of these funds are used for childhood immunization, but adolescent and adult programs may be supported as well. Section 317 funds may also be used to support infrastructure and programmatic activities such as quality assurance, immunization information systems (IISs), disease surveillance, and school- or community-based delivery services. The main intent of the 317 program is to provide vaccines to individuals who fall outside of the VFC program. The problem is that this program—in contrast to VFC—represents *discretionary* federal spending. The amount allocated by Congress, therefore, varies from year to year, and as the costs of vaccination have increased, so has the financing gap.

• *State and Local Funds*—States may appropriate funds to support both childhood and adult immunizations, but in general the contribution of this source to the whole funding picture is small (**Figure 2.6**). The State Children's Health Insurance Program (SCHIP), enacted in 1997, is a federal block grant program targeted to low-income children who are not eligible for Medicaid and are otherwise uninsured. States can use SCHIP funds to expand Medicaid or to create separate, freestanding children's insurance programs.

Table 2.4 shows various models that states have developed to pay for childhood vaccination. As of 2006, 18 states and territories had some type of universal purchase policy. Under these plans, federal, state, and local monies are used to purchase recommended childhood vaccines at the CDC-negotiated price. The vaccines are then distributed to providers free of charge for administration to children, regardless of insurance status. Providers may still charge administration fees but reimbursement varies. Supporters argue that universal purchase removes financial barriers to immunization, improves coverage rates, reinforces the concept of the medical home, increases immunization rates, improves efficiency, reduces overhead at the provider level, and facilitates participation in IISs. Detractors argue that public funds should not be used to pay for vaccines that insurers would otherwise cover. In addition, concerns have been raised about potential restrictions on product choice and provider autonomy,

TABLE 2.4 — State Vaccine Financing Models[a]

Policy	Description
Universal	State provides all routine childhood vaccines for all children in all settings
Universal select	State provides some routine childhood vaccines for all children in all settings
VFC-enhanced	State provides all routine childhood vaccines for VFC-eligible[b] and under-insured[c] children in all settings
VFC-enhanced select	State provides some vaccines for under-insured[c] children and all routine childhood vaccines for VFC-eligible[b] children in all settings
VFC only	State provides all routine childhood vaccines for VFC-eligible[b] children only

[a] In general, these models only cover the costs of the vaccines themselves and not the costs of administration.
[b] Under 19 years of age and Medicaid-eligible, uninsured, American Indian/Alaska Native, or underinsured and receiving vaccines through a federally qualified health center or rural health center.
[c] Insured but coverage does not include vaccines.

Stokley S, et al. *Am J Pub Health*. 2006;96:1308-1313.

as well as loss of financial incentives for manufacturers to bring new vaccines to market.

The current system for funding vaccine services has achieved high levels of childhood immunization, but new challenges exist, including the increased number of recommended vaccines, high prices, disparities in coverage, low levels of adult immunization, the growing burden of vaccine practice on clinicians, shortages, and the increased costs of bringing new products to market. With these factors in mind, the CDC asked the IOM in 2002 to study vaccine financing. The final report of the Committee on the Evaluation of Vaccine Purchase Financing in the United States, released in 2003, recommended replacement of existing government vaccine purchasing programs with a new vaccine insurance mandate, subsidy, and voucher plan. The principal recommendations are summarized below:

- Legislation requiring vaccination coverage by all public and private health plans
- A federal subsidy to reimburse health plans and providers for mandated vaccine costs and administration fees
- A voucher system for vaccines and administration fees for designated uninsured populations
- Principal application of the insurance mandate, subsidy, and voucher system to vaccines with substantial societal benefits

- Determination of the amount of subsidies and vouchers for current vaccines as well as those not yet available, taking into account the calculated societal benefit
- Changes in the procedures and membership of the ACIP to ensure that vaccine coverage decisions are associated with societal benefits and costs, including the impact of the price of a vaccine with recommendations for its use
- Stakeholder deliberations on the administrative, technical, and legislative issues surrounding a shift to a mandatory system, as well as postimplementation studies

In 2005, the NVAC issued a response to the IOM report. It agreed with IOM on many points, including the need for action in ensuring easy access to vaccines, stabilizing the market so that it remains attractive to manufacturers, and the need for additional funding. However, NVAC suggested incremental improvements in the current system rather than replacing it with something else. The principal recommendations are summarized below:

- Expansion and stabilization of funding through Section 317 for immunization program infrastructure and operations, as well as for vaccine purchase, within existing guidelines
- Expansion of funding through Section 317 to support adolescent and adult immunization programs including vaccine purchase
- Rapid appropriation of new funds through Section 317 when new vaccines are recommended for universal use
- Expansion of VFC to include underinsured children in all public health clinics, removal of price caps, and giving all providers and clinics a choice of vaccines
- Regulatory harmonization to facilitate introduction of vaccines licensed in other countries that are in compliance with FDA-approved standards
- Further exploration of regulatory and other factors impeding vaccine research and development
- Increased communication between industry and the FDA throughout the process of vaccine research and development
- Promotion of "first-dollar" insurance coverage for immunization and promoting prompt coverage and recalculation of capitation rates when new vaccines are recommended
- Assurance of adequate reimbursement for administration of vaccines
- Expanded discussion about the possibility of a vaccines for adults or vaccines for all program to ensure that adults have access to vaccines, even if they do not have insurance

Supply

The last decade has seen unique and unprecedented shortages in the supply of many routinely used vaccines. The impact of these shortages has included frequent and sometimes confusing changes in the recommended immunization schedule, temporary revision of state school entry requirements, parental frustration, and a burden placed on providers to track interrupted schedules and recall patients when vaccine supplies returned to sufficiency. To date, there is no evidence that shortages have caused disease outbreaks.

Shortages result from a convergence of factors, such as:

- *Fewer manufacturers*—Vaccines are low-profit products compared with other pharmaceuticals. The costs of development have skyrocketed, the time line from preclinical testing to market may be longer than a decade, and the risks are substantial—a licensed vaccine may or may not be recommended for use in large numbers of people. Moreover, the risk of failure persists for some time after marketing—the low tolerance for adverse events leaves manufacturers vulnerable to market failure after millions of doses have been distributed. In the late 1960s, there were >20 vaccine manufacturers licensed in the United States; today, there are only six—GlaxoSmithKline, MedImmune, Merck, Novartis, Sanofi Pasteur, and Wyeth. Some of this decrease was due to mergers but some resulted from companies simply getting out of the business. With so few manufacturers, disruptions at one company can have a major effect on supply. For single-source products like PCV7 and varicella vaccine, the effect is magnified.
- *Business decisions*—Some companies have chosen to pull products from the market rather than invest in costly changes in manufacturing processes or facilities. Such changes might be mandated in order to adhere to GMPs; others might be prompted by new recommendations. An example of the latter was the 1999 recommendation to remove thimerosal from childhood vaccines (see Chapter 8, *Addressing Concerns About Vaccines*), which led some companies to pull out rather than retool their manufacturing and packaging processes (ie, to make single-dose vials or prefilled syringes) and demonstrate equivalency of the reformulated products in lot-comparison trials.
- *Production problems*—Production problems may have a biologic basis. For example, the influenza A (H3N2) strain used for the 2000-2001 vaccine grew slowly in culture, delaying vaccine production. Similarly, a low yield of vaccine strain varicella zoster virus in culture led to shortages of MMRV. Production problems can also result from routine physical plant maintenance activities.
- *Underestimated demand*—The recommendation in April 2000 to decrease the age for routine influenza vaccination from 65 to 50 years compounded production problems by increasing demand. Similarly, greater-than-expected demand for PCV7 and MCV4 after each of these vaccines was licensed contributed to shortages.

Recent vaccine shortages are summarized in **Table 2.5**. This table also describes the issues leading to the shortage and the associated CDC recommendations. In instances when deferral is recommended, providers should keep lists of patients who will need to be recalled once supplies improve. Current information about vaccine shortages can be found at http://www.cdc.gov/vaccines/vac-gen/shortages/default.htm (Accessed August 15, 2008).

The CDC has maintained stockpiles of vaccines since 1983. These might be more accurately termed *storage and rotation contracts* or *dynamic strategic inventories*—some portion of vaccine production lots enters the stockpile, and older vaccine with at least 12 months of shelf life left is released onto the market. Between 1983 and 2002, only single-source vaccines were stockpiled. Since 2002, the goal has been to stockpile 6 months' worth of each routine childhood vaccine (except for influenza vaccine, which changes in composition from year to year). The stockpile has been accessed on at least 8 occasions because of supply issues.

In 2003, the NVAC suggested the following short-term measures to improve vaccine supply:

- Increase funding for vaccine stockpiles that would include all routinely administered vaccines
- Increase support for CBER in order to enhance review of the scientific evidence supporting the safety, efficacy, and quality of vaccines
- Highlight the function of NVPO and NVAC in identifying vaccine priorities
- Maintain and strengthen the National Vaccine Injury Compensation Program (see *Chapter 3*), which removes liability concerns as a barrier to manufacturers; include coverage for injuries due to preservatives, additives, and excipients, not just the vaccine antigens
- Require manufacturers to warn HHS of intent to withdraw a product from the market
- Improve availability of accurate supply information for opinion leaders and consumers
- Enhance the valuation of vaccines through educational campaigns

Bioterrorism

Bioterrorism refers to the deliberate release of a harmful biological agent to intimidate civilians and their government (biowarfare more accurately refers to the use of such agents by warring parties to inflict mass casualties). The discovery in the 1990s that the Soviet Union and Iraq had well-established bioweapons development programs, and the occurrence of high-profile domestic and international terrorist events, combined to raise alarm that governments, individuals, or small groups could mount effective biological attacks. This fear was realized in the US anthrax attacks of September and October 2001.

The following characteristics make certain biological agents ideal for use as agents of terrorism:

- Ability to cause high morbidity and mortality
- Potential for person-to-person transmission
- Low infective dose
- Infectious by aerosol dissemination
- Effective vaccine unavailable or in short supply
- Absence of natural immunity
- Availability of the agent and feasibility of large-scale production
- Environmental stability
- Ability to induce panic based on historical fears of infectious diseases

Agents that are currently considered potential threats are listed in **Table 2.6**; many of these agents have already been weaponized in several countries. Vaccines (and passive immunoprophylactics) have a role in biodefense, but that role is complicated by a number of factors. First, until recently there have been few incentives to develop vaccines against many of these agents. In addition, the development process is long and arduous, and great forethought is needed to anticipate which vaccines might become necessary. Second, there are few if any historical precedents for the use of vaccines in biodefense. Third, for many diseases efficacy cannot be tested directly and surrogate markers of protection are not known. Fourth, biological agents can be genetically manipulated to change their antigenicity and render conventional vaccines less useful. Finally, the balance between the benefits of pre-exposure vaccination and safety concerns must be addressed. The infrastructure for large-scale postexposure vaccination must be developed, although for some agents with short incubation periods, postexposure vaccination would not be useful.

TABLE 2.5 — Recent Vaccine Shortages[a]

Vaccine	Date	Issue	Principal Recommendations	Reference
DTaP	March 2001	Wyeth Lederle and Baxter Hyland stopped production	Defer dose 4 for infants if necessary Continue dose at 4 to 6 years of age	*MMWR.* 2001;50:189-190
	January 2002	Continued shortage	Prioritize primary series in infants Defer doses 4 and 5 if necessary	*MMWR.* 2002;50:1159
HepA	July 2002	Supply sufficient	Resume routine schedule	*MMWR.* 2002;51:598-599
	August 2007	Regulatory review of manufacturing change for Vaqta (Merck)	No new recommendations	CDC[a]
Hib	December 2007	PedvaxHIB and Comvax (Merck) recalled because of potential for bacterial contamination	Defer routine booster dose at 12 to 15 months of age	*MMWR.* 2007;56:1318-1320
Influenza	July 2000	Potential shortage for 2000-2001 season	Delay implementation of organized campaigns until November Continue vaccination of high-risk individuals Develop contingency plans	*MMWR.* 2000;49:619-622
	July 2001	Potential shortage for 2001-2002 season	Target vaccine in September and October to high-risk individuals Include healthy individuals 50 to 64 years of age, and others wishing to	*MMWR.* 2001;50:582-585

78

Vaccine	Date	Status	Recommendation	Reference
			reduce their risk, in November	
			Delay workplace and public campaigns until November	
	August 2003	Supply sufficient	Resume routine vaccination	MMWR. 2003;52:796-797
	October 2004	License to manufacture Fluvirin (Chiron) suspended for 2004-2005 season	Prioritize vaccine to high-risk groups, including children 6 to 23 months of age, pregnant women, and health care workers	MMWR. 2004;53:923-924
			Encourage use of LAIV	
MCV4	May 2006	Supply outpaced by demand	Defer vaccination of individuals 11 to 12 years of age	MMWR. 2006;55:567-568
	November 2006	Supply sufficient	Resume routine vaccination	MMWR. 2006;55:1177
MMR	March 2002	Voluntary interruptions in manufacturing operations (Merck)	Defer second MMR dose at 4 to 6 years of age if necessary	MMWR. 2002;51:190-193
	July 2002	Supply sufficient	Resume routine schedule	MMWR. 2002;51:598-599
PCV7	September 2001	Delayed delivery	Defer vaccination of children >2 years of age except those 2 to 5 years of age who are high-risk	MMWR. 2001;50:783-784
	December 2001	Duration and severity of shortage worse than anticipated	For severe shortage: • <6 months of age: defer doses 3 and 4 • 7 to 12 months of age: defer dose 3	MMWR. 2001;50:1140-1142

Continued

2

TABLE 2.5 — *Continued*

Vaccine	Date	Issue	Principal Recommendations	Reference
PCV7 *(continued)*			• 12 to 23 months of age: defer dose 2 • >24 months of age: no vaccination unless high-risk Report invasive pneumococcal disease in vaccinees	
	May 2003	Supply sufficient	Resume routine schedule	*MMWR.* 2003;52:446
	December 2003	Production constraints	Manufacturer to implement an allocation plan	*MMWR.* 2003;52:1234
	February 2004	Shortage	Defer dose 4	*MMWR.* 2004;53:108-109
	March 2004	Continued shortage	Defer doses 3 and 4	*MMWR.* 2004;53:177-178
	July 2004	Supply improved	Reinstitute dose 3	*MMWR.* 2004;53:589-590
	September 2004	Supply sufficient	Resume routine vaccination	*MMWR.* 2004;53:851-852
Td	November 2000	Decreased release by Wyeth and prolonged maintenance on production facilities at Aventis Pasteur	Prioritize: • Individuals traveling to diphtheria-endemic areas • Wound management • Individuals with incomplete primary series • Pregnant women, individuals with occupational risk, adolescents, and	*MMWR.* 2000;49:1029-1030

	Date	Status	Recommendation	Reference
			adults who have not received Td in the last 10 years	
	May 2001	Continued shortage	Defer routine boosters in adults and adolescents	MMWR. 2001;50:418-427
	June 2002	Supply sufficient	Resume routine boosters	MMWR. 2002;51:529-530
	March 2002	Voluntary interruptions in manufacturing operations (Merck)	Delay vaccination until 18 to 24 months of age Prioritize: • Health care workers, contacts of immunocompromised persons, adolescents, adults, high-risk children • Susceptible children 5 to 12 years of age • Children 2 to 4 years of age	MMWR. 2002;51:190-193
Varicella	August 2002	Supply sufficient	Resume routine schedule	MMWR. 2002;51:679
	February 2007	Low yield of varicella resulted in suspension of MMRV production	Use monovalent vaccine	MMWR. 2007;56:146-147

[a] Current Vaccine Shortages & Delays. Centers for Disease Control and Prevention Web site. http://www.cdc.gov/vaccines/vac-gen/shortages/default.htm. Accessed August 15, 2008.

TABLE 2.6 — Potential Agents of Bioterrorism

Category	Characteristics	Disease/Condition	Agent	US Vaccine Status
A	Highest priority Easily disseminated or transmitted from person to person High mortality Potential for major public health impact Potential for public panic and social disruption Require specpial action for preparedness	Anthrax	*Bacillus anthracis*	Licensed (see Chapter 10, *Specialized Vaccines*)
		Botulism	*Clostridium botulinum* toxin	Pentavalent toxoid vaccine available through CDC
		Plague	*Yersinia pestis*	Formalin-inactivated whole-cell vaccine no longer available
		Smallpox	Variola virus	Licensed (see *Chapter 10*)
		Tularemia	*Francisella tularensis*	Live-attenuated vaccine (used for laboratory workers) no longer available
		Viral hemorrhagic fevers	Filoviruses (eg, Ebola, Marburg), arenaviruses (eg, Lassa fever, Machupol)	No licensed vaccine
B	Second highest priority Moderately easy to disseminate Moderate morbidity and low mortality	Brucellosis	*Brucella* sp	No licensed vaccine
		Epsilon toxin	*Clostridium perfringens*	No licensed vaccine
		Food safety threats	*Salmonella* sp, *Escherichia coli*	Typhoid vaccine licensed (see *Chapter 10*)

Category	Disease	Agent	Vaccine
Require specific enhancements of diagnostic capacity and surveillance		O157:H7, *Shigella*	No licensed vaccine
	Glanders	*Burkholderia mallei*	No licensed vaccine
	Melioidosis	*Burkholderia pseudomallei*	No licensed vaccine
	Psittacosis	*Chlamydophila psittaci*	No licensed vaccine
	Q fever	*Coxiella burnetii*	No licensed vaccine
	Ricin toxin	Derived from castor beans (*Ricinus communis*)	No licensed vaccine
	Enterotoxin B	*Staphylococcus aureus*	No licensed vaccine
	Typhus fever	*Rickettsia prowazekii*	No licensed vaccine
	Viral encephalitis	Alphaviruses (eg, Venezuelan equine encephalitis, eastern equine encephalitis, western equine encephalitis)	No licensed vaccine
	Water safety threats	*Vibrio cholerae*, *Cryptosporidium parvum*	Phenol-inactivated cholera vaccine no longer available
C	Emerging infectious diseases	Nipah virus, hantavirus	No licensed vaccine
	Could be used in the future		

Bioterrorism Agents/Diseases. Centers for Disease Control and Prevention Web site. http://www.bt.cdc.gov/agent/agentlist-category.asp. Accessed August 15, 2008; and Biodefense Information & Resources. Infectious Diseases Society of America Web site. http://www.idsociety.org/bt/toc.htm. Accessed August 15, 2008.

Vaccine Development and Licensure

US Food and Drug Administration. Good Clinical Practice in FDA-Regulated Clinical Trials. http://www.fda.gov/oc/gcp. Accessed August 15, 2008.

Monitoring Delivery

Centers for Disease Control and Prevention (CDC). National, state, and local area vaccination coverage among children aged 19–35 months—United States, 2006. *MMWR Morb Mortal Wkly Rep.* 2007;56:880-885.

Centers for Disease Control and Prevention (CDC). National vaccination coverage among adolescents aged 13–17 years—United States, 2006. *MMWR Morb Mortal Wkly Rep.* 2007;56:885-888.

Centers for Disease Control and Prevention (CDC). State-specific influenza vaccination coverage among adults aged > or =18 years—United States, 2003-04 and 2005-06 influenza seasons. *MMWR Morb Mortal Wkly Rep.* 2007;56:953-959.

Centers for Disease Control and Prevention (CDC). Vaccination coverage among children in kindergarten—United States, 2006–07 school year. *MMWR Morb Mortal Wkly Rep.* 2007;56:819-821.

Immunization Coverage in the U.S. Centers for Disease Control and Prevention Web site. http://www.cdc.gov/vaccines/stats-surv/imz-coverage.htm#nis. Accessed August 15, 2008.

Luman ET, Barker LE, McCauley MM, et al. A measure of success: findings from the National Immunization Survey. *Am J Prev Med.* 2001;20(suppl 4):1-154.

Luman ET, Barker LE, Shaw KM, McCauley MM, Buehler JW, Pickering LK. Timeliness of childhood vaccinations in the United States: days undervaccinated and number of vaccines delayed. *JAMA.* 2005;293:1204-1211.

Monitoring Effectiveness

Active bacterial core surveillance. Centers for Disease Control and Prevention Web site. http://www.cdc.gov/ncidod/dbmd/abcs/index.htm. Accessed August 15, 2008.

New vaccine surveillance network. Centers for Disease Control and Prevention Web site. http://www.cdc.gov/vaccines/stats-surv/nvsn/default.htm. Accessed August 15, 2008.

Wharton M, Hughes H, Reilly M, eds. *Manual for the Surveillance of Vaccine-Preventable Diseases.* 3rd ed, 2002. http://www.cdc.gov/vaccines/pubs/surv-manual/default.htm#compressed. Accessed August 15, 2008.

The Vaccine Safety Net

Bonhoeffer J, Kohl KS, Chen R, et al. The Brighton Collaboration: addressing the need for standardized case definitions of adverse events following immunization (AEFI). *Vaccine.* 2002;21:298-302.

Chen RT. Evaluation of vaccine safety after the events of 11 September 2001: role of cohort and case-control studies. *Vaccine*. 2004;22:2047-2053.

Chen RT, Glasser JW, Rhodes PH, et al. Vaccine Safety Datalink project: a new tool for improving vaccine safety monitoring in the United States. The Vaccine Safety Datalink Team. *Pediatrics*. 1997;99:765-773.

National Institute of Allergy and Infectious Diseases; National Institutes of Health. Task Force on Safer Childhood Vaccines: Final Report and Recommendations. http://www.niaid.nih.gov/publications/vaccine/safervacc.htm. Accessed August 15, 2008.

Peter G, Myers MG; National Vaccine Advisory Committee; National Vaccine Program Office. Intussusception, rotavirus, and oral vaccines: summary of a workshop. *Pediatrics*. 2002;110:e67.

Varricchio F, Iskander J, Destefano F, et al. Understanding vaccine safety information from the Vaccine Adverse Event Reporting System. *Pediatr Infect Dis J*. 2004;23:287-294.

Zhou W, Pool V, Iskander JK, et al. Surveillance for safety after immunization: Vaccine Adverse Event Reporting System (VAERS)—United States, 1991-2001. *MMWR Surveill Summ*. 2003;52:1-24.

Financing

Committee on the Evaluation of Vaccine Purchase Financing in the United States, Board on Health Care Services, Institute of Medicine of the National Academes. Financing Vaccines in the 21st Century: Assuring Access and Availability. http://www.nap.edu/catalog.php?record_id=10782. Accessed August 15, 2008.

Hinman AR; National Vaccine Advisory Committee. Financing vaccines in the 21st century: recommendations from the National Vaccine Advisory Committee. *Am J Prev Med*. 2005;29:71-75.

Hinman AR, Orenstein WA, Rodewald L. Financing immunizations in the United States. *Clin Infect Dis*. 2004;38:1440-1446.

Lee GM, Santoli JM, Hannan C, et al. Gaps in vaccine financing for underinsured children in the United States. *JAMA*. 2007;298:638-643.

Orenstein WA, Mootrey GT, Pazol K, Hinman AR. Financing immunization of adults in the United States. *Clin Pharmacol Ther*. 2007;82:764-768.

Supply

Hinman AR, Orenstein WA, Santoli JM, Rodewald LE, Cochi SL. Vaccine shortages: history, impact, and prospects for the future. *Annu Rev Public Health*. 2006;27:235-259.

Klein JO, Myers MG. Vaccine shortages: why they occur and what needs to be done to strengthen vaccine supply. *Pediatrics*. 2006;117:2269-2275.

Klein JO, Myers MG. Strengthening the supply of routinely administered vaccines in the United States: problems and proposed solutions. *Clin Infect Dis*. 2006;42(suppl 3):S97-S103.

Santoli JM, Peter G, Arvin AM, et al; National Vaccine Advisory Committee. Strengthening the supply of routinely recommended vaccines in the United States: recommendations from the National Vaccine Advisory Committee. *JAMA*. 2003;290:3122-3128.

Sloan FA, Berman S, Rosenbaum S, Chalk RA, Giffin RB. The fragility of the U.S. vaccine supply. *N Engl J Med*. 2004;351:2443-2447.

Standards, Principles, and Regulations

Healthy People 2010

Healthy People 2010: Objectives for Improving Health, issued January 25, 2000, is a comprehensive set of health objectives for the first decade of the new century issued by the US Department of Health and Human Services (HHS). An extension of the 1979 Surgeon General's Report entitled *Healthy People* and *Healthy People 2000: National Health Promotion and Disease Prevention Objectives*, the updated *Healthy People 2010* identifies the most significant preventable threats to health and focuses public and private efforts to address those threats. The agenda was developed over several years by scientists, federal and state agencies, and national professional organizations, with input from the public.

Healthy People 2010 has two overarching goals: to increase quality and years of healthy life and to eliminate health disparities. Twenty-eight focus areas are identified, one of which is Immunization and Infectious Diseases, wherein the following aspects of vaccines are emphasized:

- Vaccines can prevent disease and death from infectious diseases, but they do not necessarily eliminate the causative organisms; by extension, decreased vaccine coverage can lead to reemergence of disease.
- Vaccines protect individuals, and vaccinated individuals protect society through herd immunity.
- Vaccines provide significant cost-benefits.

Tremendous progress in reducing indigenous cases of vaccine-preventable diseases is noted, successes mediated by outreach to underserved populations, expansion of school entry requirements, public financing of childhood vaccinations, and the widespread use of novel, highly effective vaccines such as Hib. However, the report highlights the persistence of underserved groups and the fact that most vaccine-preventable diseases in the United States occur in adults, who are much less likely to be appropriately immunized.

The following strategies are given to continue protecting people from vaccine-preventable diseases:

- Improving the quality and quantity of vaccine delivery services
- Minimizing financial barriers
- Increasing community participation, education, and partnership
- Improving the monitoring of disease and vaccine coverage
- Developing new or improved vaccines and improving vaccine use

The report sets general objectives for prevention of disease through universal and targeted vaccination programs; these are summarized in **Table 3**.**1**. The report also sets the goal for coverage with universally recommended vaccines at 90%. Baseline rates for 3 doses of Hib, 1 dose of MMR, and 3 doses of polio vaccine in 1998 actually exceeded that mark, whereas the rates for 4 doses of DTaP and 3 doses of HepB were slightly below. The rate for varicella vaccine at that time was only 43%. **Table 3**.**2** gives the specific *Healthy People 2010* goals for vaccine-preventable diseases.

In August 2007, HHS announced the establishment of the Secretary's Advisory Committee on National Health Promotion and Disease Prevention Objectives for 2020. The framework for *Healthy People 2020* is expected to be released by early 2009, with a final set of objectives by January 2010.

Standards for Pediatric Immunization Practices

In 1992, a working group convened by the National Vaccine Advisory Committee developed a set of standards for pediatric immunization practices, largely in response to the measles resurgence in the late 1980s. These standards were revised and updated in 2002 and have been endorsed by most professional organizations that deal with pediatric immunization. Rather than setting a mark for the minimum standard of care, the standards represent the most desirable practices that pediatric health care professionals should strive to achieve.

Key elements of each standard are listed below. The means to implement many of these standards are elaborated upon elsewhere in this book.

- *Standard 1—Vaccination services are readily available.* Routinely recommended vaccines should always be part of primary care. Vaccination status should be assessed at all points of contact with the health care system, including subspecialty practices, schools, and specialty clinics. If vaccines cannot be offered at these sites, patients should be referred elsewhere for vaccination. Primary care providers should be notified about vaccines given outside the medical home.
- *Standard 2—Vaccinations are coordinated with other health care services and provided in a medical home when possible.* Vaccinations should be coordinated with routine well-child visits or other visits. Patients who receive vaccines outside the medical home should be encouraged to receive subsequent vaccines from their primary care provider. Those who do not have a primary care provider should receive assistance in finding one.
- *Standard 3—Barriers to vaccination are identified and minimized.* Vaccine visits should be scheduled promptly

and, if necessary, independently of visits for other well-child services. Long waiting periods in the office should be avoided and culturally and age-appropriate educational materials should be available. A physical examination is not required for immunization—observation and screening are sufficient (see Chapter 4, *Vaccine Practice*). Providers should ask parents and patients how they can make vaccinations more accessible.

• *Standard 4—Patient costs are minimized.* Money should not be a barrier to vaccination. Free vaccines are available through public programs like the Vaccines for Children (VFC) Program, Public Health Service Section 317 grants to states, and state and local programs (see Chapter 2, *Vaccine Infrastructure in the United States*). Providers utilizing these resources should make it clear that even though the patient may be charged fees for administration of the vaccines, they will not be denied vaccination because of inability to pay. Health and insurance plans should cover all routinely recommended vaccines and reimbursement to providers should be enough to cover all expenses associated with delivering vaccines in practice.

• *Standard 5—Health care professionals review the vaccination and health status of patients at every encounter to determine which vaccines are indicated.* Any and all health care visits afford an opportunity to review vaccination status and minimize missed opportunities (see *Chapter 4*). This might include, for example, emergency room visits, hospitalizations, and appointments with specialists. Undervaccination should be documented in the patient's chart. Providers who do not give vaccines should refer patients to a primary care provider who does.

• *Standard 6—Health care professionals assess for and follow only medically accepted contraindications.* There are very few true contraindications to vaccination (see Chapter 5, *General Recommendations*). Decisions to withhold vaccination should be supported by published guidelines and should be documented in the medical record.

• *Standard 7—Parents/guardians and patients are educated about the benefits and risks of vaccination in a culturally appropriate manner and in easy-to-understand language.* Sufficient time should be allowed to discuss the benefits of vaccines, the diseases they prevent, and the known risks. The schedule should be reviewed and the importance of bringing the hand-held vaccination record should be emphasized. Parents should be told how to report adverse events. Vaccine Information Statements (VISs) should be provided and supplemented by oral or visual explanations when appropriate, and the parent's questions and concerns should be addressed. Reporting of adverse events should be encouraged.

TABLE 3.1 — Selected *Healthy People 2010* General Objectives for Immunization

Metric/Group	Vaccine or Vaccine Series	Pre-2000 Baseline	2010 Target
Coverage rates/children 19 to 35 months of age	4 DTaP	84	90
	3 IPV	91	90
	1 MMR	92	90
	3 Hib	93	90
	3 HepB	87	90
	1 varicella vaccine	43	90
	4 DTaP; 3 IPV; 1 MMR; 3 Hib; 3 HepB	73	80
Coverage rates/adolescents 13 to 15 years of age	≥3 HepB	48	90
	≥2 MMR	89	90
	≥1 Td	93	90
	≥1 varicella vaccine	45	90
Noninstitutionalized adults ≥65 years of age	Yearly TIV	64	90
	Ever received PPSV23	46	90
Noninstitutionalized high-risk adults 18 to 64 years of age	Yearly TIV	26	60
	Ever received PPSV23	13	60
Proportion of public providers measuring vaccination coverage in their practice in the last 2 years		66	90

Proportion of private providers measuring vaccination coverage in their practice in the last 2 years	6	90
Proportion of children <6 years of age participating in registries	32	95

Centers for Disease Control and Prevention. Healthy People 2010. Healthy People Web site. http://www.healthypeople.gov/Publications/. Accessed August 15, 2008.

TABLE 3.2 — Selected *Healthy People 2010* Objectives For Vaccine-Preventable Diseases

Disease	Group	Annual Cases or Incidence Pre-2000 Baseline	Target	Comments
Diphtheria	<35 years	1	0	Disease extremely rare
Tetanus	<35 years	14	0	Herd immunity not applicable
Pertussis	<7 years	3417	2000	Adults are a major reservoir[a]
Hepatitis A	All ages	11.3/100,000	4.5/100,000	Children are primary source of new infections in communities
Hepatitis B (acute)	2 to 18 years	945	9	Target high-risk groups
	19 to 24 years	24.0/100,000	2.4/100,000	Universal vaccination anticipated[b]
	25 to 39 years	20.2/100,000	5.1/100,000	Infection will decrease as universally-immunized infants reach adolescence and adulthood
	≥40 years	15.0/100,000	3.8/100,000	High-risk groups should be targeted
	IV drug users	7232	1808	
	Heterosexuals	15,225	1240	
	Men who have sex with men	7232	1808	
	Occupational	249	62	
(perinatal)	<2 years	1682	400	95% of perinatal infections are preventable by appropriate maternal screening and infant care[c]
Haemophilus influenzae type b	<5 years	163	0	Conjugate vaccines have resulted in near elimination

Neisseria meningitidis	All ages	1.3/100,000	1.0/100,000	Target high-risk groups
Streptococcus pneumoniae	<5 years	76.0/100,000	46.3/100,000	Conjugate vaccines anticipated[d] Reduced penicillin-resistant infections will accompany general reduction in cases
	≥65 years	62.0/100,000	42.3/100,000	
Meningitis (bacterial)	1 to 23 months	13.0/100,000	8.6/100,000	Widespread use of Hib and pneumococcal conjugates expected
Measles	All ages	74	0	Transmission in United States interrupted multiple times since 1993[e]
Mumps	All ages	666	0	Interruption of spread feasible with 2 doses
Rubella	All ages	364	0	Interruption of spread feasible with 2 doses[e]
Rubella (congenital)	<1 years	7	0	Focus on women of childbearing age and foreign-born adults[e]
Polio	All ages	0	0	Eliminated in the United States
Varicella	<18 years	4,000,000	400,000	Monitoring effect of vaccine difficult because varicella not uniformly reportable[f]

[a] Booster vaccination for adolescents and adults became available in 2005.

[b] Immunization of all children in the second year of life was recommenced in 2006.

[c] Since 2006, the routine childhood schedule has stated that the birth dose of HepB can be deferred only with a physician's order and a copy of the mother's negative HBsAg test result on the infant's chart.

[d] MCV4 was licensed in 2005 and recommended for universal use at 11 to 12 years of age. In 2007, the recommendation was expanded to all individuals 11 to 18 years of age.

[e] By 2004, measles, mumps, rubella, and congenital rubella syndrome were no longer endemic in the United States.

[f] In 2003, varicella was added to the list of Nationally Notifiable Infectious Diseases, although reporting by states to the CDC is voluntary.

Centers for Disease Control and Prevention. Healthy People 2010. Healthy People Web site. http://www.healthypeople.gov/Publications/. Accessed August 15, 2008.

- *Standard 8—Health care professionals follow appropriate procedures for vaccine storage and handling*. Recommendations for storage and handling, as well as emergency procedures, are found in *Chapter 4*.
- *Standard 9—Up-to-date, written vaccination protocols are accessible at all locations where vaccines are administered*. Protocols should detail vaccine storage and handling; the recommended schedule; contraindications; administration technique; treatment and reporting of adverse events; risk-benefit communication; and record maintenance and accessibility.
- *Standard 10—People who administer vaccines and staff who manage or support vaccine administration are knowledgeable and receive ongoing education*. Vaccine recommendations change frequently, and all personnel involved in the process of vaccine delivery should remain abreast of these changes. Many resources are available for this purpose, including free e-mail listservs and CDC-sponsored distance-based training opportunities.
- *Standard 11—Health care professionals simultaneously administer as many indicated vaccine doses as possible*. There are essentially no routine vaccines that cannot be administered at the same time at separate sites. When vaccines are not given simultaneously, arrangements should be made for the patient's earliest return to receive the needed vaccines. Although not specifically mentioned in the standard, combination vaccines allow delivery of multiple antigens with fewer shots and are preferred to separately administered components (see Chapter 9, *Routine Vaccines*).
- *Standard 12—Vaccination records for patients are accurate, complete, and easily accessible*. This standard goes beyond the record keeping mandated by law. It calls for a permanent record that the parents carry with them and verification of vaccines received from other providers. All vaccinations should be reported to state or local immunization information systems (registries). Vaccine refusal also should be documented.
- *Standard 13—Health care professionals report adverse events after vaccination promptly and accurately to the Vaccine Adverse Events Reporting System (VAERS) and are aware of a separate program, the National Vaccine Injury Compensation Program (VICP)*. These programs are described below. Reporting of certain events is required by law, and reporting of all significant events is encouraged, even if causality is not established. Health care professionals should be aware that parents and patients may report adverse events to VAERS on their own.
- *Standard 14—All personnel who have contact with patients are appropriately vaccinated*. Offices and clinics should have policies to review and maintain the vaccination status of their staff. Vaccination of health care personnel is discussed in Chapter 7, *Vaccination in Special Circumstances*.

- *Standard 15—Systems are used to remind parents/guardians, patients, and health care professionals when vaccinations are due and to recall those who are overdue.* Computerized or manual tracking, recall, and reminder systems should be in place (see *Chapter 4*).
- *Standard 16—Office- or clinic-based patient record reviews and vaccination coverage assessments are performed annually.* A simple random survey of patient records can yield information about coverage rates, missed opportunities, and record quality; in general, physicians will find that they overestimate the proportion of their patients who are appropriately immunized. *Chapter 4* offers strategies for systematic assessments. Feedback and incentives are important elements of quality improvement.
- *Standard 17—Health care professionals practice community-based approaches.* Providers should be responsive to the needs of their patients, but it should be recognized that high coverage rates protect the entire community. Partnering with other service providers, such as the US Department of Agriculture's Special Supplemental Nutrition Program for Women, Infants, and Children (WIC), advocacy groups, schools, and service organizations should be encouraged.

In 1996, the ACIP, AAP, AAFP, and AMA called for routine health care visits for all children at 11 to 12 years of age. Before 2005, vaccinations during adolescence consisted for the most part of catch-up, with the exception of the Td booster. Since then, new vaccines (MCV4, Tdap, and HPV vaccine) have been recommended for adolescents, and since 2006, the National Immunization Survey has reported coverage rates for adolescents. In 2007, the routine schedule for the first time included a stand-alone chart for older children and adolescents. While there are as yet no adolescent standards per se, it is worth emphasizing that optimally immunizing adolescents represents a special set of challenges for providers, not the least of which is the fact that adolescents make infrequent visits for preventive health services.

Standards for Adult Immunization Practices

The National Coalition for Adult Immunization first offered standards for adult immunization practices in 1990. These standards were revised in 2003 by a working group of the National Vaccine Advisory Committee to reflect changes in the health care system and new information regarding adult vaccine coverage. Many of the standards, given in **Table 3.3**, parallel the pediatric standards.

Annual mortality from vaccine-preventable diseases among adults reaches into the tens of thousands; hospitalizations reach into the hundreds of thousands and societal costs into the billions

TABLE 3.3 — Standards for Adult Immunization Practices

Standard 1—Adult vaccination services are readily available

Standard 2—Barriers to receiving vaccines are identified and minimized

Standard 3—Patient "out-of-pocket" vaccination costs are minimized

Standard 4—Health care professionals routinely review the vaccination status of patients

Standard 5—Health care professionals assess for valid contraindications

Standard 6—Patients are educated about risks and benefits of vaccination in easy-to-understand language

Standard 7—Written vaccination protocols are available at all locations where vaccines are administered

Standard 8—Persons who administer vaccines are properly trained

Standard 9—Health care professionals recommend simultaneous administration of indicated vaccine doses

Standard 10—Vaccination records for patients are accurate and easily accessible

Standard 11—All personnel who have contact with patients are appropriately vaccinated

Standard 12—Systems are developed and used to remind patients and health care professionals when vaccinations are due and to recall patients who are overdue

Standard 13—Standing orders for vaccinations are employed

Standard 14—Regular assessments of vaccination coverage levels are conducted in a provider's practice

Standard 15—Patient-oriented and community-based approaches are used to reach target populations

Poland GA, et al. *Am J Prev Med.* 2003;25:144-150.

of dollars. Yet historically, adult and adolescent immunization rates have lagged behind childhood rates. In June 2007, the IDSA published a set of principles—billed as a "call to action"—designed to rectify this situation. Some of the principles reiterate the adult practice standards; others extend into the area of policy. The document can be downloaded at: http://www.journals.uchicago.edu/doi/pdf/10.1086/519541?cookieSet=1 (Accessed August 15, 2008).

National Childhood Vaccine Injury Act

In response to growing public concern about vaccine safety and the effects that liability issues were having on the pharmaceutical industry, Congress passed the National Childhood Vaccine Injury

Act of 1986 (NCVIA, P.L. 99-660). The NCVIA established two important programs that providers need to be familiar with, the VICP and VAERS. In addition, the NCVIA required providers to give adult vaccine recipients or the parents or guardians of minors receiving vaccines a VIS for each vaccine received.

■ The National Vaccine Injury Compensation Program (VICP)

The VICP, which went into effect on October 1, 1988, is a no-fault alternative to the tort system for resolving claims that result from adverse reactions to mandated childhood vaccines. It is administered jointly by the Health Resources and Services Administration of HHS, the US Court of Federal Claims (the Court), and the Department of Justice (DOJ), and is funded by an excise tax levied on every dose of vaccine that is purchased.

Anyone who feels they were injured by a covered vaccine must first pursue a remedy through the VICP. In order to receive compensation, petitioners must show that any one of the following occurred: 1) they incurred an injury found in the Vaccine Injury Table (VIT); 2) the vaccine caused the injury; or 3) the vaccine significantly aggravated a pre-existing condition. The VIT, which lists specific injuries or conditions and the time frames in which they must have occurred, serves as a basis for presumption of causation (updated versions can be found at http://www.hrsa. gov/vaccinecompensation/table.htm. Accessed August 15, 2008). Individuals can file claims for injuries not listed in the VIT, but *proof of causation* must be given. In recent years, the standard for proof has shifted from a preponderance of the evidence to biologic plausibility.

In order for a claim to be filed, the injury must have lasted for at least 6 months following vaccination, resulted in hospitalization and surgery, or resulted in death. In order to be paid, the petitioners must prove that a) they received a vaccine listed on the VIT, and b) the first signs of injury occurred within the specified time frame, or the vaccine caused the injury or caused an existing illness to get worse (it must also be determined that the injury or death did not have another cause). When a claim is filed, HHS reviews the medical aspects and makes recommendations to a DOJ lawyer representing the Secretary of Health and Human Services, who reviews the legal aspects of the case. The HHS and DOJ reviews are then forwarded to the Court, wherein a Special Master (a lawyer appointed by the Court) decides if the claim will be paid and how much money will be offered. If the medical case is straightforward—for example, an individual develops chronic arthritis (not otherwise explained) within 7 to 42 days after receiving a rubella-containing vaccine—HHS may concede the case in its review, acknowledging that the injury fits the VIT definition (this is often referred to as a "Table injury"). In this instance, the Special Masters will usually pay the claim. If it is not a Table injury and HHS contests the claim, hearings may be held. The decision of the Special Masters can be appealed by either party (HHS or the petitioner) to a judge of the Court, then to the US Court of Appeals for the Federal Circuit, and ultimately to the US Supreme Court.

Vaccines recommended by the ACIP for routine use in children are automatically covered under the VICP. Advise regarding the VICP and recommended changes to the VIT comes from the Advisory Commission on Childhood Vaccines, which consists of 9 members (3 health care professionals, 3 members of the general public, and 3 attorneys) who meet at least quarterly. Nonvoting, ex-officio members include the Director of the National Institutes of Health, the Assistant Secretary for Health, the Director of the CDC, and the Commissioner of the FDA, or their designees.

Important points about the VICP include:

- Covered vaccines as of October 2008 include DT, DTaP, HepA, HepB, Hib, HPV vaccine, HRV, IPV, LAIV, measles vaccine, MCV4, MMR, MPSV4, MR, PCV7, PRV, rubella vaccine, Td, Tdap, TIV, TT, varicella vaccine, and any combination of these. DTwP and OPV are covered but are no longer used in the United States. Additional vaccines may be added in the future.
- Claims can be filed by individuals, parents, legal guardians, trustees, legal representatives of the estate of deceased persons, non-US citizens, and, under certain conditions, individuals vaccinated outside of the United States.
- Adults are covered under the program if they receive one of the covered vaccines.
- After adjudication, petitioners are free to reject the decision of the Court and pursue civil litigation.
- Compensation is available for past and future nonreimbursable medical, custodial, and rehabilitation costs and lost earnings. There are no limits on compensation for attorney's fees; petitioners representing themselves can only recover legal costs, not fees. Compensation for pain and suffering, and compensation to the estate in the case of death, is capped at $250,000.

■ **The Vaccine Adverse Event Reporting System (VAERS)**

VAERS, in operation since 1990, is a passive surveillance program that collects and analyzes postmarketing information about adverse vaccine events. Any event following vaccination can be reported, with no restriction on the interval between vaccination and the onset of illness and no requirement for medical care having been rendered. Anyone can submit a report, including health care professionals, pharmaceutical companies, parents, and patients. However, health care providers are *required* to report events that are listed by the manufacturer as a contraindication to subsequent doses as well as events listed in the Reportable Events Table (RET, **Table 3.4**), which is similar to but not identical with the VIT. Reports can be submitted directly on the Internet (https://secure.vaers.org/VaersDataEntryintro.htm. Accessed August 15, 2008) or forms can be downloaded (http://vaers.hhs.gov/pdf/vaers_form.pdf. Accessed August 15, 2008) and mailed in. VAERS data are available to the public for analysis, although caveats regarding interpretation are offered (see *Chapter 2*).

■ Vaccine Information Statements (VISs)

A VIS is a concise (1-page, 2-sided) description of the risks and benefits of a given vaccine written for lay people and published by the CDC. A VIS for each vaccine can be downloaded from the Internet free of charge at http://www.cdc.gov/vaccines/pubs/vis/default.htm (Accessed August 15, 2008).

Some important things to keep in mind about VISs and providers' obligations under the NCVIA are:

- The VIS must be physically given (and explained) to the parent or patient prior to the vaccination. Providers should intend for the family to take the VIS home with them, although parents or patients may chose not to take it.
- All providers, whether public or private, must use the VIS published by the CDC.
- Use of the VIS is mandatory for all vaccines covered by the VICP and listed on the VIT; the basis for this is the NCVIA. VISs are also mandated for any vaccine purchased through a CDC contract; the basis for this is the "duty to warn" clause in CDC contracts. Although technically not required, use of the VIS is strongly encouraged for all other vaccines.
- A VIS should be given before each dose of each vaccine, every time the child is immunized. In January 2008, a multiple-vaccines–VIS was released that covers all of the vaccines in the first 6 months of life.
- If a combination vaccine is used and a single VIS is not available, providers should give the individual VISs corresponding to the components of the combination.
- The provider should record in the medical record which VIS was given, its publication date, and the date it was given to the patient.
- The VIS should be supplemented as needed with oral discussions, videotapes, other printed material, and whatever else is needed for the parent or patient to gain understanding. The information on the VIS must still be conveyed to the vaccinee even if he or she is blind, deaf, or cannot read. VIS translations are available in many languages.
- Providers do not need to withhold a vaccine if a VIS for it does not yet exist. In this situation, the package insert or a homemade information sheet can be used until the official VIS is available. At that point, the VIS should be used.
- The VIS published by the CDC should not be altered, although the name, address, and phone number of the practice may be added.

TABLE 3.4 — Reportable Events Table[a]

Note: For all vaccines in the table, events listed in the package insert as contraindications to additional doses are considered reportable events, even if they are not listed here.

Vaccine	Event[b]	Interval From Vaccination When Event Occurs
Tetanus in any combination	Anaphylaxis or anaphylactic shock	7 days
	Brachial neuritis	28 days
Pertussis in any combination	Anaphylaxis or anaphylactic shock	7 days
	Encephalopathy or encephalitis	7 days
MMR in any combination	Anaphylaxis or anaphylactic shock	7 days
	Encephalopathy or encephalitis	15 days
Rubella in any combination	Chronic arthritis	42 days
Measles in any combination	Thrombocytopenic purpura	7 to 30 days
	Vaccine-strain measles virus infection in an immunodeficient recipient	6 months
Oral polio	Paralytic polio	Immunocompetent: 30 days
		Immunocompromised: 6 months
		Community case: not applicable
	Vaccine-strain polio virus infection	Immunocompetent: 30 days
		Immunocompromised: 6 months
		Community case: not applicable

Vaccine	Event	Interval
IPV	Anaphylaxis or anaphylactic shock	7 days
HepB	Anaphylaxis or anaphylactic shock	7 days
Hib	No condition specified	
Varicella	No condition specified	
Rotavirus	Intussusception	30 days
PCV7	No condition specified	
HepA	No condition specified	
Influenza	No condition specified	

[a] Effective July 1, 2005.
[b] See reference below for event definitions. Any acute complications or sequelae of these events, including death, are also reportable, with no applicable interval from vaccination.

VAERS Table of Reportable Events Following Vaccination. Vaccine Adverse Event Reporting System Web site. http://vaers.hhs.gov/pdf/Reportable EventsTable.pdf. Accessed August 15. 2008.

- The VIS may be given out at other times in addition to (but not in place of) the day of vaccination. An example of this might be a prenatal visit.
- VISs are not consent forms. There is no federal requirement for a signature signifying informed consent for vaccination, although this may be required by some states.
- VISs are only updated when new information needs to be added.
- The information in the VIS parallels the information in the ACIP recommendations rather than the package insert (sometimes the two differ).
- If immunizations are to be given when the parent is not present, for example during a school-based program, the following options can be exercised:
  – *Consent prior to administration of each dose of a series.* The VIS is mailed to the family or sent home with the student prior to each dose. A consent form is signed and returned before vaccination, and the form is placed in the medical record.
  – *Single signature for series.* Some states permit the parents to sign a single consent form for the entire vaccine series. They first receive a copy of the VIS and sign a statement acknowledging receipt of the VIS and authorizing the complete series. A VIS is still sent home prior to each dose in the series.

Table 3.5 summarizes the federal obligations that are binding on vaccine providers. Keep in mind that there may be state laws that supplement these national requirements.

Occupational Safety and Health Administration (OSHA)

Because most vaccines are injected percutaneously, vaccine providers and their employees are at risk for needlestick injuries. As such, all facilities where vaccinations are given, including doctor's offices, public health clinics, and hospitals, fall under OSHA regulations designed to minimize occupational exposure to bloodborne pathogens. Some states may have OSHA plans that exceed the federal requirements discussed below, but those plans cannot be less stringent.

In 1991, under authority of the Occupational Safety and Health Act of 1970, OSHA promulgated the Bloodborne Pathogens Standard (29 CFR 1910.1030), which mandated that employers establish and implement an exposure-control plan for their employees. This plan had to include work-practice controls, procedures for handling exposures, personal protective clothing and equipment, training, medical surveillance, HepB vaccination, signs, and labels. In addition, engineering controls designed to isolate or remove hazards, such as sharps-disposal containers, self-sheathing needles, and plastic capillary tubes, were mandated. In 2000, recognizing that occupational exposure to blood-borne pathogens was a continuing concern and that newer preventive technologies were available, Congress passed the Needlestick Safety and Prevention Act (P.L. 106-430), which directed OSHA to revise the blood-borne pathogens standard. This act called for more detail in the requirements for engineered devices, added new elements to the exposure-control plan, including documentation of employee input, and required the creation of a sharps-injury log. The revised standard went into effect on April 18, 2001.

The basic elements of the Bloodborne Pathogens Standard, as revised, are listed below. With respect to vaccinations, the most important element is the use of engineered sharps protections on needles and the proper disposal of sharps. However, most physicians' offices perform other procedures, such as phlebotomy, wound cleansing, and suturing, necessitating attention to many other areas of the standard.

- *Exposure-control plan*—A *written* plan needs to be in place that details all of the elements listed below. In addition, the procedures and job classifications where exposure to blood might occur should be delineated. An annual review and update must be conducted that takes into account innovations in medical procedures and new technological developments that reduce the risk of exposure.

- *Sharps-injury log*—Employers must maintain a log of percutaneous injuries from contaminated sharps. It must include, at a minimum, the type and brand of device, department or work area where the incident occurred, and an explanation of how the incident occurred (including, for example, the procedure being performed and the body part affected). In addition, it must protect the confidentiality of the injured employee. The log should serve as a tool to identify high-risk areas and evaluate devices.

- *Engineered sharps protections*—Devices with built-in safety features or mechanisms that effectively reduce the risk of exposure must be used for procedures that will have contact with blood. Such features should be an integral part of the device, allow the worker's hands to remain behind the needle at all times, remain in effect after the procedure and during disposal, and should be as simple as possible. Examples pertinent to immunizations include syringes with sheaths that slide forward by a single-handed operation to cover the attached needle after use, as well as retractable needles. Documentation must be provided in the exposure-control plan that appropriate, commercially available, engineered devices are evaluated each year, and justification must be provided for selecting a particular device (*not* selecting an engineered device is *not* an option). In addition, it must be documented

TABLE 3.5 — Federal Requirements Regarding Vaccination

Requirement	Details
Give a VIS	Give a current, *take-home* copy of the relevant VIS to the parent, legal representative, or adult recipient before *each* dose of *each* vaccine
	Use the VIS published by the CDC[a]
	Mandatory for vaccines covered under the National Vaccine Injury Compensation Program[b]
	Mandatory for vaccines purchased under a federal (CDC) contract
	Encouraged for all other vaccines
	Provide VIS for each component of a combination vaccine if there is no VIS for the combination
	Use visual or oral supplements for illiterate or blind patients
	Translations are available[c]
Document in the permanent medical record or office log	Name of the VIS, publication date, and date it was given to the recipient[d]
	Name and title of the individual who administered the vaccine
	Address where the permanent record is kept
	Date of administration
	Manufacturer
	Lot number
Report to VAERS	Any event listed by the manufacturer as a contraindication to subsequent doses of the vaccine
	Any event listed in the Reportable Events Table (**Table 3.4**) that occurs within the specified time period after vaccination

[a] Vaccine Information Statements. Centers for Disease Control and Prevention Web site. http://www.cdc.gov/vaccines/pubs/vis/default.htm. Accessed August 15, 2008.

[b] As of October 2008, includes DT, DTaP, HepA, HepB, Hib, HPV, HRV, IPV, LAIV, measles, MCV4, MMR, MPSV4, MR, PCV7, PRV, rubella, Td, Tdap, TIV, TT, varicella, and any combination of these vaccines. DTwP and OPV are covered but are no longer used in the United States.

[c] The California and Minnesota state immunization programs have translated the VISs into 30 different languages. These are considered *de facto* equivalents of the English versions and are available from the Immunization Action Coalition Web site. http://www.immunize.org. Accessed August 15, 2008.

[d] The patient's signature is *not* required and the VIS should not be construed as informed consent, which may be required in certain states.

that nonmanagerial, front-line employees with direct patient care responsibilities had input into the selection (this can take the form of meeting minutes or written evaluations filled out by employees). Selected devices must not jeopardize patient or employee safety or be medically inadvisable. Since sheaths and the like are considered temporary measures, even sharps with engineered protections must be disposed of in an approved container.

- *Universal precautions*—All blood and body fluids must be treated as if infectious for hepatitis B, hepatitis C, and HIV, even if they are from low-risk individuals. Facilities for hand-washing and personal protective equipment (eg, gloves, gowns, masks, mouthpieces, and resuscitation bags) must be available at no cost to employees. Lab coats and scrubs, if used as protective equipment, must be laundered by the employer at no cost; home laundering is not permitted. Gloves (hypoallergenic if necessary) must be available and hand-washing is required after use. However, use of gloves is *not* required when administering intramuscular or subcutaneous injections as long as bleeding is not anticipated.
- *Procedures*—Detailed protocols must be given for all procedures with risk, including decontamination of equipment, handling of sharps-disposal containers and other regulated waste, broken glassware, and laundry. Routine cleaning of work sites should be described.
- *Sharps handling*—A protocol for handling of sharps needs to be in the exposure-control plan. Recapping contaminated needles is prohibited but this should not be an issue since needles will have engineered controls. If recapping is necessary for uncontaminated needles, such as those used to draw vaccine from a vial into a syringe, the cap should be scooped up from a flat surface using the hand that is holding the syringe and needle. Disposal containers should be closable, puncture resistant, leak proof, labeled appropriately, and located where procedures are performed. The protocol should specify how the containers are handled once they are filled.
- *Warning labels*—Orange or orange-red biohazard labels must be affixed to containers of regulated waste and refrigerators and freezers containing blood or infectious materials (labeled bags may also be used).
- *HepB vaccination*—Vaccination should be available at no cost to all employees with potential blood contact. The employee's health insurance cannot be used to pay this expense unless the employer routinely pays the entire premium. Employees must sign a declination form if they choose to opt out.
- *Postexposure evaluation*—Specific procedures should be outlined for the handling of exposures. Baseline and follow-up laboratory tests should be done after consent is obtained and must be provided free of charge. Provisions for confidential

medical follow-up must be made. Postexposure HIV prophylaxis should be offered if indicated in accord with current guidelines. The source individual's blood should be tested for blood-borne pathogens after consent is obtained; if consent is not given, this needs to be documented. Medical records on employees must be kept for the duration of employment plus 30 years.

- *Training*—Training that includes background information and the exposure-control plan must be provided upon assignment and annually thereafter. Documentation of training sessions, including the dates, content, trainer, and attendees must be maintained.

Checklists, model exposure-control plans, and lists of commercially available safety-engineered sharp devices can be obtained from the International Health Care Worker Safety Center at the University of Virginia at http://www.healthsystem.virginia.edu/internet/epinet/home.cfm (Accessed August 15, 2008). In addition, many vaccines are now available from manufacturers in prefilled syringes and needles with engineered protections.

School Mandates and State Legislation

There are no federal laws specifying which vaccines civilians must receive. There are, however, state laws specifying which vaccines must be received before attendance at day care, preschool, school, or college is allowed. These requirements have been instrumental in the eradication or near-eradication of many diseases. The courts have repeatedly upheld the legal basis for these statutes, which include the societal mandate to protect nonenfranchised individuals (children who do not have a vote) and the rights of others to be protected from harm (transmission of disease from unimmunized individuals). The case for vaccination that mandates the prevention of highly contagious diseases such as measles, which are spread in schools, is relatively straightforward. The situation becomes more complicated when considering infections such as HBV and HPV, which are arguably not spread in schools and which can largely be prevented by avoidance of high-risk behaviors.

There are few laws that apply to adults other than college students, those entering military service, and immigrants. However, some states, employers, or institutions might require certain vaccines or proof of immunity for selected individuals. Examples include influenza vaccine and HepB for health care workers, influenza and pneumococcal vaccines for residents and employees of long-term care facilities, vaccines for laboratory workers who work with specific pathogens, and rabies vaccine for animal handlers.

The CDC recommends a 4-day grace period for specific age requirements. For example, a child who receives the MMR 3 days before his first birthday should be considered effectively immunized. However, some local school districts may not accept this, so the best advice is to give vaccines at the recommended ages. Practitioners may have to balance the liabilities of giving a vaccine before the exact specified age with the risk that the patient may not return to be vaccinated at the appropriate time.

All states allow either temporary or permanent exemption from school immunization requirements for medical reasons. As of 2006, some form of religious exemption was granted by 48 states, and 20 granted some form of philosophical exemption. The AAP emphasizes the need for sensitivity and flexibility in dealing with parents' religious beliefs. While it also supports the repeal of religious-exemption laws, it does not advocate the stringent application of medical-neglect laws when parents refuse the recommended childhood immunizations. Philosophical exemptions are more problematic because the level of proof can be minimal (it may be minimal for religious exemptions as well), amounting simply to parents being "opposed to immunization." In some cases, parents request philosophical exemptions as a matter of convenience when their children's immunizations are not up-to-date. Physicians, public health providers, and school officials should not grant philosophical exemptions in such circumstances, and in general should work toward the repeal of philosophical exemption laws. Importantly, the risk of pertussis has been shown to increase with the availability of philosophical exemptions and the ease with which these are granted. For parents considering exemption, physicians should emphasize that disease rates among exemptors are higher than among vaccinated individuals; in addition, large numbers of exemptors in a community put everyone at risk, including vaccinated children. Chapter 8 (*Addressing Concerns About Vaccines*) has a more in-depth discussion of vaccine refusal.

The best centralized sources for information about state requirements are the National Network for Immunization Information (www.immunizationinfo.org/vaccineInfo) and the Immunization Action Coalition (www.immunize.org/laws). For the most up-to-date information, it is best to contact your state health department (see Chapter 12, *Vaccine Resources*).

Healthy People 2010

US Department of Health and Human Services. *Healthy People 2010, Volume I (2nd edition)*. http://www.healthypeople.gov/Document/HTML/Volume1/14Immunization.htm#_Toc494510239. Accessed August 15, 2008.

Standards for Pediatric Immunization Practices

Gardner P, Pickering LK, Orenstein WA, Gershon AA, Nichol KL; Infectious Diseases Society of America. Guidelines for quality standards for immunization. *Clin Infect Dis*. 2002;35(5):503-511.

National Vaccine Advisory Committee. Standards for child and adolescent immunization practices. National Vaccine Advisory Committee. *Pediatrics*. 2003;112(4);958-963.

Standards for pediatric immunization practices. Recommended by the National Vaccine Advisory Committee. *MMWR Recomm Rep*. 1993;42(RR-5):1-10.

Standards for Adult Immunization Practices

Hinman AR, Orenstein WA. Adult immunization: what can we learn from the childhood immunization program? *Clin Infect Dis*. 2007;44(12):1532-1535.

Poland GA, Shefer AM, McCauley M, Webster PS, Whitley-Williams PN, Peter G; National Vaccine Advisory Committee, Ad Hoc Working Group for the Development of Standards for Adult Immunization Practices. Standards for adult immunization practices. *Am J Prev Med*. 2003;25(2):144-150.

National Childhood Vaccine Injury Act

Centers for Disease Control and Prevention. Vaccine information statements. http://www.cdc.gov/vaccines/pubs/vis/default.htm. Accessed August 15, 2008.

Health Resources and Services Administration. National Vaccine Injury Compensation Program (VICP). http://www.hrsa.gov/vaccinecompensation. Accessed August 15, 2008.

US Department of Health and Human Services. Vaccine Adverse Event Reporting System. http://vaers.hhs.gov. Accessed August 15, 2008.

Occupational Safety and Health Administration (OSHA)

Occupational Safety & Health Administration. Bloodborne pathogens and needlestick prevention. http://www.osha.gov/SLTC/bloodborne-pathogens/index.html. Accessed August 15, 2008.

School Mandates and State Legislation

Feikin DR, Lezotte DC, Hamman RF, Salmon DA, Chen RT, Hoffman RE. Individual and community risks of measles and pertussis associated with personal exemptions to immunization. *JAMA*. 2000;284(24):3145-3150.

Horlick G, Shaw FE, Gorji M, Fishbein DB; Working Group on Legislation, Vaccination and Adolescent Health. Delivering new vaccines to adolescents: the role of school-entry laws. *Pediatrics.* 2008;121(suppl 1):S79-S84.

Omer SB, Pan WK, Halsey NA, et al. Nonmedical exemptions to school immunization requirements: secular trends and association of state policies with pertussis incidence. *JAMA.* 2006;296(14):1757-1763.

Orenstein WA, Hinman AR. The immunization system in the United States—the role of school immunization laws. *Vaccine.* 1999;17(suppl 3):S19-S24.

Religious objections to medical care. American Academy of Pediatrics Committee on Bioethics. *Pediatrics.* 1997;99(2):279-281.

Salmon DA, Haber M, Gangarosa EJ, Phillips L, Smith NJ, Chen RT. Health consequences of religious and philosophical exemptions from immunization laws: individual and societal risk of measles. *JAMA.* 1999;282(1):47-53.

4 Vaccine Practice

Vaccine Handling

Mishandling of vaccines can reduce potency and leave vaccinated individuals susceptible to disease. **Table 4.1** describes the recommended handling and storage of commonly used vaccines, and the following list provides some general rules:

- Designate one person (and a backup) to be in charge of inventory, handling, and storage.
- Maintain an inventory log, including product name, manufacturer, lot number, doses received, date received, condition on arrival, and expiration date.
- Inspect products on delivery, including the integrity of containers and cold chain monitoring devices.
- Store vaccines immediately under appropriate conditions.
- Discard mishandled and expired vaccines (vaccines can be used until the last day of the month indicated on the expiration date).
- Consider as invalid any doses that were inadvertently given with mishandled or expired vaccine.
- Do not open more than 1 multidose vial at a time.
- Be aware that for some multidose vials, there is a limited recommended shelf life after the vial is first entered.
- Do not prefill syringes with vaccines that are supplied in vials.

There are also some general rules regarding refrigerators and freezers:

- A freezer used for vaccines should not be a compartment within a refrigerator (as in a "dormitory" unit). It should be a separate sealed unit and should have a separate external door.
- Do not store food in the vaccine refrigerator or freezer (frequent opening of the door can cause temperature fluctuations).
- Do not store vaccines in shelves on the refrigerator door.
- Vaccines that need to be refrigerated but protected from freezing should be stored in the middle of the refrigerator, away from the freezer portion of the unit.
- Use clearly labeled, color-coded trays for each product and include separate compartments for unopened and opened vials (record the date of opening or reconstitution directly on the label).
- Rotate stock (place newly received vaccines behind current supplies).
- Post a sign that specifies which vaccines are stored in the refrigerator and which are stored in the freezer.
- Keep a thermometer in the refrigerator and one in the freezer and record the temperatures on a log when the office opens

TABLE 4.1 — Handling of Commonly Used Vaccines[a]

Vaccine	Shipping[b]	Storage[c]	Comments
DT	Refrigerated[d]	Refrigerate	Do not freeze[e]
Td	Refrigerate	Refrigerate	Do not freeze
DTaP	Refrigerate	Refrigerate	Do not freeze
DTaP-HepB-IPV	Refrigerate	Refrigerate	Do not freeze
DTaP/Hib	Refrigerate	Vaccine (Hib): refrigerate	Requires reconstitution[f]
		Diluent (DTaP): refrigerate	Do not freeze vaccine or diluent
			Administer within 30 minutes of reconstitution
DTaP-IPV	Refrigerate	Refrigerate	Do not freeze
DTaP-IPV/Hib	Refrigerate	Vaccine (Hib): refrigerate	Requires reconstitution
		Diluent (DTaP-IPV): refrigerate	Do not freeze vaccine or diluent
			Administer immediately after reconstitution
HepA	Refrigerate	Refrigerate	Do not freeze
HepB	Refrigerate	Refrigerate	Do not freeze
HepA-HepB	Refrigerate	Refrigerate	Do not freeze
HepB-Hib	Refrigerate	Refrigerate	Do not freeze
Hib (PRP-OMPC)	Refrigerate	Refrigerate	Do not freeze
Hib (PRP-T)	Refrigerate	Vaccine: refrigerate	Requires reconstitution[f]
		Diluent: refrigerate or keep at room temperature	Do not freeze vaccine or diluent
			Administer within 30 minutes of reconstitution

112

Vaccine	Storage	Storage detail	Notes
HRV	Refrigerate	Vaccine: refrigerate Diluent: room temperature	Requires reconstitution[f] Do not freeze vaccine or diluent Administer within 24 hours of reconstitution (store in refrigerator or at room temperature) Protect from light
HPV	Refrigerate	Refrigerate	Do not freeze Protect from light
IPV	Refrigerate	Refrigerate	Do not freeze
LAIV	Refrigerate	Refrigerate	Do not freeze
MMR	≤50°F (10°C)	Vaccine: freeze or refrigerate Diluent: refrigerate or keep at room temperature	Requires reconstitution[f] Do not freeze diluent Administer as soon as possible after reconstitution or in the refrigerator up to 8 hours Protect from light
MMRV	Freeze	Vaccine: freeze (may be stored in the refrigerator for 72 hours before reconstitution)[g] Diluent: refrigerate or keep at room temperature	Requires reconstitution[f] Do not freeze diluent Administer within 30 minutes of reconstitution Protect from light
MCV4	Refrigerate	Refrigerate	Do not freeze
MPSV4	Refrigerate	Vaccine: refrigerate Diluent: refrigerate or keep at room temperature	Requires reconstitution[f] 1-dose vial: administer within 30 minutes of reconstitution 10-dose vial: refrigerate up to 35 days

Continued

113

4

TABLE 4.1 — *Continued*

Vaccine	Shipping[b]	Storage[c]	Comments
PCV7	Refrigerate	Refrigerate	Do not freeze
PPSV23	Refrigerate	Refrigerate	Do not freeze
PRV	Refrigerate	Refrigerate	Do not freeze
			Administer as soon as possible after removing from the refrigerator
			Protect from light
Tdap	Refrigerate	Refrigerate	Do not freeze
TIV	Refrigerate	Refrigerate	Do not freeze
			Afluria, Fluarix, and FluLaval should be protected from light
Varicella	Freeze	Vaccine: freeze (may be stored in the refrigerator for 72 hours before reconstitution)[g]	Requires reconstitution[f]
		Diluent: refrigerate or keep at room temperature	Do not freeze diluent
			Administer within 30 minutes of reconstitution
			Protect from light
Zoster	Freeze	Vaccine: freeze	Requires reconstitution[f]
		Diluent: refrigerate or keep at room temperature	Do not freeze diluent
			Administer within 30 minutes of reconstitution
			Protect from light

[a] Note: all vaccine materials should be disposed of using medical waste disposal procedures, including sharps/biohazard containers. Remember that materials coming in contact with live vaccines carry the risk of contagion.

114

[b] If there are questions about a vaccine's condition at delivery, store the vaccine under the recommended conditions and contact the manufacturer's quality-control office or the state immunization program for advice.

[c] See text for refrigerator and freezer rules.

[d] Refrigerate means a temperature between 35°F and 46°F (2°C and 8°C).

[e] Freeze means a temperature ≤5°F (-15°C).

[f] Do not freeze after reconstitution.

[g] Refrigerator-stable formulations of MMRV and varicella vaccine have been licensed but are not distributed in the United States.

Individual vaccine package inserts and vaccine management: recommendations for storage and handling of selected biologicals, November 2007. Centers for Disease Control and Prevention Web site. http://www.cdc.gov/vaccines/pubs/downloads/bk-vac-mgt.pdf. Accessed August 15, 2008.

in the morning and when it closes in the evening. Appropriate ranges are 35°F to 46°F (2°C to 8°C) for the refrigerator and ≤5°F (-15°C) for the freezer. Alternatively, a recording thermometer can be used.

- Keep large jugs of water in the refrigerator and ice packs in the freezer to help maintain a steady temperature. This also helps maintain the temperature in the event of a power outage.
- Place a "DO NOT UNPLUG" sign near the outlet for the refrigerator and freezer units. Mark other points along the circuit (eg, fuses, circuit breakers) in a similar fashion.
- Do not use an outlet with a ground fault circuit interrupter (ie, one with test and reset buttons) or one connected to a wall switch.
- Use plug guards to prevent accidental dislodging.
- If possible, use an outlet connected to an auxiliary power source.

Table 4.2 gives some suggestions for managing the vaccine inventory in the event of a power failure or weather emergency.

Improving Vaccine Delivery

Many of the following strategies for improving immunization rates are emphasized in the Standards for Immunization Practices outlined in Chapter 3, *Standards, Principles, and Regulations*.

■ Reminder, Recall, and Tracking Systems

Reminders are messages that immunizations are due. They may be directed at parents in the form of telephone calls (by humans or computers) or mailings (simple postcards or letters), or they may be directed at physicians, nurses, or other staff members in the form of chart or electronic medical record flags saying "vaccines are due." Recall messages are notices to parents that vaccinations are overdue. Tracking systems, which can be manual or computerized, allow each child's immunization status to be followed precisely.

Studies have consistently shown improvements in immunization rates for both children and adults if tracking and messaging systems are used, whether it be in the public or private sectors. The AAP has offered the following guidelines (among others):

- Goals should include documenting immunization status, increasing immunization rates, decreasing costs of immunization, and facilitating immunization opportunities.
- There should be accurate documentation of each child's immunization status.
- Confidentiality should be preserved.
- Immunization information should be available at all times to ensure that all opportunities to immunize are used.
- Information on coverage rates should not be used to sanction health care workers.

TABLE 4.2 — Power Outages and Weather Emergencies

Power Outages
- Do not open refrigerators and freezers until power is restored
- Record temperature after power is restored and note duration of outage (do not open to monitor temperature during outage)
- Transfer to alternative storage with reliable power source if possible, maintaining cold chain and monitoring temperature
- If there is *any* question about the potential potency of exposed vaccine, contact state or local public health authorities or the vaccine manufacturer before considering administration
- Label exposed vaccine and keep it separated from new stock
- Live vaccines are the most susceptible to inactivation by warming

Weather Emergencies
- Suspend vaccination and implement emergency procedures in advance of the event
- Identify alternative storage facilities with backup power
- Ensure availability of staff to package and transport vaccine
- Maintain appropriate packing materials
- Ensure availability of transportation
- Standard operating procedures should include the following:
  - Emergency phone numbers for power company, equipment repair, alarm monitoring companies, backup storage facility, dry ice vendor, generator repair company, National Weather Service, and vaccine manufacturers
  - Working agreements with hospitals, health departments, or other facilities to serve as emergency vaccine storage facilities
  - Procedures for entering facilities and storage areas during emergency or after hours, including location of emergency equipment and packing materials, as well as phone numbers for responsible individuals
  - Procedures for packaging (including inventory documentation and cold-chain monitoring) and transporting vaccines (including preferred and alternative routes)
  - Priority list for vaccine rescue, aiming to minimize dollar loss but ensure ability to deliver the routine schedule in the short term

Impact of power outage on vaccine storage. Centers for Disease Control and Prevention Web site. http://www.cdc.gov/vaccines/recs/storage/poweroutage.htm. Accessed August 15, 2008; and Emergency procedures for protecting vaccine inventories. Centers for Disease Control and Prevention Web site. http://www.cdc.gov/vaccines/recs/storage/vacc-weather-emerg.htm. Accessed August 15, 2008.

- Data input and access should be easy.
- Incomplete immunization status should not be used to deny any child access to care or eligibility for insurance benefits.
- Collaboration between public and private initiatives should include the ability to link databases.

Reminder and recall systems are particularly difficult to implement in practices with high patient turnover or in populations that change residence frequently. Keep in mind that in some areas, bilingual reminders may be necessary.

■ Missed Opportunities

Providers should utilize all clinical encounters to assess immunization status and administer vaccines for which the child is eligible, as long as true contraindications do not exist. The idea is to prevent contacts with the health care system from becoming *missed opportunities* for vaccination. Common reasons why opportunities are missed are listed below:
- Failure of providers to consider acute care visits as a time to catch up on immunizations
- Inability to determine immunization status through parent recall, shot cards, or contact with primary care providers
- Adherence to erroneous contraindications (**Table 5.4**)
- Failure to give all needed vaccines simultaneously

Additional barriers may exist in emergency departments and other acute care facilities, including time constraints, insurance reimbursement, and the perception that by giving routine immunizations, the patient's relationship with his primary care provider will be disrupted. Immunization Information Systems (IISs) and standing orders can help prevent missed opportunities.

■ Expanding Access

After-hours or weekend clinics may help boost coverage rates by making it more convenient for parents to bring their children in or for adults to stop by after work. In addition, access to vaccination once a patient enters the office can be facilitated through the use of "vaccination express lanes" and drop-in clinics. With proper vaccine storage and handling, there is no reason why home visits could not be used for vaccination of those individuals who are receiving home health services for other reasons.

■ Standing Orders

Standing orders enable nonphysician personnel, such as nurses and pharmacists, to prescribe or deliver vaccinations by protocol without direct physician involvement at the time of the encounter. This is one of the most consistently effective interventions for increasing adult immunization rates, and recent studies even show that the entire process can be computerized—that is, patients can be screened for eligibility electronically and the orders can be generated automatically, without investment of personnel time. Employing standing orders in nursing homes, hospitals, clinics, physicians' offices, and other institutional settings can increase coverage rates. In fact, standing orders for adult pneumococcal and influenza vaccination are recommended. Standing orders are also applicable to pediatric patients. In fact, it is recommended that all birthing hospitals have standing orders in place for HepB immunization of newborns (see Chapter 9, *Routine Vaccines*). Standing orders could be employed for influenza immunization of children 6 months of age or older who are hospitalized in the fall for any reason.

■ Immunization Information Systems

IISs, formerly known as registries, are confidential, population-based, centralized computerized systems that maintain information about children's immunizations. The ideal registry contains all children in a geographic area and receives vaccination data from all regional providers. The need for registries is driven by a simple fact: an increasingly complex vaccine schedule must be administered to children who frequently relocate and change health care providers. This results in vaccination histories that are incomplete and fragmented, as well as a spectrum of errors ranging from missed opportunities to unnecessary duplication. For these reasons, one of the *Healthy People 2010* (see *Chapter 3*) goals is for at least 95% of children <6 years of age to participate in a fully operational population-based IIS. As of 2006, approximately 65% of US children in this age group participated in an IIS. CDC survey data indicated that the majority of IISs had the capacity to track vaccinations for persons of all ages and that for more than two thirds of children, vaccine information was entered within 30 days of administration. However, many records were incomplete, particularly for core elements like vaccine manufacturer and lot number.

Table 4.3 summarizes potential benefits of IISs as well as potential barriers from the provider's point of view. Organizations such as the American Immunization Registry Association, in collaboration with the CDC, have worked on defining best practices to help overcome these barriers and ensure that IISs can support required core program activities at the state and local levels.

The CDC has supported the development of state registries since 1993 through Section 317 Public Health Service grants. Additional support has come from organizations such as the Robert Wood Johnson Foundation. In 1998, the National Vaccine Advisory Committee launched the Initiative on Immunization Registries to facilitate community- and state-based registries. Four major challenges were identified:

- *Protecting confidentiality*—The need to gather and share information must be balanced with the family's right to privacy. Minimum specifications include executing written

TABLE 4.3 — Immunization Information Systems (Registries)

Benefits
- Ensure that patients remain current with recommendations
- Provide recalls and reminders
- Ensure timely vaccination after changes in location or provider
- Prevent unnecessary immunization
- Provide official, accurate documentation of immunization history
- Assess coverage rates
- Identify high-risk populations
- Prevent disease outbreaks
- Link with other databases (eg, newborn screening)
- Streamline immunization program management
- Reduce provider paperwork
- Facilitate introduction of new vaccines
- Integrate vaccinations with other public health services
- Facilitate monitoring of adverse events

Barriers
- Cost and/or time of data entry (which may be duplicative) and retrieval
- Practices are too busy to adopt a new procedure, resist change, and expect difficulty integrating IIS use into existing business practices and work flow
- Cost and time of staff training
- Difficulties and costs of interfacing with other systems, including electronic medical records and billing systems (and their vendors)
- Concerns about privacy, confidentiality, and HIPAA
- Difficulty coordinating the efforts of clinical, administrative, and information systems departments
- Perception of minimal value-added for participation

Centers for Disease Control and Prevention. *MMWR*. 2001;50(RR-17): 1-17; and Turning barriers into opportunities: survey and best practice report. American Immunization Registry Association Web site. http://www.immregistries.org/pdf/Provider_Participation_Final_2005.pdf. Accessed August 15, 2008.

confidentiality policies, notifying parents of the existence of the registry and allowing them to opt out, and defining who has access and what can be done with the information.

- *Participation by providers and recipients*—Because the majority of vaccine delivery has shifted to the private sector, efforts to recruit private providers are essential. Part of what makes a registry attractive to providers is simplicity, minimization of administrative burden, high quality of data, and functionality (eg, ability to generate reminders).

- *Operational challenges*—The functional capabilities of registry hardware and software differ from community to community; this is not conducive to the overall goal of seamless information exchange. For this reason, the CDC developed the following operational standards. IISs should:
  - Electronically store core data elements: name, birth date, sex, birth state, mother's name, vaccine type, manufacturer, lot number, and immunization date
  - Record initiation within 6 weeks of birth
  - Make information available at each health visit
  - Receive and process information within 1 month of vaccination
  - Protect confidentiality of medical information
  - Protect security of medical information
  - Exchange information using accepted communication standards (Health Level 7)
  - Automatically identify vaccines needed at each visit
  - Automatically identify persons due for immunizations and produce recall and reminder notices
  - Produce official coverage reports
  - Produce authorized shot records
  - Promote accuracy and completion
- *Resources to maintain registries*—Registries are likely to result in cost savings by reducing the manual labor involved in pulling medical records for provider visits, managed care reporting, and school system review. Additional cost savings should accrue from eliminating duplicate immunizations and reducing disease burden. It costs about $5 or $6 per child per year to maintain a registry, and in 1999 only 40% of this cost was covered by federal sources. Since 2000, the Centers for Medicare and Medicaid Services (formerly the Health Care Financing Administration) has provided funding to state programs for the development of IISs in the context of the Medicaid Management Information System.

The AAP has strongly supported the development of IISs and has suggested that research be done into their cost-effectiveness in increasing immunization rates. In addition, the AAP has called for a critical examination of the cost and benefits for the practicing physician and has suggested that physicians be reimbursed for entering historical information into databases. Finally, it has cautioned that the data in IISs be used to improve quality, not to penalize poor performers.

■ Other Strategies
Parent and community education regarding the importance of immunizations can improve coverage rates by increasing demand. Physician and staff education is equally important, and it helps to designate an "Immunization Tsar" (or Tsarina) in the practice who can champion all issues related to vaccination, from decreasing

missed opportunities to scanning for new recommendations to preparing talking points that address the latest parental concerns. Regular, systematic assessment and feedback can identify problem areas and evaluate the effectiveness of new interventions.

Along these lines, the CDC has developed a quality improvement methodology called AFIX, for Assessment (of a provider's vaccination coverage levels and practices), Feedback (of results to the provider along with suggestions for improvement), Incentives (to reward improved performance), and eXchange (of information and resources to facilitate improvement). Traditionally used to evaluate immunization delivery systems for children, AFIX can be generalized to apply to any age group. The data used in AFIX assessments come from IISs or from chart reviews. A software application called CoCASA, for Comprehensive Clinic Assessment Software Application, is available from the CDC to assess immunization practices in clinics, private practices, or other sites where immunizations are given. More information on these programs is available at http://www.cdc.gov/vaccines/programs/default.htm. Accessed August 15, 2008.

Screening

Screening patients for contraindications, precautions, and other problems before every dose of a vaccine is an important part of preventing adverse events. This can be effectively accomplished by asking the simple questions shown in **Table 4.4**, which are applicable to both children and adults. The issues addressed by these questions are also indicated in the table. Standardized forms for screening can be downloaded from the Immunization Action Coalition website free of charge (http://www.immunize.org. Accessed August 15, 2008).

Vaccine Administration

■ General Issues

During well care visits, it is probably most efficient to bring the vaccines to the examination room rather than have the patient move to a designated shot area. If reconstitution is needed, it should be done for each individual patient, rather than in batches, in order to reduce the risk of confusion and wastage. Young infants may do better if held on the parent's lap, while older children may prefer to sit on the edge of the examining table and hug their parent. Health care workers should wash their hands or use antiseptic hand gel before each patient, and sterile technique should be used, including swiping of the injection site with alcohol and allowing it to dry. Gloves are not required unless the individual administering the vaccine has open skin lesions and is likely to come in contact with body fluids. The needle should not be changed after withdrawing vaccine from the vial and before injecting it into the patient. A direct, rapid plunge of the needle through the skin is recommended followed by a rapid withdrawal after delivering the vaccine. Aspirating back on the syringe after penetration in order to look for blood return is not necessary, although many nurses feel uncomfortable injecting before they can confirm that the needle is not resting in a vessel. Importantly, a recent study showed that the slow aspiration technique is more painful than the "jab" technique. Multiple vaccines can be given in the same limb but should be separated by 1" to 2". It has been suggested that multiple injections can be given simultaneously by different personnel in order to minimize anticipatory anxiety.

Smallpox vaccine is the only one that is given by an entirely unique method (see Chapter 10, *Specialized Vaccines*). This live vaccine is administered intradermally with a bifurcated needle that punctures the skin and draws a small amount of blood. As such, *gloves should be worn* and the site should be covered with gauze and a semipermeable dressing. Skin preparation is not required unless there is gross contamination, in which case soap and water should be used for cleansing. If alcohol is used, the skin must dry thoroughly before inoculation to prevent inactivation of the vaccine virus.

■ Intramuscular Administration
The needle should enter the skin at a 90° angle, penetrating deep enough to hit the muscle (**Figure 4.1**). Traction can be applied to the skin and subcutaneous tissue before injection and released after injection. Preferred sites, which differ by age, include the anterolateral aspect of the upper thigh (vastus lateralis muscle) and the upper, outer part of the arm above the armpit and below the acromion (deltoid muscle); the required needle length will also vary by patient age (**Table 4.5**). The buttocks should not be used because the fat layer is too thick and damage to the sciatic nerve is possible. An exception can be made for large-volume passive immunization (eg, immune globulin), but here the site should be the upper, outer mass of the gluteus maximus and the needle should be directed perpendicular to the table while the patient is lying prone. Alternatively, the injection can be given in the center of the triangle formed by the anterior superior iliac spine, the tubercle of the iliac crest, and the upper border of the greater trochanter. No more than 5 mL should be given to an adult at a single site.

■ Subcutaneous Administration
For subcutaneous injections, the skin and subcutaneous tissue should be pinched-up, and the needle directed at a 45° angle (**Figure 4.1**). The preferred sites and needle length again vary with age (**Table 4.5**).

■ Oral Administration
For infants, oral administration of PRV or HRV is best accomplished with the child lying in the feeding position in the parent's

TABLE 4.4 — Screening Questions

Question	Issue Addressed
Is the patient sick today?	Moderate-to-severe illness is a precaution for all vaccines
Does the patient have severe allergies to medicines, foods, drugs, or vaccines?	Severe allergy or anaphylaxis to vaccine components or previous doses is a contraindication for all vaccines
	Severe egg allergy is a contraindication for LAIV, TIV, and YF vaccine
Has the patient had serious reactions to previous vaccinations?	Various contraindications and precautions for further doses
Has the patient had a seizure, brain, or neurologic problem?	Evolving neurologic disorder is a contraindication for pertussis-containing vaccines
	Patients who are susceptible to febrile seizures may benefit from fever prophylaxis
	Guillain-Barré syndrome within 6 weeks of previous influenza or tetanus vaccination is a precaution for further doses
	Personal history of Guillain-Barré syndrome is a contraindication for LAIV and a precaution for MCV4
Does the patient have asthma or another chronic medical condition?	LAIV may be contraindicated
	Certain nonroutine vaccines may be recommended
If the patient is a child between 2 and 4 years of age, has a health care provider diagnosed wheezing or asthma in the past year?	LAIV may be contraindicated

Does the patient have cancer, leukemia, a blood disorder, HIV infection, AIDS, tuberculosis, or any problem with the immune system?	Live vaccines are generally contraindicated in patients with immune impairment MMR can cause thrombocytopenia Active untreated tuberculosis is a precaution for MMR and zoster vaccine
In the last 3 months, has the patient received any treatments that might weaken his or her immune system, such as steroids, cancer chemotherapy, or radiation?	Live vaccines are generally contraindicated in patients with immune impairment Patient may respond poorly to vaccination
Are there any family members who have problems with their immune system?	The patient might be at risk for a heritable immune deficiency, which could contraindicate live vaccines
Has the patient received blood transfusions or immune globulin in the past year?	Receipt of antibody-containing products is a precaution for most live vaccines Undisclosed serious underlying illness may be discovered
Is the patient pregnant or is there a chance she could become pregnant in the next 3 months?	Live vaccines are generally contraindicated during pregnancy, as is HPV vaccine
Has the patient received any other vaccines in the last 4 weeks?	Live vaccines not given on the same day need to be separated by 1 month The AAP (but not the ACIP) recommends that if Tdap and MCV4 are not given on the same day, they need to be separated by 1 month Violating the minimum interval between doses in a series may result in invalid doses

Centers for Disease Control and Prevention. General recommendations on immunization. In: Atkinson W, Hamborsky J, McIntyre L, Wolfe C, eds. *Epidemiology and Prevention of Vaccine-Preventable Diseases*. 10th ed. Washington, DC: Public Health Foundation; 2007:27-29; Screening questionnaire for child and teen immunization. Immunization Action Coalition Web site. http://www.immunize.org/catg.d/p4060.pdf. Accessed August 15, 2008; Screening questionnaire for adult immunization. Immunization Action Coalition Web site. http://www.immunize.org/catg.d/p4065.pdf. Accessed August 15, 2008.

4

FIGURE 4.1 — Injection Technique

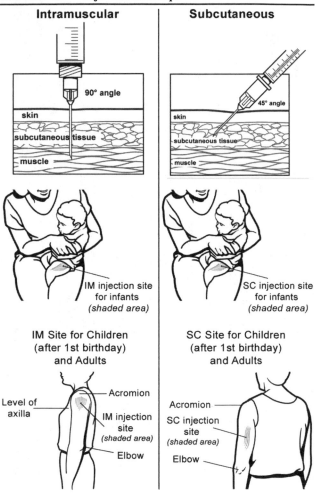

Modified from: The Minnesota Department of Health Web site. http://www
.immunize.org/catg.d/p2020.pdf. Accessed August 15, 2008.

arms. The tip of the applicator is placed in the infant's mouth toward the inner cheek and slowly emptied until all of the liquid is dispensed. If the infant spits or regurgitates, the dose is counted and not repeated.

■ Intranasal Administration

LAIV is supplied in a sprayer that resembles a syringe. The recipient should be in the upright position. The tip of the sprayer is inserted just inside the nose and the plunger is rapidly depressed until the dose-divider clip stops the plunger. The clip is then removed and the remainder of the dose is given in the other nostril. Sneezing or leakage of some of the liquid from the nose is not a reason to repeat the dose.

■ Intravenous Immune Globulin Administration

In rare situations, intravenous immune globulin products may be needed as part of a prophylactic strategy for a vaccine-preventable disease. For example, immune globulin intravenous (IGIV) can be used to prevent varicella in high-risk individuals if VariZIG, an investigational high-titer, polyclonal, immune globulin product, cannot be obtained. To administer IGIV, a temporary peripheral intravenous catheter should be inserted; for short infusions, a butterfly needle may suffice (the antecubital vein should be used for more concentrated solutions). In-line filtering is acceptable, but pore sizes >15 microns should be used so as not to impede flow. Patients can be premedicated with acetaminophen, 10 to 15 mg/kg orally, and diphenhydramine, 1 to 1.25 mg/kg orally, intramuscularly, or intravenously to avoid systemic reactions. Infusions are usually started slowly and the rate is increased if tolerated, but protocols differ based on the product, concentration, and total volume infused. If flushing or changes in heart rate or blood pressure occur, slowing the infusion rate will usually ameliorate these symptoms. Infusions should be done in a medical observation unit in case anaphylaxis or other severe reactions occur.

■ Dealing With Anxiety, Pain, and Fever

Vaccinations induce significant levels of stress and anxiety in children. To some extent this can be ameliorated by truthfully informing them what to expect before the visit occurs and by parental endorsement of vaccination as being valuable. Oral sucrose solution (50%) given directly into the mouth with a small syringe or administered on a pacifier seems to work well for infants <6 months of age and should be considered routinely. Parents should be allowed to comfort young children (rather than assist in restraining them) and should try to distract them by telling stories, playing music, or having them blow into pinwheels or imaginary candles. Topical anesthetics, such as eutectic mixture of local anesthetic (EMLA cream) or vapocoolant sprays, should be considered for patients who are phobic or extremely anxious about the injection. Manual pressure applied to the site for about 10 seconds prior to the injection seems to be effective in reducing pain. Finally, it is reasonable to administer acetaminophen, 10 to 15 mg/kg orally at the time of vaccination and at 4 and 8 hours afterwards; this is particularly useful for DTaP vaccination. Samples should be kept in the office, and prescriptions should be on hand for patients who must purchase drugs through medical assistance.

TABLE 4.5 — Needle Type and Injection Site

Age	Intramuscular[a] (22- to 25-gauge) Site	Needle (inch)	Subcutaneous[b] (23- to 25-gauge) Site	Needle[e] (inch)
0 to 28 days (including premature infants)	Anterolateral aspect of upper thigh	⅝[c]	Fatty part of upper anterolateral thigh	⅝ to ¾
1 to 12 months	Anterolateral aspect of upper thigh	1	Fatty part of upper anterolateral thigh	⅝ to ¾
1 to 2 years	Anterolateral aspect of upper thigh[d]	1 to 1¼	Fatty part of upper outer triceps area of arm or upper anterolateral thigh	⅝ to ¾
	Deltoid	⅝[c] to 1		
3 to 18 years	Deltoid[d]	⅝[c] to 1	Fatty part of upper outer triceps area of arm or upper anterolateral thigh	⅝ to ¾
	Anterolateral aspect of upper thigh	1 to 1¼		
≥19 years	Deltoid	Male or female <60 kg: 1 Female 60 to 90 kg: 1 to 1½ Male 60 to 118 kg: 1 to 1½ Female >90 kg: 1½ Male >118 kg: 1½	Fatty part of upper outer triceps area of arm or upper anterolateral thigh	⅝ to ¾

128

[a] The needle is inserted at a 90° angle.

[b] Skin and subcutaneous tissue are bunched up and the needle is inserted at a 45° angle.

[c] When using a short needle, the skin should be stretched tight to ensure that the muscle is reached.

[d] Preferred site.

[e] CDC recommends a ⅝-inch needle; AAP recommends a ⅝- to ¾-inch needle.

Centers for Disease Control and Prevention. *MMWR*. 2006;55(RR-15):1-48 and American Academy of Pediatrics. Active immunization. In: Pickering LK, ed. *2006 Red Book: Report of the Committee on Infectious Diseases*. 27th ed. Elk Grove Village, IL: American Academy of Pediatrics; 2006:19-22.

Dealing with Emergencies

■ Preparation

Acute emergencies after vaccine administration are rare—the risk for children and adolescents is estimated at less than one episode per million doses. The AAP suggests that when possible, patients should be observed in the office for 15 to 20 minutes after vaccination; the ACIP has never recommended a specific waiting period. In actual fact, life-threatening emergencies, such as anaphylaxis, usually occur within minutes when the patient is still likely to be within reach of medical personnel. The benefits of rapid, mass vaccination programs, such as drive-by influenza vaccine clinics, probably far outweigh the risks of curtailing any medical observation period.

Standing orders for emergencies should be in place in the office, and **Table 4.6** lists supplies that should be available in the event they are needed.

■ Syncope

Vasovagal reactions are most common in adolescents and young adults, particularly females. About 60% occur within 5 minutes of vaccination and approximately 90% occur within 15 minutes. Between 1990 and 2001, slightly over 2200 reports of syncope were made to the VAERS. Approximately 12% of cases resulted in hospitalization, and there are some reports of serious injury such as skull fracture. Since the advent of the adolescent vaccine platform—Tdap and MCV4 in 2005 and especially HPV vaccine in 2006—there has been a sharp increase in reported syncopal episodes related to vaccination. However, the absolute number of reported episodes remains low—463 VAERS reports between 2005 and 2007, most of them in female adolescents. Health care workers should be aware of predisposing conditions (eg, needle phobia) and presyncopal symptoms (eg, light-headedness or dizziness). At-risk individuals should be encouraged to sit or lie down, and consideration should be given to observing all patients for 15 minutes after vaccination. If syncope does occur, the patient should be protected as much as possible from fall injury and should be placed supine with the legs raised until symptoms abate.

■ Anaphylaxis

Anaphylaxis occurs rapidly and is a medical emergency. Signs and symptoms include:
- Flushing, warmth, urticaria, erythema, soft tissue edema, pruritus
- Dry mouth, swelling of the lips, tongue and throat, sneezing, congestion, rhinorrhea
- Hoarseness, stridor, cough, dyspnea, chest tightness, wheezing, cyanosis
- Tachycardia, hypotension, weak pulse, dizziness, shock, cardiovascular collapse
- Crampy abdominal pain, nausea, vomiting, diarrhea

For patients with mild symptoms, the initial approach is to administer epinephrine 1:1000 (aqueous) at a dose of 0.01 mL/kg intramuscular (the maximum dose is 0.5 mL). Injection should be to the lateral thigh. A dose can be repeated every 10 to 20 minutes if necessary for up to 3 total doses. In addition, an antihistamine such as diphenhydramine can given at a dose of 1-2 mg/kg (maximum 100 mg per dose) orally, intramuscularly, or intravenously every 4 to 6 hours; an alternative antihistamine is hydroxyzine, 0.5-1 mg/kg (maximum 100 mg per dose) orally or intramuscularly every 4 to 6 hours. The patient should be observed for several hours, and if improved and stable, can be given a prescription for an autoinjector of epinephrine and sent home on an oral antihistamine for the next 24 hours. Additional therapies may include a short course of oral steroids and the addition of an H_2 blocker (cimetidine or ranitidine).

For more severe cases, the emergency medical system should be activated immediately. Patients may require intensive emergency management, including airway maintenance, oxygen, and blood pressure support with isotonic intravenous fluids and vasopressors. Biphasic reactions may account for up to 50% of fatal cases. Asymptomatic intervals vary widely and can be as long as 24 hours. All patients with mild or severe anaphylaxis reactions should be referred to an allergist prior to future vaccinations.

Coding, Billing, and Vaccine Costs

Billing third-party payers for immunization services (and all other health services) is based on two systems:

• *Current Procedural Terminology (CPT) Codes*—These describe the *procedures* or *services* performed during a visit. The *visit itself* usually falls under evaluation and management codes for preventive medicine services performed in the outpatient setting, provided the immunization occurs in the context of a comprehensive "checkup." These codes, which vary by age and whether the person is new to the practice or established as a patient, are given in **Table 4.7**. There are corresponding codes for the *vaccines themselves*, which are given in **Table 4.8** (this table includes the codes for immune globulin products as well). There are also codes for the *administration* of the vaccines, given in **Table 4.9**, and *administration* of immune globulins, given in **Table 4.10**. If the visit is *only* for immunization (eg, before travel), most offices bill only for the vaccine and the administration, using the specific codes listed in **Tables 4.8** and **4.9**.

If evaluation and management services unrelated to vaccination are performed during the vaccine visit, those services receive separate CPT and ICD-9-CM codes. Some payers may require that the modifier "-25" be attached to the CPT code to indicate that the service was separate from

TABLE 4.6 — Emergency Office Supplies for Vaccination

Drugs and Fluids
- Oxygen
- Albuterol for inhalation
- Epinephrine (1:1000)
- Activated charcoal
- Antibiotics
- Anticonvulsant agents (diazepam, lorazepam)
- Corticosteroids (parenteral/oral)
- Dextrose (25%)
- Diphenhydramine (parenteral, 50 mg/mL)
- Epinephrine (1:10,000)
- Atropine sulfate (0.1 mg/mL)
- Naloxone (0.4 mg/mL)
- Sodium bicarbonate (4.2%)
- Normal saline solution or lactated Ringer's solution (500 mL-bags)
- 5% Dextrose, 0.45 normal saline (500-mL bags)

Equipment
- Airway management:
  - Oxygen delivery system
  - Bag-valve-mask (450 and 1000 mL)
  - Clear oxygen masks, breather and nonrebreather, with reservoirs (infant, child, adult)
  - Suction device, tonsil tip, bulb syringe
  - Nebulizer (or metered-dose inhaler with spacer/mask)
  - Oropharyngeal airways (sizes 00 to 5)
  - Pulse oximeter
  - Nasopharyngeal airways (sizes 12F to 30F)
  - Magill forceps (pediatric, adult)
  - Suction catheters (sizes 5F to 16F) and Yankauer suction tip
  - Nasogastric tubes (sizes 6F to 14F)
  - Laryngoscope handle (pediatric, adult) with extra batteries, bulbs
  - Laryngoscope blades (0 to 2 straight; 2 to 3 curved)
  - Endotracheal tubes (uncuffed 2.5 to 5.5; cuffed 6.0 to 8.0)
  - Stylets (pediatric, adult)
  - Esophageal intubation detector or end-tidal carbon dioxide detector
- Vascular access and fluid management:
  - Butterfly needles (19 to 25 gauge)
  - Catheter-over-needle device (14 to 24 gauge)
  - Arm boards, tape, tourniquet
  - Intraosseous needles (16 and 18 gauge)
  - Intravenous tubing, microdrip

Continued

TABLE 4.6 — *Continued*

• Miscellaneous equipment and supplies:
  – Color-coded tape or preprinted drug doses
  – Cardiac arrest board/backboard
  – Sphygmomanometer (infant, child, adult, thigh cuffs)
  – Splints, sterile dressings
  – Automated external defibrillator with pediatric capabilities
  – Spot glucose test
  – Stiff neck collars (small/large)
  – Heating source (overhead warmer/infrared lamp)

4

Adapted from: American Academy of Pediatrics Committee on Pediatric Emergency Medicine, Frush K. *Pediatrics.* 2007;120:200-212.

immunization but delivered by the same physician on the same day. A relatively minor, incidental problem discovered by the nurse who is giving the immunizations could lead to use of CPT code 99211 (office or other outpatient services, established patient) along with the ICD-9 code describing the reason for the incremental service. To use this code, the presence of a physician is not required, but the presenting problem should be minimal and the time taken should be on the order of 5 minutes. Importantly, the service performed must be medically necessary and must be separate from the vaccine administration. An example is an incidental runny nose discovered during a routine vaccine visit and diagnosed as a mild upper respiratory viral infection.

• *International Classification of Diseases, Ninth Revision, Clinical Modification (ICD-9-CM) Codes*—These describe the *reason* for the service. The *visit itself* usually falls under V20.2 (health supervision of infant or child, routine infant or child health check; ages 0-17 years) or V70.0 (general medical examination, routine general medical examination at a health care facility; adults). Most vaccines and immune globulins *themselves* have specific ICD-9-CM codes, given in **Table 4.8**.

Many payers are now requiring that National Drug Codes (NDCs) for vaccines be submitted along with CPT and ICD-9-CM codes. The Drug Listing Act of 1972 required registered drug establishments to provide the FDA with a current list of all drugs manufactured, prepared, propagated, compounded, or processed for commercial distribution. The NDC is a unique 10-digit, 3-segment number. The first segment identifies the company that makes, repacks, or distributes the product. The second segment identifies the product, strength, dosage form, and formulation. The third segment identifies the package size and type. Sometimes an asterisk appears as a place holder. NDCs can easily be found by searching the National Drug Code Directory (http://www.fda.

**TABLE 4.7 — CPT Codes for
Preventive Medicine Services, 2008[a]**

Age (years)	New Patient[b]		Established Patient[c]	
	CPT	ICD-9-CM	CPT	ICD-9-CM
<1	99381	V20.2	99391	V20.2
1 to 4	99382	V20.2	99392	V20.2
5 to 11	99383	V20.2[d]	99393	V20.2[d]
12 to 17	99384	V20.2[d]	99394	V20.2[d]
18 to 39	99385	V70.0	99395	V70.0
40 to 64	99386	V70.0	99396	V70.0
≥65	99387	V70.0	99397	V70.0

[a] If vaccinations are scheduled but not carried out, the following set of ICD-9-CM codes can be used to indicate the reason:

V64.00, vaccination not carried out, unspecified reason

V64.01, vaccination not carried out because of acute illness

V64.02, vaccination not carried out because of chronic illness or condition

V64.03, vaccination not carried out because of immune compromised state

V64.04, vaccination not carried out because of allergy to vaccine or component

V64.05, vaccination not carried out because of caregiver refusal

V64.06, vaccination not carried out because of parental refusal

V64.07, vaccination not carried out for religious reasons

V64.08, vaccination not carried out because patient had disease being vaccinated against

V64.09, vaccination not carried out for other reason.

[b] Initial comprehensive preventive medicine.

[c] Periodic comprehensive preventive medicine.

[d] If the visit is for a school physical, V70.3 (general medical examination for adoption, camp, school admission, etc) can be used.

Beebe M, et al. *CPT 2008 Professional Edition.* Chicago, IL: AMA Press; 2007; Hart AC, Stegman MS. *ICD-9-CM Professional: International Classification of Diseases—9th Revision—Clinical Modification 2008.* 6th ed. Salt Lake City, UT: Ingenix, Inc; 2007.

gov/cder/ndc/database/default.htm. Accessed August 15, 2008) by proprietary name, active ingredient, or company name. It is also found on the package insert in the "How Supplied" section.

A routine visit for a 6-month-old infant might be coded as shown in **Table 4.11**. Remember, all components of all services should be clearly documented in the medical record. If the practice receives vaccines free-of-charge through the VFC Program, it cannot bill for the *vaccine itself*, but it can bill for *administration of the vaccine* and for the *visit itself*.

Table 4.12 provides information on the purchase price for commonly used vaccines. The public sector cost is the contracted price between the CDC and the manufacturer, which changes from year to year. The private sector cost is based on the direct purchase price from the manufacturer. Because contractual and buying arrangements may vary for individual practices, the table is most useful in highlighting relative differences between products. In negotiating contract prices with private payers, physicians must consider all of the costs involved in providing vaccines. **Table 4.13** lists some of those costs for consideration.

ADDITIONAL READING

Improving Vaccine Delivery

American Immunization Registry Association. Registry standards of excellence in support of an immunization program. http://www.immregistries.org/pdf/PROWstandardscomp1.pdf. Accessed August 15, 2008.

Briss PA, Rodewald LE, Hinman AR, et al. Reviews of evidence regarding interventions to improve vaccination coverage in children, adolescents, and adults. The Task Force on Community Preventive Services. *Am J Prev Med.* 2000;18(suppl 1):97-140.

Centers for Disease Control and Prevention (CDC). Immunization information systems progress—United States, 2006. *MMWR Morb Mortal Wkly Rep.* 2008;57(11):289-291.

Centers for Disease Control and Prevention (CDC). Impact of missed opportunities to vaccinate preschool-aged children on vaccination coverage levels—selected U.S. sites, 1991-1992. *MMWR Morb Mortal Wkly Rep.* 1994;43(39):709-718.

Centers for Disease Control and Prevention. IIS: 2001 minimum functional standards for registries. http://www.cdc.gov/vaccines/programs/iis/stds/min-funct-std-2001.htm. Accessed August 15, 2008.

Committee on Practice and Ambulatory Medicine; Yasuda K. Immunization information systems. *Pediatrics.* 2006;118(3):1293-1295.

Daley MF, Beaty BL, Barrow J, et al. Missed opportunities for influenza vaccination in children with chronic medical conditions. *Arch Pediatr Adolesc Med.* 2005;159(10):986-991.

Development of community- and state-based immunization registries. CDC response to a report from the National Vaccine Advisory Committee. *MMWR Recomm Rep.* 2001;50(RR-17):1-17.

Dexter PR, Perkins SM, Maharry KS, Jones K, McDonald CJ. Inpatient computer-based standing orders vs physician reminders to increase influenza and pneumococcal vaccination rates: a randomized trial. *JAMA.* 2004;292(19):2366-2371.

Hinman AR. Tracking immunization. *Pediatr Ann.* 2004;33(9):609-615.

Jacobson VJC, Szilagyi P. Patient reminder and recall systems to improve immunization rates. Cochrane Review Web site. http://www.cochrane.org/reviews/en/ab003941.html. Accessed August 15, 2008.

McKibben LJ, Stange PV, Sneller VP, Strikas RA, Rodewald LE; Advisory Committee on Immunization Practices. Use of standing orders

TABLE 4.8 — Codes for Vaccines and Immune Globulins, 2008

	Trade Name	Manufacturer/Distributor	CPT Code	ICD-9-CM[a]
Vaccines				
Anthrax, SC	Biothrax	Bioport	90581	V03.89
DT, <7 years, IM	Tetanus and Diphtheria Toxoids Adsorbed USP for Pediatric Use	Sanofi Pasteur	90702	V06.5
DTaP, <7 years, IM	Daptacel	Sanofi Pasteur	90700	V06.1
	Infanrix	GlaxoSmithKline		
	Tripedia	Sanofi Pasteur		
DTaP-HepB-IPV, IM	Pediarix	GlaxoSmithKline	90723	V06.8
DTaP/Hib, IM	TriHIBit	Sanofi Pasteur	90721	V06.8
DTaP-IPV, 4 to 6 years, IM	Kinrix	GlaxoSmithKline	90696	V06.8
DTaP-IPV/Hib, IM	Pentacel	Sanofi Pasteur	90698	V06.8
HepA, adult, IM	Havrix	GlaxoSmithKline	90632	V05.3
	Vaqta	Merck		
HepA, pediatric/adolescent, 2 dose, IM	Havrix	GlaxoSmithKline	90633	V05.3
	Vaqta	Merck		
HepA, pediatric/adolescent, 3 dose, IM	Havrix	GlaxoSmithKline	90634	V05.3
HepA-HepB, adult, IM	Twinrix	GlaxoSmithKline	90636	V06.8
HepB, adolescent, 2 dose, IM	Vaqta	Merck	90743	V05.3

Description	Vaccine	Manufacturer	Code	ICD
HepB, adult, IM	Engerix-B	GlaxoSmithKline	90746	V05.3
	Recombivax HB	Merck		
HepB, dialysis or immunosuppressed, 3 dose, IM	Recombivax HB	Merck	90740	V05.3
HepB, dialysis or immunosuppressed, 4 dose, IM	Engerix-B	GlaxoSmithKline	90747	V05.3
HepB, adolescent, 2 dose, IM	Recombivax HB	Merck	90743	V05.3
HepB, pediatric/adolescent, 3 dose, IM	Engerix-B	GlaxoSmithKline	90744	V05.3
	Recombivax HB	Merck		
HepB-Hib, IM	Comvax	Merck	90748	V06.8
Hib, PRP-OMPC conjugate, 3 dose, IM	PedvaxHIB	Merck	90647	V03.81
Hib, PRP-T conjugate, 4 dose, IM	ActHIB	Sanofi Pasteur	90648	V03.81
HPV4, types 6, 11, 16, 18 (quadrivalent), 3 dose, IM	Gardasil	Merck	90649	V04.89
HPV2, types 16, 18 (bivalent), 3 dose, IM	Cervarix[b]	GlaxoSmithKline	90650	V04.89
Influenza, split virus, 6 to 35 months, IM	Fluzone	Sanofi Pasteur	90657	V04.8
Influenza, split virus, preservative-free, 6 to 35 months, IM	Fluzone	Sanofi Pasteur	90655	V04.81
Influenza, split virus, ≥3 years, IM	Afluria	CSL Biotherapies	90658	V04.81
	Flulaval	GlaxoSmithKline		
	Fluvirin	Novartis		
	Fluzone	Sanofi Pasteur		
Influenza, split virus, preservative-free, ≥3 years, IM	Afluria	CSL Biotherapies	90656	V04.81
	Fluarix	GlaxoSmithKline		
	Fluvirin	Novartis		
	Fluzone	Sanofi Pasteur		

4

Continued

TABLE 4.8 — *Continued*

	Trade Name	Manufacturer/ Distributor	CPT Code	ICD-9-CM[a]
Influenza, live, intranasal	FluMist	MedImmune	90660	V04.81
Influenza, subunit, cell culture-derived, preservative- and antibiotic-free, IM			90661	V04.81
Influenza, split virus, preservative-free, enhanced immunogenicity via increased antigen content, IM			90662	V04.81
Influenza, pandemic formulation			90663	V04.81
IPV, SC or IM	IPOL	Sanofi Pasteur	90713	V04.0
Japanese encephalitis, SC	JE-Vax	Sanofi Pasteur	90735	V05.0
Japanese encephalitis, inactivated, IM[b]			90738	V05.0
Measles, live, SC	Attenuvax	Merck	90705	V04.2
MMR, live, SC	M-M-R II	Merck	90707	V06.4
MMRV, live, SC	ProQuad	Merck	90710	V06.8
Mumps, live, SC	Mumpsvax	Merck	90704	V04.6
MCV4, serogroups A, C, Y, W-135, IM	Menactra	Sanofi Pasteur	90734	V03.89
MPSV4, any serogroups, SC	Menomune– A/C/Y/W-135	Sanofi Pasteur	90733	V03.89
PCV7, <5 years, IM	Prevnar	Wyeth	90669	V03.82
PPSV23, adult or immunosuppressed, ≥2 years, SC or IM	Pneumovax 23	Merck	90732	V03.82

Continued

Vaccine	Trade name	Manufacturer	CPT	V code
Rabies, IM	Imovax Rabies	Sanofi Pasteur	90675	V04.5
	RabAvert	Novartis		
Rotavirus, pentavalent, live, 3 dose, PO	RotaTeq	Merck	90680	V04.89
Rotavirus, human, attenuated, live, 2 dose, PO	Rotarix	GlaxoSmithKline	90681	V04.89
Rubella, live, SC	Meruvax II	Merck	90706	V04.3
Smallpox	ACAM2000	Acambis	90749c	V04.1
	Dryvax	Wyeth		
Td, ≥7 years, IM	Tetanus and Diphtheria Toxoids Adsorbed for Adult Use	Sanofi Pasteur and Massachussetts Public Health Biologic Laboratories	90718	V06.5
Td, preservative-free, ≥7 years, IM	Decavac	Sanofi Pasteur	90714	V06.5
Tdap, ≥7 years, IM	Adacel	Sanofi Pasteur	90715	V06.1
	Boostrix	GlaxoSmithKline		
Tetanus toxoid, adsorbed, IM	Tetanus Toxoid Adsorbed	Sanofi Pasteur	90703	V03.7
Typhoid, live, PO	Vivotif	Berna	90690	V03.1
Typhoid, Vi capsular polysaccharide, IM	Typhim Vi	Sanofi Pasteur	90691	V03.1
Varicella, live, SC	Varivax	Merck	90716	V05.4
Yellow fever, live, SC	YF-Vax	Sanofi Pasteur	90717	V04.4
Zoster, live, SC	Zostavax	Merck	90736	V05.8
Unlisted vaccine/toxoid			90749	

TABLE 4.8 — *Continued*

	Trade Name	Manufacturer/Distributor	CPT Code	ICD-9-CM[a]
Need for prophylactic vaccination and inoculation against:				
Other specified single bacterial disease				V03.89
Unspecified single bacterial disease				V03.9
Other viral disease				V04.89
Other specified single disease				V05.8
Unspecified single disease				V05.9
Other combination of diseases				V06.8
Unspecified combined vaccine				V06.9
Immune Globulins				
Immune globulin, human, IM	GamaSTAN S/D	Talecris	90281	V07.2[d]
Immune globulin, human, IV	Gammagard Liquid	Baxter	90283	V07.2
	Gammagard S/D	Baxter		
	Iveegam E/N	Baxter		
	Polygam S/D	Baxter		
	Carimune NF	CSL Behring		
	Gammar-P I.V.	CSL Behring		
	Panglobulin NF	CSL Behring		

Description	Product	Manufacturer	Code	ICD
	Privigen	CSL Behring		
	Flebogamma DIF 5%	Grifols		
	Venoglobulin-S	Grifols		
	Octagam	Octapharma		
	Gamimune N	Talecris		
	Gamunex	Talecris		
Immune globulin, human, 100 mg, each, SC	Vivaglobin	CSL Behring	90284	V07.2
Botulinum antitoxin, equine, any route			90287	V07.2
Botulism immune globulin, human, IV	BabyBIG	Massachussetts Public Health Biologic Laboratories and Cangene	90288	V07.2
CMV immune globulin, human, IV	CytoGam	CSL Behring	90291	V04.89
Diphtheria antitoxin, equine, any route			90296	V07.2
Hepatitis B immune globulin, human, IM	HepaGam B	Apotex	90371	V05.3
	HyperHEP B S/D	Talecris		
	Nabi-HB	Nabi		
Rabies immune globulin, human, IM and/or SC	HyperRAB	Talecris	90375	V04.5
Rabies immune globulin, heat-treated, human, IM and/or SC	Imogam Rabies–HT	Sanofi Pasteur	90376	V04.5
RSV immune globulin, monoclonal, IM	Synagis	MedImmune	90378	V04.82
RSV immune globulin, IV	RespiGam	MedImmune	90379	V04.82

4

Continued

TABLE 4.8 — Continued

	Trade Name	Manufacturer/ Distributor	CPT Code	ICD-9-CM[a]
Tetanus immune globulin, human, IM	HyperTET	Talecris	90389	V07.2
Vaccinia immune globulin, human, IM			90393	V04.1
Varicella immune globulin, human, IM	VariZIG[b]	Cangene	90396	V05.4
Unlisted immune globulin			90399	V07.2

[a] The ICD-9-CM codes specify the reason for the vaccine or immune globulin. For example, the ICD-9-CM code that accompanies DTaP vaccination is V06.1, "need for prophylactic vaccination and inoculation against combinations of diseases, diphtheria-tetanus-pertussis." ICD-9-CM codes in addition to those listed may be submitted. For example, a visit for a DiGeorge syndrome patient for administration of varicella immune globulin might be coded as V05.4, "need for other prophylactic vaccination and inoculation against single diseases, varicella", as well as 279.11, "disorders involving the immune mechanism, deficiency of cell-mediated immunity, DiGeorge's syndrome." In some cases, the diagnosis codes are sufficiently ambiguous as to allow several options. For example, although the table shows the code V05.8 ("need for other prophylactic vaccination and inoculation against single diseases, other specified disease") for zoster vaccine, the code V04.89 ("need for other prophylactic vaccination and inoculation against certain viral diseases, other viral diseases") might also be appropriate.

[b] Not licensed as of October 2008.

[c] Unlisted vaccine/toxoid (there is currently no specific CPT code for smallpox vaccine).

[d] Indicates prophylactic immunotherapy.

Beebe M, et al. *CPT 2008 Professional Edition.* Chicago, IL: AMA Press; 2007; Hart AC, Stegman MS. *ICD-9-CM Professional: International Classification of Diseases—9th Revision—Clinical Modification 2008.* 6th ed. Salt Lake City, UT: Ingenix, Inc; 2007.

programs to increase adult vaccination rates. *MMWR Recomm Rep.* 2000;49(RR-1):15-16.

Policy on the development of immunization tracking systems. American Academy of Pediatrics Committee on Practice and Ambulatory Medicine. *Pediatrics.* 1996;97:927.

Szilagyi PG, Bordley C, Vann JC, et al. Effect of patient reminder/recall interventions on immunization rates: a review. *JAMA.* 2000;284(14): 1820-1827.

Walton S, Elliman D, Bedford H. Missed opportunities to vaccinate children admitted to a paediatric tertiary hospital. *Arch Dis Child.* 2007;92(7):620-622.

Wood DL; American Academy of Pediatrics Committee on Community Health Services, American Academy of Pediatrics Committee on Practice and Ambulatory Medicine. Increasing immunization coverage. *Pediatrics.* 2003;112(4):993-996.

Vaccine Administration

Schechter NL, Zempsky WT, Cohen LL, McGrath PJ, McMurtry CM, Bright NS. Pain reduction during pediatric immunizations: evidence-based review and recommendations. *Pediatrics.* 2007;119(5):e1-184-e1198.

Dealing With Emergencies

Bohlke K, Davis RL, Marcy SM, et al; Vaccine Safety Datalink Team. Risk of anaphylaxis after vaccination of children and adolescents. *Pediatrics.* 2003;112(4):815-820.

Centers for Disease Control and Prevention. Syncope after vaccination—United States, January 2005-July 2007. *MMWR Morb Mortal Wkly Rep.* 2008;57:457-460.

Coding, Billing, and Vaccine Costs

Tuck RH. Coding and payment for immunizations. *Pediatr Ann.* 2006;35(7):507-512.

TABLE 4.9 — CPT Codes for Vaccine Administration, 2008[a]

Procedure	Code	Example
***Pediatric-Specific Codes*[b,c]**		
Immunization administration <8 years of age (includes percutaneous, intradermal, SC, and IM) when the physician counsels the patient/family; *first injection*[d] (single or combination vaccine/toxoid), per day	90465 • Do not report in conjunction with 90467	DTaP given as the first injection of that day for a child <8 years of age, where the physician performs face-to-face counseling in conjunction with the administration
Immunization administration <8 years of age (includes percutaneous, intradermal, SC, and IM) when the physician counsels the patient/family; *each additional injection* (single or combination vaccine/toxoid), per day	+90466 • List separately in addition to code for primary procedure • Use in conjunction with 90465 or 90467	PCV7 given as the second injection of that day for a child <8 years of age, where the physician performs face-to-face counseling in conjunction with the administration
Immunization administration <8 years of age (includes intranasal and oral) when the physician counsels the patient/family; *first administration*[d] (single or combination vaccine/toxoid), per day	90467 • Do not report in conjunction with 90465	PRV given as the first vaccine of that day for a child <8 years of age, where the physician performs face-to-face counseling in conjunction with the administration

| | PRV given as the second vaccine of that day for a child <8 years of age, where the physician performs face-to-face counseling in conjunction with the administration |

Immunization administration <8 years of age (includes intranasal and oral) when the physician counsels the patient/family; *each additional administration* (single or combination vaccine/toxoid), per day

+90468
• List separately in addition to code for primary procedure
• Use in conjunction with 90465 or 90467

Non–Age-Specific Codes[e]

Immunization administration (includes percutaneous, intradermal, SC, and IM); one vaccine[d] (single or combination vaccine/toxoid)

90471
• Do not report in conjunction with 90473

DTaP given as the first injection of that day

Immunization administration (includes percutaneous, intradermal, SC, and IM); each additional vaccine (single or combination vaccine/toxoid)

+90472
• List separately in addition to code for primary procedure
• Use in conjunction with 90471 or 90473

PCV7 given as the second injection of that day

Immunization administration by intranasal or oral route; one vaccine[d] (single or combination vaccine/toxoid)

90473
• Do not report in conjunction with 90471

PRV given as the first vaccine of that day

Immunization administration by intranasal or oral route; each *additional* vaccine (single or combination vaccine/toxoid)

+90474
• List separately in addition to code for primary procedure
• Use in conjunction with 90471 or 90473

PRV given as the second vaccine of that day

Continued

145

TABLE 4.9 — *Continued*

a Each code covers all services associated with giving the vaccine, including making the appointment, preparing the chart, billing, filing, receptionist activities, taking vital signs, screening, reviewing the Vaccine Information Statement, answering questions, administering the vaccine, documenting the administration, and observing after administration. The CPT code for administration and the CPT code for the vaccine (listed in **Table 4.8**) are each reported along with the ICD-9-CM code corresponding to the vaccine (also listed in **Table 4.8**).

b These codes should be used when the patient is <8 years of age *and the physician* performs face-to-face counseling associated with administration of the vaccine. Vaccine counseling includes obtaining information related to contraindications, reviewing the *Vaccine Information Statement*, discussing risks and benefits, obtaining consent, addressing parents' concerns, and entering information into immunization information systems (registries). The physician does not have to actually perform the administration. An advanced nurse practitioner who performs the counseling can report these codes as "incident to" a physician, provided the state allows this under the nurse practitioner's scope of practice. Medicare requires that in this situation, the patient must be an established patient and the service must be performed under the direct supervision of the physician (at the very least, he or she must be immediately available in the office suite).

c The RVUs assigned to these families of codes are the same; therefore, reimbursement is likely to be the same (except, perhaps, for some private payers). However, it is important to point out that the RVUs for all administration codes more than doubled between 2004 and 2007. In essence, the valuation of practice expenses and physician work that was inherent in the pediatric-specific codes was also incorporated into the non-age-specific codes.

d The idea here is that there can only be one "first" vaccine given during a particular visit. It does not matter which of the day's vaccines are reported as the first one; all other vaccines given at that visit, however, must be reported using an "additional vaccine" administration code.

e These codes should be used when neither of the requirements for pediatric-specific codes (90465–90468) are met.

Comprehensive overview: immunization administration. American Academy of Pediatrics Web site. http://www.aap.org/visit/OverviewImmunization Administration2008.pdf. Accessed August 15, 2008.

TABLE 4.10 — CPT Codes for Immune Globulin Administration, 2008

Procedure	Code	Example
IV infusion, for therapy, prophylaxis, or diagnosis (specify substance or drug); initial, up to 1 hour	90765	IV immune globulin given as prophylaxis against varicella
IV infusion, for therapy, prophylaxis, or diagnosis (specify substance or drug); each additional hour	+90766 • List separately in addition to code for primary procedure • Use in conjunction with 90765	Prolonged IV immune globulin infusion
SC infusion, for therapy or prophylaxis (specify substance or drug); initial, up to 1 hour, including pump set-up and establishment of SC infusion site(s)	90769	SC immune globulin for a child with hypo-gammaglobulinemia
SC infusion, for therapy or prophylaxis (specify substance or drug); each additional hour	+90770 • List separately in addition to code for primary procedure • Use in conjunction with 90769	Prolonged SC immune globulin infusion
Therapeutic, prophylactic, or diagnostic injection (specify substance or drug); SC or IM	90772	RSV mAB (palivizumab), IM

Beebe M, et al. *CPT 2008 Professional Edition*. Chicago, IL: AMA Press; 2007.

TABLE 4.11 — Coding for a Routine Visit at 6 Months of Age, 2008[a]

Procedure	Visit		Vaccine		Vaccine Administration	
	CPT	ICD-9-CM	CPT	ICD-9-CM	CPT	ICD-9-CM
Checkup	99391[b]	V20.2[c]	—	—	—	—
DTaP	—	—	90700	V06.1	90465[d]	V06.1
Hib, PRP-T conjugate	—	—	90648	V03.81	90466	V03.81
PCV7	—	—	90669	V03.82	90466	V03.82
HepB	—	—	90744	V05.3	90466	V05.3
PRV	—	—	90680	V04.89	90468	V04.89

[a] The billing rules for particular insurance companies may vary.
[b] Established patient, periodic comprehensive preventive medicine, under 1 year of age.
[c] Routine infant or child health check.
[d] This series of codes is used if the requirements for pediatric-specific codes are met (see **Table 4.9**).

TABLE 4.12 — Vaccine Costs, 2007

Vaccine	Trade Name	Age Indication	Manufacturer/ Distributor	How Supplied (No. in Package)	Cost/Dose (US$)	
					CDC	Private Sector
DTaP	Tripedia	6 weeks to 6 years	Sanofi Pasteur	1-dose vial (10)	12.65	21.40
	Daptacel	6 weeks to 6 years	Sanofi Pasteur	1-dose vial (10)	13.25	22.04
	Infanrix	6 weeks to 6 years	GlaxoSmithKline	1-dose vial (10)	13.25	20.96
				Prefilled syringe (5)	13.25	21.44
DTaP-HepB-IPV	Pediarix	6 weeks to 6 years	GlaxoSmithKline	1-dose vial (10)	47.25	70.72
				Prefilled syringe (5)	47.25	70.72
DTaP-Hib	Trihibit	15 to 18 months	Sanofi Pasteur	1-dose vial (5)	25.91	42.89
HepA	Vaqta (Pediatric)	12 months to 18 years	Merck	1-dose vial (10)	12.25	30.37
	Vaqta (Adult)	≥19 years	Merck	1-dose vial (1)	18.85	63.51
				1-dose vial (10)	18.85	59.99
	Havrix (Pediatric)	12 months to 18 years	GlaxoSmithKline	1-dose vial (10)	12.25	28.74
				Prefilled syringe (5)	12.25	28.74
	Havrix (Adult)	≥19 years	GlaxoSmithKline	1-dose vial (10)	18.86	58.28
				Prefilled syringe (5)	18.86	58.29
HepA-HepB	Twinrix	≥18 years	GlaxoSmithKline	1-dose vial (10)	37.64	83.10
				Prefilled syringe (5)	37.64	82.83

Continued

149

TABLE 4.12 — Continued

Vaccine	Trade Name	Age Indication	Manufacturer/ Distributor	How Supplied (No. in Package)	Cost/Dose (US$) CDC	Cost/Dose (US$) Private Sector
HepB	Engerix-B (Pediatric)	<20 years	GlaxoSmithKline	1-dose vial (10)	9.10	21.37
				Prefilled syringe (5)	9.10	21.37
	Engerix -B (Adult)	≥20 years	GlaxoSmithKline	1-dose vial (10)	24.73	50.35
				Prefilled syringe (5)	24.73	50.35
	Recombivax HB (Pediatric/Adolescent)	<20 years	Merck	1-dose vial (10)	9.50	23.20
	Recombivax HB (Adolescent)	11 to 15 years	Merck	1-dose vial (10)	24.25	59.09
	Recombivax HB (Adult)	≥20 years	Merck	1-dose vial (1)	23.78	59.70
				1-dose vial (10)	23.78	59.09
HepB-Hib	Comvax	6 weeks to 15 months	Merck	1-dose vial (10)	27.75	43.56
Hib	PedvaxHIB	2 to 71 months	Merck	1-dose vial (10)	10.83	22.77
	ActHIB	2 to 18 months	Sanofi Pasteur	1-dose vial (5)	8.12	21.78
HPV	Gardasil	9 to 26 years	Merck	1-dose vial (10)	96.75	120.50
IPV	IPOL	≥6 weeks	Sanofi Pasteur	10-dose vial (1)	11.06	22.80
				Prefilled syringe (10)	11.06	26.34
LAIV	FluMist	2 to 49 years	MedImmune	1-dose sprayer (10)	17.65	17.95

150

MCV4	Menactra	2 to 55 years	Sanofi Pasteur	1-dose vial (1)	73.09	89.43
				1-dose vial (5)	73.09	89.43
MMR	M-M-R II	$\geq$12 months	Merck	1-dose vial (10)	17.60	44.84
MMRV	ProQuad	12 months to 12 years	Merck	1-dose vial (10)	77.75	124.37
PCV7	Prevnar	6 weeks to 9 years	Wyeth	Prefilled syringe (10)	62.14	79.19
PPSV23	Pneumovax 23	$\geq$2 years	Merck	5-dose vial (1)	14.86	26.08
				1-dose vial (10)	16.91	29.28
PRV	RotaTeq	6 to 32 weeks	Merck	1-dose tube (10)	55.05	66.94
Td	Decavac	$\geq$7 years	Sanofi Pasteur	1-dose vial (10)	17.38	19.14
				Prefilled syringe (10)	17.38	19.14
	Tetanus and Diphtheria Toxoids Adsorbed for Adult Use	$\geq$7 years	Massachusetts Biologic Labs	15-dose vial (1)	9.86	19.19
Tdap	Boostrix	10 to 18 years	GlaxoSmithKline	1-dose vial (10)	30.75	36.25
				Prefilled syringe (5)	30.75	36.25
	Adacel	11 to 64 years	Sanofi Pasteur	1-dose vial (10)	30.75	37.43
TIV	Fluzone	$\geq$6 months	Sanofi Pasteur	10-dose vial (1)	10.153	11.72
	Fluzone (preservative-free)	6 to 35 months	Sanofi Pasteur	1-dose vial (10)	12.77	14.26
	Fluzone (preservative-free)	$\geq$36 months	Sanofi Pasteur	1-dose vial (10)	13.751	15.36
				Prefilled syringe (10)	13.751	15.36

Continued

4

151

TABLE 4.12 — *Continued*

Vaccine	Trade Name	Age Indication	Manufacturer/ Distributor	How Supplied (No. in Package)	Cost/Dose (US$) CDC	Cost/Dose (US$) Private Sector
	Fluvirin	≥4 years	Novartis	10-dose vial (1)	10.16	12.48
	Fluvirin (preservative-free)	≥4 years	Novartis	Prefilled syringe (10)	12.61	15.54
	Fluarix	≥18 years	GlaxoSmithKline	Prefilled syringe (5)	12.00	13.25
Varicella	Varivax	≥12 months	Merck	1-dose vial (10)	59.15	74.56
Zoster	Zostavax	≥60 years	Merck	1-dose (1)	113.24	152.50
			Merck	1-dose vial (10)	107.93	145.35

CDC vaccine price list. Centers for Disease Control and Prevention Web site. http://www.cdc.gov/vaccines/programs/vfc/cdc-vac-price-list.htm. Accessed August 15, 2008.

TABLE 4.13 — Provider Costs for Vaccination Services

Direct Costs
- Vaccine purchase (including excise tax)
- Sales or usage tax

Overhead
- Personnel time to order and inventory vaccines, negotiate prices, track unpaid claims, immunization information system data entry
- Storage (includes refrigerator and associated maintenance, portion of rent and electric bill, etc)
- Insurance against vaccine loss
- Wastage and nonpayment
- Lost opportunity costs (eg, use of rooms for counseling parents about vaccines that could have been used for other income-generating activities, money tied up in inventory that could have been gaining interest, etc)

Administration Expenses
- Physician work
- Staff time
- Medical supplies (eg, gloves, exam table paper, syringes, needles, alcohol swabs, emergency response items, etc)
- Professional liability insurance

Vaccines: a survival guide for pediatric practices. American Academy of Pediatrics Web site. http://www.cispimmunize.org/pro/pdf/Vacc_survival_insert.pdf. Accessed August 15, 2008.

5

General Recommendations

Rules by Which to Vaccinate

Vaccine recommendations have become very complex. The following general rules are offered as a guide to providers in day-to-day practice. Remember, however—there are exceptions to every rule.

■ **Any Vaccines Can Be Given at the Same Time**
EXCEPTION: *Varicella and smallpox vaccines.*

Simultaneous administration of all vaccines for which a child is eligible at a given visit is encouraged for two reasons: achievement of optimal protection is not delayed and completion of all recommended vaccine series is more likely. There are no vaccines that cannot be given at the same time, considering both reactogenicity and immunogenicity, except for varicella and smallpox vaccines. However, the vaccines must be given at separate sites and should never be mixed in the same syringe unless the products are specifically labeled for this purpose. Licensed combination vaccines can reduce the high number of shots that are now unavoidable at certain visits.

■ **Live Vaccines Not Given at the Same Time Should Be Separated by at Least 4 Weeks**
EXCEPTIONS: *1) Yellow fever vaccine may be given at any time after single-antigen measles vaccine; 2) Live oral vaccines (PRV, HRV, and typhoid Ty21a) may be given at any time in relation to any other live vaccines.*

Different live vaccines can be given simultaneously (except for varicella and smallpox vaccines) at different sites. If live vaccines are to be given sequentially, they should be separated by at least 4 weeks so that replication of the first vaccine does not interfere with replication of the second. Any timing sequence between live vaccines and inactivated vaccines is acceptable.

■ **Different Inactivated Vaccines May Be Given at Any Time With Respect to Each Other**
EXCEPTIONS: *None.*

Simultaneous administration, or better yet the use of combination vaccines, is preferred because of improved compliance. However, there is no evidence that sequential administration of *different* inactivated vaccines at any time interval interferes with immunogenicity or increases reactogenicity. The case of sequential administration of Tdap and MCV4 is a little tricky. While these are ostensibly *different* vaccines, they both contain diphtheria toxoid (it is the carrier protein for the polysaccharide in MCV4). The AAP suggests a minimum interval of 1 month between Tdap and MCV4 if the vaccines are not given on the same day—the concern is that too many doses of diphtheria toxoid in sequence can cause increased reactogenicity). The ACIP, however, does not recommend a minimum interval.

■ **There are Minimum Acceptable Intervals Between Doses of the Same Vaccine**
   EXCEPTIONS: *1) The 4-day grace period; 2) Early, accelerated, or compressed schedules in certain situations.*

Proper spacing of doses within a given vaccine series is essential for optimal immune responses. For this reason, doses of the same vaccine administered sooner than the specified minimum interval are considered invalid. The CDC suggests a "grace period" wherein a dose given up to 4 days before the recommended interval should be counted as valid (the exception to this is rabies vaccine, which has very specific timing requirements). However, some states and local jurisdictions may not accept this interpretation for school entry requirements, so the best advice is to give the vaccine at the recommended minimum age and interval. Invalid doses should be repeated, but the minimum interval should elapse between the invalid dose and the repeat dose. There are circumstances where early, accelerated, or compressed schedules can be used, such as for catch-up immunization or impending international travel. However, even here the minimum intervals should be followed. **Table 5.1** shows the recommended minimum ages and intervals for routinely used vaccines.

■ **There Are Minimum Ages for Administration of All Vaccines**
   EXCEPTIONS: *BCG, HepB, and rabies vaccine.*

For live parenteral vaccines, the issue is inactivation of the vaccine by circulating maternal antibody, which can persist for as long as a year. PRV and HRV, live oral vaccines, have not been studied in children <6 weeks of age. For other vaccines such as Hib, the issue is that administration in the first 6 weeks of life might induce immunologic tolerance. HepB and BCG may be given at birth. During measles outbreaks when cases are occurring in infants under a year of age, and for impending travel outside the United States, measles vaccine can be given before the recommended minimum age of 12 months (and as early as 6 months). Doses given under 12 months of age, however, are not counted as part of the routine series.

■ **Partial or Fractional Doses of a Vaccine Should Never Be Used**
   EXCEPTIONS: *None.*

In the past, some practitioners have "split" doses of vaccines (particularly DTwP) into multiple smaller shots in order to minimize potential reactions. There is no support for this practice, even in premature infants. Less than full doses of vaccines should not be counted as valid.

■ **A Multidose Vaccine Series Should Not Be Restarted if the Recommended Dosing Interval Is Exceeded**
EXCEPTION: *Oral typhoid Ty21a.*

If there is a lapse in the administration of sequential doses of a given series, simply begin where the series was suspended, keeping in mind the minimum intervals between doses. The only exception to this rule is the oral typhoid Ty21a vaccine, for which some experts recommend repeating the series if all 4 doses are not given within 3 weeks.

■ **Similar Vaccines Made by Different Manufacturers Are Interchangeable**
EXCEPTION: *There is a preference for using the same DTaP and rotavirus vaccine products for the entire series.*

Vaccines from different manufacturers differ in composition, formulation, and content. However, sufficient data exist to consider many of the vaccines made by different manufacturers interchangeable in a given vaccine series, including diphtheria toxoid, tetanus toxoid, HepA, HepB, and IPV. Hib vaccines are also interchangeable, but if ActHIB (PRP-T) is used as the first or second dose, the primary series should include 3 doses (an all-PedvaxHIB [PRP-OMPC] schedule requires only 2 doses for the primary series). All types (TIV and LAIV) and brands of influenza vaccine are considered interchangeable, provided the products are used in the appropriate age groups. Because of limited data, the ACIP has expressed a preference for the same DTaP product for the entire series. Practically speaking, however, this recommendation is difficult to implement, and the ACIP states that vaccination *should not be deferred* if the same product is not immediately available or if the previous products are not known. Similarly, rotavirus vaccination should not be deferred if the same product as the previous dose is not available; however, if any one of the doses in the series was PRV, 3 total doses should be given (an all-HRV schedule requires only 2 doses).

It should be mentioned that vaccines for the same disease are not strictly interchangeable if they are fundamentally different vaccines. For example, both MCV4 and MPSV4 protect against meningococcal disease. However, the former is a conjugate vaccine and the latter is a pure polysaccharide vaccine, and the recommendations for each differ. The same is true for PCV7 and PPSV23. The varicella and zoster vaccines contain the exact same live-attenuated varicella virus, although in differing amounts, and the two vaccines are used for entirely different purposes. Likewise, DTaP and Tdap may contain the same antigens but are used for different purposes.

TABLE 5.1 — Minimum Ages and Intervals for Routine Vaccines

Vaccine	Dose Number	Age		Interval to Next Dose	
		Recommended	Minimum	Recommended	Minimum
HepB	1	Birth[a]	Birth[a]	1 to 4 months	4 weeks
	2	1 to 2 months	4 weeks	2 to 17 months	8 wk[b]
	3	6 to 18 months	24 weeks	—	—
DTaP	1	2 months	6 weeks	2 months	4 weeks
	2	4 months	10 weeks	2 months	4 weeks
	3	6 months	14 weeks	6 to 12 calendar months	6 calendar months[c]
	4	15 to 18 months	12 months	3 years	6 calendar months
	5	4 to 6 years	4 years	—	—
Hib	1[d]	2 months	6 weeks	2 months	4 weeks
	2	4 months	10 weeks	2 months	4 weeks
	3[e]	6 months	14 weeks	6 to 9 calendar months	8 weeks
	4	12 to 15 months	12 months	—	—
HRV[f]	1	2 months	6 weeks	2 months	4 weeks
	2	4 months	10 weeks	—	—
IPV	1	2 months	6 weeks	2 months	4 weeks
	2	4 months	10 weeks	2 to 14 months	4 weeks
	3	6 to 18 months	14 weeks	3 to 5 years	4 weeks
	4	4 to 6 years	18 weeks	—	—

Vaccine	Dose				
PCV7	1[d]	2 months	6 weeks	2 months	4 wk[g]
	2	4 months	10 weeks	2 months	4 wk[g]
	3	6 months	14 weeks	6 months	8 wk[g]
	4	12 to 15 months	12 months	—	—
MMR	1	12 to 15 months	12 months	3 to 5 years	4 wk[h]
	2	4 to 6 years	13 months	—	—
VAR	1	12 to 15 months	12 months	3 to 5 years	12 wk[i]
	2	4 to 6 years	15 months	—	—
HepA	1	12 to 23 months	12 months	6 to 18 calendar months	6 calendar months
	2	18 to 41 months	18 months	—	—
TIV	1[j]	Annual	6 months[k]	1 month	4 weeks
LAIV	1[j]	Annual	2 years	1 month	4 weeks
MCV4	1	11 to 12 years	2 years	—	—
MPSV4[l]	1	—	2 years	5 years	5 years
	2[m]	—	7 years	—	—
Td	1	11 to 12 y[n]	7 years	10 years	5 years
Tdap	1	≥11 years	10 y[k]	—	—
PPSV23	1	—	2 years	5 years	5 years
	2[o]	—	7 years	—	—

Continued

TABLE 5.1 — *Continued*

Vaccine	Dose Number	Age Recommended	Age Minimum	Interval to Next Dose Recommended	Interval to Next Dose Minimum
HPV[p]	1	11 to 12 years	9 years	2 months	4 weeks
	2	11 to 12 years (plus 2 months)	109 months	4 months	12 weeks[q]
	3	11 to 12 years (plus 6 months)	112 months	—	—
PRV[f]	1	2 months	6 weeks	2 months	4 weeks
	2	4 months	10 weeks	2 months	4 weeks
	3	6 months	14 weeks	—	—
Zoster	1	60 years	60 years	—	—

See *Conventions Used in This Book* for definitions of ages and time intervals.

a Combination products cannot be used for the birth dose.
b Dose 3 should be given at least 16 weeks after dose 1.
c Dose 4 need not be repeated if given at least 4 months after dose 3.
d Children receiving dose 1 after 6 months of age require fewer doses.
e A dose at 6 months of age is not necessary if PRP-OMPC (PedvaxHIB; Merck) is used for doses 1 and 2.
f According to the package insert, dose 1 of HRV can be given between 6 and 20 weeks of age, but no doses should be given after 24 weeks. The package insert for PRV says dose 1 should be given at 6 to 12 weeks, and no doses should be given after 32 weeks. Provisional ACIP recommendations (July 2008) set dose 1 of both vaccines at 6 weeks to 14 weeks 6 days and the last dose before 8 months 0 days.
g At <12 months of age, the minimum interval between doses of PCV7 is 4 weeks. At ≥12 months of age, the minimum interval is 8 weeks.
h The minimum interval is 3 months if MMRV (ProQuad; Merck) is used.

i If the second dose is given ≥28 days after the first dose, this should be considered valid and should not be repeated. The minimum interval is 4 weeks if the series is initiated after 12 years of age.

j Two doses separated by at least 4 weeks are required for children <9 years of age who are being immunized for the first time, as well as children <9 years of age who were immunized for the first time in the prior year and only received 1 dose.

k The minimum age differs by product.

l MCV4 is preferred for individuals 2 to 55 years of age.

m Dose 2 is recommended for individuals who remain at high risk.

n Tdap is preferred for routine use at 11 to 12 years of age.

o Dose 2 is recommended for individuals at highest risk; consider giving dose 2 after 3 years for high-risk children who would be <10 years of age at revaccination.

p This vaccine is only recommended for females.

q Dose 3 should be given at least 24 weeks after dose 1.

Centers for Disease Control and Prevention. *MMWR.* 2006;55(RR-15):1-48, with modifications based on recommendations released since 2006.

■ **There Is No Harm in Vaccinating a Person Who Has Already Had the Disease or the Vaccine**

EXCEPTION: *Administering too many doses of PPSV23 or tetanus or diphtheria toxoid-containing vaccines can cause increased reactogenicity.*

For some diseases, vaccination is *indicated* even if the person has had the disease. For example, infants <2 years of age who had invasive *H influenzae* infection should still be vaccinated because infection at that age does not confer effective immunity. The zoster vaccine is specifically designed to be given to people who have had the (varicella zoster virus) infection. For *S pneumoniae*, the vaccine protects against multiple serotypes, so prior infection with a particular serotype does not obviate the need for vaccination. The same reasoning holds true for HPV vaccine. Influenza vaccine *must* be given each year whether or not the person has had influenza in the past. Some experts recommend pertussis vaccine for children who have had well-documented pertussis (culture positive or epidemiologically linked to a culture-positive case) because the duration of natural immunity is not known. Clinicians often wonder if a child with a questionable history of chickenpox or varicella vaccination should receive the vaccine. The motto here is—*when in doubt, vaccinate*! With chickenpox, as with most other diseases, there is no evidence of harm if a person who has had the disease or the vaccine receives another dose of the vaccine.

■ **Live Vaccines Should be Deferred After Receipt of Antibody-Containing Blood Products**

EXCEPTIONS: *1) Yellow fever vaccine, oral typhoid Ty21a, LAIV, and zoster vaccine; 2) MMR and varicella vaccine should not be deferred in postpartum women who received antibody-containing blood products during pregnancy, including anti-Rho(D) globulin; 3) Rotavirus vaccine should not be deferred if deferral would cause the first dose to be given beyond the recommended age.*

Antibodies contained in blood products can inactivate live vaccines and reduce effectiveness or "take." Several factors play into whether or not deferral is recommended and determine the time interval after which a vaccine can be given. One factor is the product itself—immune globulin intravenous is likely to contain more antibody than packed red cells, hence necessitating a longer delay. Another factor is the specific antibody content of the product; for example, blood products in the United States are unlikely to contain antibodies to yellow fever virus and *S typhi*, so these vaccines can be given at any time with respect to blood products. Finally, the route of administration of the vaccine is a factor—parenteral vaccines are more likely to be inactivated by circulating, passively transferred antibodies than are oral or intranasal vaccines (the rationale for deferral of rotavirus vaccine is not clear). **Table 5.2** shows the recommended intervals between blood product administration and certain live vaccines. Keep in mind that the antibodies in blood products do not interfere with inactivated vaccines. Three other caveats deserve mention: 1) if a child has already received MMR, varicella vaccine, or MMRV, 2 weeks should elapse before an antibody-containing blood product is given, because the vaccine viruses must still replicate in order to induce immunity; 2) if a pregnant woman receives a blood product, that should not result in deferral of her infant's first dose of rotavirus vaccine; and 3) monoclonal antibody products such as RSV-mAB (Synagis) do not interfere with (heterologous) live vaccines.

■ **More Vaccination Pearls**

• Invalid doses can arise from specific circumstances other than those mentioned above.

– *Route of administration*: A dose of HepB that is mistakenly given subcutaneously (the recommended route is intramuscular) is considered invalid, whereas a dose of MCV4 that is mistakenly given subcutaneously (the recommended route is also intramuscular) is considered valid. Doses of subcutaneously administered vaccines (varicella vaccine, MMR, MMRV, yellow fever vaccine, MPSV4, anthrax) that are mistakenly given intramuscularly are considered valid. Remember that IPV and PPSV23 can be given either subcutaneously or intramuscularly.

– *Site of administration*: Intramuscular injections should be given in the anterolateral thigh in infants and the deltoid in older children and adults (see Chapter 4, *Vaccine Practice*). The gluteal muscle should not be used because of the thick fat layer over the muscle. For HepB and rabies vaccine, avoidance of the gluteal muscle is critical; doses of HepB given to adults in the gluteal region, and doses of rabies vaccine given to persons of any age in the gluteal region, are considered invalid.

– *Expired or damaged vaccine*: Doses of vaccines that have passed their expiration date and vaccines that have been damaged (eg, inadequate storage conditions) are considered invalid. Doses of expired inactivated vaccines should be repeated as soon as possible with nonexpired vaccine—do not wait for the minimum interval to elapse after the invalid dose. Doses of expired live vaccines should be repeated in 4 weeks using nonexpired vaccine.

– *Vaccine mix-ups*: Similar vaccines may be confused with one another. Here are examples of vaccine mix-ups and how to handle them.

• If DTaP (which is labeled for children ≤6 years of age) is inadvertently given to an adolescent or adult instead of Tdap, the dose is valid. On the other hand, if Tdap (which is labeled for adults and/or adolescents) is inadvertently given to an infant as part of the 3-dose primary series, the

163

TABLE 5.2 — Interval Between Receipt of Antibody-Containing Products and Administration of Live Vaccines

Product (Route of Administration)	Indication	Usual Dose	Live Vaccine — MMR, Varicella, or MMRV[c]	Live Vaccine — Rotavirus[a]	Live Vaccine — LAIV, Ty21a, YF, Zoster[b]
RSVmAB (IM) Synagis	Prevention of RSV disease	15 mg/kg	None[c]	None	None
IGIM	Pre- or postexposure prophylaxis for hepatitis A	0.02 or 0.06 mL/kg	3 months	42 days	None
	Postexposure prophylaxis for measles:				
	Standard	0.25 mL/kg	5 months	42 days	None
	Immunocompromised[d]	0.5 mL/kg	6 months	42 days	None
IGIV	Replacement therapy for immune deficiency[d]	400 mg/kg	8 months	42 days	None
	Postexposure prophylaxis for varicella	400 mg/kg	8 months	42 days	None
	Immune thrombocytopenic purpura	400 mg/kg	8 months	42 days	None
	Kawasaki disease	1 g/kg	10 months	42 days	None
		2 g/kg	11 months	42 days	None
Blood transfusion (IV)	Red blood cells:				
	Washed	—	None	None	None
	Adenine-saline added	10 mL/kg	3 months	42 days	None
	Packed	10 mL/kg	6 months	42 days	None
	Whole blood	10 mL/kg	6 months	42 days	None

Product	Dose			
Plasma or platelet products	10 mL/kg	7 months	42 days	None
CMV-IGIV	Prevention of CMV disease in transplant patients[d]	150 mg/kg	6 months	42 days	None
HBIG (IM)	Postexposure prophylaxis for hepatitis B	0.06 mL/kg	3 months	42 days	None
HRIG (IM and intrawound)	Postexposure prophylaxis for rabies	20 IU/kg	4 months	42 days	None
RhoGAM (IM)	Prevention of maternal Rh isoimmunization	300 mcg	None[e]	None[e]	None
TIG (IM)	Postexposure prophylaxis for tetanus	250 units	3 months	42 days	None
VariZIG (IM)[f]	Postexposure prophylaxis for varicella	125 units/10 kg	5 months	42 days	None

[a] Rotavirus vaccine should be given if deferral would cause the first dose to be given outside the recommended age range.

[b] Blood products in the United States are unlikely to contain substantial amounts of antibody to *Salmonella typhi* and YFV. Even if antibodies to the current circulating strain of influenza virus were present, they would be unlikely to inactivate LAIV, which is administered on a mucosal surface. Zoster vaccine is normally given to individuals who already have circulating antibodies to VZV.

[c] Vaccine may be given at any time.

[d] Live viral vaccines may be contraindicated in these patients.

[e] Administration of live vaccines, if indicated, to postpartum women should not be delayed if antibody-containing products were given during the last trimester (this includes RhoGAM). Likewise, the infant's immunization with rotavirus vaccine should not be delayed.

[f] This product is licensed in Canada and is available in the United States under an investigational new-drug application expanded-access protocol.

Centers for Disease Control and Prevention. *MMWR*. 2006;55(RR-15):1-48.

dose is considered invalid and should be repeated with DTaP, either at the same visit or as soon as possible. If Tdap is given by mistake to a child ≤6 years of age as dose-4 or dose-5, it is considered valid.

- If zoster vaccine (which is labeled for adults ≥60 years of age) is inadvertently given to a child, it should be counted as a single valid dose of varicella vaccine. If varicella vaccine is mistakenly given to an adult for protection against zoster, the dose is considered invalid and should be repeated with zoster vaccine at the same visit or at ≥28 days form the invalid dose (this prevents interference between the vaccines).

- Serology is of limited utility in vaccine practice. Testing for varicella antibodies before vaccination might be cost-effective in adults who have a negative personal history of chickenpox. However, in most other circumstances vaccines should just be given without testing for immunity. This would include internationally adopted children with a questionable vaccination history—it is probably simpler just to reimmunize than to test for immunity to multiple antigens. For the most part, immunity is presumed to result from appropriate vaccine schedules and doses. Testing for seroconversion is indicated only rarely, such as in high-risk health care workers or dialysis patients given HepB, laboratory workers receiving pre-exposure rabies vaccination, and in some cases where individuals received invalid doses.

- A physical examination is not required for vaccination of healthy individuals.

- Gloves are not routinely needed to administer vaccines, but should be worn if the vaccinator may come in contact with body fluids or has open lesions on his or her hands.

- It is not necessary to change the needle after withdrawing a vaccine from the vial and before administering it to the patient. This only increases the risk of sharps injury and bacterial contamination.

- Aspirating back on the syringe after insertion but before injection is not necessary. There are no large vessels in the anatomic areas that are recommended for vaccine injection.

- Injections in the same area should be separated by at least 1 inch.

- Syringes should not be prefilled by the end user. This increases the risk of administration error and raises stability and storage issues. The one exception is mass influenza immunization campaigns where only one vaccine type is being used. In this situation, a small number of syringes can be prepared and labeled in advance; they should be used soon after filling, and unused syringes should be discarded. Many vaccines are now supplied by manufacturers in single-use, prefilled syringes.

A *contraindication* is a condition that *increases the likelihood of a serious adverse event*; when present, the vaccine in question should not be given. The only true permanent contraindication for all routine vaccines, based on a definitive risk, is severe allergy or anaphylaxis to the vaccine or any of its components. In this regard, it should be mentioned that most vaccines contain buffers as well as excipients, which are substances other than the vaccine that are included in the manufacturing process or added to the final product (excipients are listed in the relevant vaccine sections; a complete list is available at http://www.cdc.gov/vaccines/pubs/pinkbook/downloads/appendices/B/excipient-table-2.pdf [Accessed August 15, 2008]). In addition, there may be contaminating substances that carry over from early steps in processing, and some vial stoppers and syringes contain latex, which can carry over to the patient during injection. Both excipients and contaminants can be triggers for allergic reactions in sensitized patients. The best advice is to check the package insert before administering any vaccine to a person with a relevant allergy history.

A permanent contraindication for DTaP and Tdap is acute encephalopathy within 7 days of receipt of a pertussis-containing vaccine, based on the theoretic possibility of exacerbation or recurrence of encephalopathy. Pregnancy is a contraindication for live vaccines based on theoretic risks to the fetus and the possibility that naturally occurring birth defects might be attributed to the vaccine (see Chapter 7, *Vaccination in Special Circumstances*). However, there is no definitive evidence of fetal damage from any live vaccine. In addition, in some circumstances, the benefits may outweigh the risks; for example, yellow fever vaccine can be considered for pregnant women traveling to high-risk areas. Although live vaccines are generally contraindicated in persons with immune incompetence, there may again be situations where the benefits outweigh the risks (see *Chapter 7*). For example, natural varicella probably represents a greater risk to a DiGeorge syndrome patient with mildly impaired cellular immunity than does the live attenuated vaccine.

A *precaution* is called for when a condition exists that *might increase the risk of a serious adverse event, compromise the immunogenicity* of the vaccine, or *be mistaken for a vaccine reaction*. Understanding what to do when a precaution is noted is sometimes difficult. Technically speaking, the default position is to defer vaccination. However, the risks of deferral (susceptibility to disease) must be weighed against the risks of vaccination (largely theoretic). In making these judgments, the provider must take into account the prevailing epidemiology of the disease, the patient's personal circumstances, and the possibility that an opportunity for vaccination will be missed. Here is an example.

A 2-month-old experiences 4 hours of inconsolable crying after receiving his first DTaP. This would constitute a precaution to the administration of a second dose of DTaP at 4 months of age. However, because the risk of a recurrence of inconsolable crying is low, the consequences of such an episode are not permanent, and the risk of pertussis is appreciable, the provider may elect to give the second dose. Here is another example. A provider may elect to give the 6-month shots to an infant with a moderate febrile illness *if* there is substantial risk that the child will not return for vaccination after the illness resolves.

Table 5.3 gives contraindications and precautions for selected vaccines, derived from the recommendations of the CDC, AAP, and vaccine manufacturers. Issues with individual vaccines generally apply to combinations.

Misconceptions about vaccine contraindications can result in missed opportunities. **Table 5.4** lists some erroneous contraindications; if present, vaccines can and should be given.

ADDITIONAL READING

Kroger AT, Atkinson WL, Marcuse EK, Pickering LK; Advisory Committee on Immunization Practices (ACIP) Centers for Disease Control and Prevention (CDC). General recommendations on immunization: recommendations of the Advisory Committee on Immunization Practices (ACIP). *MMWR Recomm Rep*. 2006;55(RR-15):1-48.

TABLE 5.3 — Contraindications and Precautions for Further Vaccine Doses

Vaccine	Contraindications[a] Condition	Risk of Giving Vaccine	Precautions[a] Condition	Risk of Giving Vaccine
All vaccines	Severe allergic reaction[b] to vaccine or vaccine component[c]	Anaphylaxis	Moderate-to-severe acute illness with or without fever	Difficulty distinguishing illness from vaccine reaction
DTaP	Encephalopathy within 7 days of vaccination with a pertussis-containing vaccine	Recurrent encephalopathy (causality not established) and difficulty distinguishing illness from vaccine reaction	Fever ≥105°F within 48 hours	Recurrent reaction
			Hypotonic hyporesponsive episode within 48 hours	Recurrent reaction
			Inconsolable crying ≥3 hours within 48 hours	Recurrent reaction
			Seizure within 3 days	Recurrent reaction
	Progressive neurologic disorder (until stabilized)	Recurrent encephalopathy (causality not established) and difficulty distinguishing illness from vaccine reaction	Guillain-Barré syndrome within 6 weeks of tetanus toxoid–containing vaccine	Recurrent Guillain-Barré syndrome
DT, Td, and TT	No specific additional contraindications[d]	—	Guillain-Barré syndrome within 6 weeks of tetanus toxoid–containing vaccine	Recurrent Guillain-Barré syndrome
			Arthus-type reaction to a tetanus or diphtheria toxoid–containing vaccine	Recurrent Arthus-type reaction

Continued

5

TABLE 5.3 — *Continued*

| Vaccine | Contraindications[a] | | Precautions[a] | |
	Condition	Risk of Giving Vaccine	Condition	Risk of Giving Vaccine
HepA	No specific additional contraindications[d]	—	Pregnancy[e]	Theoretic risk to fetus or attribution of birth defects to vaccination
HepB	Allergy to baker's yeast	Anaphylaxis	Infant weight <2000 gm unless mother is HBsAg-positive	Poor immunogenicity
Hib	Age <6 weeks	Induction of immune tolerance	No specific additional precautions[d]	
HPV	Allergy to baker's yeast No specific additional contraindications[d]	Anaphylaxis	Pregnancy[e]	Theoretic risk to fetus or attribution of birth defects to vaccination
IPV	No specific additional contraindications[d]	—	Pregnancy[e]	Theoretic risk to fetus or attribution of birth defects to vaccination
JE	Allergy to proteins of rodent or neural origin	Anaphylaxis	Pregnancy[e]	Theoretic risk to fetus or attribution of birth defects to vaccination

				Interference with vaccine delivery
LAIV	Allergy to eggs[f] Severe immune impairment[g] Chronic medical illness Pregnancy Personal history of Guillain-Barré syndrome Asthma or equivalent Children or adolescents on aspirin or other salicylates	Anaphylaxis Disease caused by live vaccine Adverse effects of live vaccine on fetus (theoretic) or attribution of birth defects to vaccination Recurrent Guillain-Barré syndrome Exacerbation of respiratory disease Reye syndrome	Severe nasal congestion	
MCV4	No specific additional contraindications[d]	—	Personal history of Guillain-Barré syndrome	Recurrent Guillain-Barré syndrome
MPSV4	No specific additional contraindications[d]	—	No specific additional precautions[d]	—
MMR	Allergy to gelatin or neomycin Severe immune impairment[d] Pregnancy	Anaphylaxis Disease caused by live vaccine Adverse effects of live vaccine on fetus (theoretic) or attribution of birth defects to vaccination	Recent receipt of antibody-containing blood product[h] History of thrombocytopenia or thrombocytopenic purpura Untreated active TB	Impaired response to vaccine Recurrent thrombocytopenia Exacerbation of TB

5

Continued

TABLE 5.3 — *Continued*

Vaccine	Contraindications[a]		Precautions[a]	
	Condition	Risk of Giving Vaccine	Condition	Risk of Giving Vaccine
PCV7	No specific additional contraindications[d]	—	No specific additional precautions[d]	—
PPSV23	No specific additional contraindications[d]	—	No specific additional precautions[d]	—
Rabies (post-exposure)	None[j]	—	Immunosuppressive therapy	Impaired response to vaccine
Rotavirus[i]	No specific additional contraindications[d]	—	Impaired immunity[g]	Disease caused by live vaccine
			Recent receipt of antibody-containing blood product[h]	Impaired response to vaccine
			Preexisting GI disease	Exacerbation of GI disease (causality not established)
			Previous history of intussusception	Recurrent intussusception (causality not established)
Smallpox (pre-event)	Eczema, atopic dermatitis, or exfoliative skin condition	Disease caused by live vaccine	Inflammatory eye disease requiring steroid therapy	Disease caused by live vaccine

Vaccine	Condition	Effect	Condition	Effect
	Immune impairment[g]	Disease caused by live vaccine		
	HIV infection	Disease caused by live vaccine		
	Household contact with certain risk factors, including pregnancy	Disease in contact caused by live vaccine		
	Breast-feeding	Disease caused by live vaccine		
	Pregnancy	Adverse effects of live vaccine (theoretical) or attribution of birth defects to vaccination		
Tdap	Encephalopathy within 7 days of vaccination with a pertussis-containing vaccine	Recurrent encephalopathy (causality not definitively established) and difficulty distinguishing illness from vaccine reaction	Guillain-Barré syndrome within 6 weeks of tetanus toxoid–containing vaccine	Recurrent Guillain-Barré syndrome
			Arthus-type reaction to a tetanus toxoid–containing vaccine or a diphtheria toxoid–containing vaccine that does not contain TT	Recurrent Arthus-type reaction
			Progressive or unstable neurologic disorder (until stabilized)	Difficulty distinguishing illness from vaccine reaction
TIV	Allergy to eggs[f]	Anaphylaxis	Guillain-Barré syndrome within 6 weeks of influenza vaccine	Recurrent Guillain-Barré syndrome

5

Continued

173

TABLE 5.3 — *Continued*

| Vaccine | Contraindications[a] | | Precautions[a] | |
	Condition	Risk of Giving Vaccine	Condition	Risk of Giving Vaccine
TViPSV (parenteral)	No specific additional contraindications[d]	—	No specific additional precautions[d]	—
Ty21a (PO)	Immune impairment[g]	Disease caused by live vaccine	Antibiotic therapy	Impaired response to vaccine
Varicella	Allergy to gelatin or neomycin	Anaphylaxis	Recent receipt of antibody-containing blood product[h]	Impaired response to vaccine
	Severe immune impairment[g]	Disease caused by live vaccine	Children or adolescents on aspirin or other salicylates	Reye syndrome
	Pregnancy	Adverse effects of live vaccine on fetus (theoretic) or attribution of birth defects to vaccination		
	Untreated active TB	Exacerbation of TB		
YF	Allergy to eggs[f]	Anaphylaxis	Pregnancy[k]	Theoretic risk to fetus or attribution of birth defects to vaccination
	Immune impairment[g]	Encephalitis		
	Age <9 months	Encephalitis		
Zoster	Immune impairment[g]	Disease caused by live vaccine	Untreated active TB	Exacerbation of TB
	Pregnancy	Adverse effects of live		

174

vaccine on fetus (theoretic) or attribution of birth defects to vaccination.

a See text for definition. Also see individual vaccine sections (Chapter 9, *Routine Vaccines* and Chapter 10, *Specialized Vaccines*) for details.

b Severe allergy is IgE-mediated, occurs in minutes to hours, and requires medical attention. Examples include generalized urticaria, facial swelling, airway obstruction, wheezing, anaphylaxis, hypotension, and shock. Delayed-type hypersensitivity is generally not a contraindication.

c Vaccines contain trace components, preservatives, other excipients, and residual media, which may differ from one manufacturer to another. The table lists particularly unusual components that may induce allergic reactions, such as traces of baker's yeast (eg, HepB and HPV), eggs (eg, TIV), and rodent or neural proteins (eg, JE vaccine). For other components that may induce allergic reactions, see individual vaccine sections. Patients with severe allergy to latex should not receive vaccines supplied in vials or syringes that contain natural rubber.

d General contraindications and precautions for all vaccines *(top row)* apply.

e The risk of adverse fetal effects from an inactivated vaccine is extremely low. It is not clear why pregnancy is listed as a precaution for some inactivated vaccines but not others.

f Being able to eat eggs (even in baked goods) without adverse effects is a reasonable indication of a very low risk of anaphylaxis. Mild or local manifestations of allergy to eggs or feathers are not a contraindication. Skin testing can be done and desensitization may be possible.

g See Chapter 7, *Vaccination in Special Circumstances*.

h Blood products, including IGIV, IGIM, and hyperimmune globulin, contain various amounts of antibodies to these live vaccine viruses. The suggested interval before vaccination depends on the product (see **Table 5.2**). This is not an issue for monoclonal antibody products like RSVmAB (Synagis).

i As of October 2008, specific ACIP recommendations regarding HRV (Rotarix) have not been published.

j Given the fact that rabies is essentially universally fatal, there are no absolute contraindications to vaccination for postexposure prophylaxis.

k Vaccination may be considered if travel cannot be postponed and if exposure is very likely.

Centers for Disease Control and Prevention. *MMWR*. 2006;55(RR-15):1-48; American Academy of Pediatrics. Guide to contraindications and precautions to immunizations, 2006. In: Pickering LK, ed. *2006 Red Book: Report of the Committee on Infectious Diseases*. 27th ed. Elk Grove Village, IL: American Academy of Pediatrics; 2006:847-851; as well as individual vaccine recommendations and package inserts. More detail can be found in individual vaccine sections.

5

TABLE 5.4 — Erroneous Contraindications to Vaccination

- Mild acute illness, with or without fever
- Mild respiratory illness (including most cases of otitis media)
- Mild gastroenteritis
- Antibiotic or antiviral therapy[a]
- Low-grade fever and/or local redness, pain, and swelling after a previous dose
- Prematurity[b]
- Pregnant, unimmunized, or immunosuppressed household contact[c]
- Breast-feeding[c]
- Convalescent phase of illness
- Exposure to an infectious disease
- Positive tuberculin skin test without active disease[d]
- Simultaneous tuberculin skin testing[e]
- Allergy to penicillin, duck meat or feathers, or environmental allergens
- Fainting after a previous dose
- Seizures, sudden infant death syndrome, allergies, or vaccine adverse events in family members
- Malnutrition
- Lack of previous physical examination in a well-appearing individual
- Stable neurologic condition (eg, cerebral palsy, well-controlled seizure disorder, developmental delay)
- Allergy shots
- Extensive limb swelling after DTwP, DTaP, or Td that is not an Arthus-type reaction
- Brachial neuritis after previous dose of tetanus toxoid–containing vaccine
- Autoimmune disease
- Having had the disease that the vaccine is designed to prevent[f]

---

[a] Antibiotics could interfere with live bacterial vaccines (eg, Ty21a), and antivirals could interfere with live viral vaccines (eg, varicella vaccine).

[b] The birth dose of HepB should be delayed (because of poor immunogenicity) in infants weighing <2000 g whose mothers are HBsAg-negative.

[c] Pre-event smallpox vaccination is an exception.

[d] Active tuberculosis is a contraindication for varicella vaccine and a precaution for MMR and zoster vaccine.

[e] Measles vaccine could temporarily suppress tuberculin reactivity. Measles-containing vaccines can be given on the same day as a tuberculin skin test is placed; if not given on the same day, the measles-containing vaccine should be delayed at least 4 weeks.

[f] Immunity from natural infection may wane with time, as in the case of pertussis. Alternatively, the vaccine (eg, HPV, MCV4, PCV7, rotavirus vaccine) might protect against serotypes to which the individual has not been previously exposed.

Continued

TABLE 5.4 — *Continued*

Centers for Disease Control and Prevention. *MMWR*. 2006;55(RR-15): 1-48; American Academy of Pediatrics. Guide to contraindications and precautions to immunizations, 2006. In: Pickering LK, ed. *2006 Red Book: Report of the Committee on Infectious Diseases*. 27th ed. Elk Grove Village, IL: American Academy of Pediatrics; 2006:847-851; as well as individual vaccine recommendations and package inserts. More detail can be found in individual vaccine sections.

5

6

Schedules

As discussed in Chapter 2, *Vaccine Infrastructure in the United States*, the Advisory Committee on Immunization Practices (ACIP) has permanent working groups that make recommendations for changes to the routine childhood/adolescent and adult vaccination schedules.

Since 1995, the childhood schedule has been "harmonized" in its current graphic layout with the recommendations of the American Academy of Pediatrics (AAP) and the American Academy of Family Physicians (AAFP). The new schedule is released in January of each year. Beginning in 2007, the schedule was split into two—one giving the routinely recommended vaccines for children 0-6 years of age (**Table 6.1**) and the other giving the recommendations for children and adolescents 7-18 years of age (**Table 6.2**). Two additional charts—the catch-up schedules (**Tables 6.3** and **6.4**)—are used to bring unimmunized and underimmunized children up-to-date as soon as possible. Catch-up can be accomplished by giving all vaccines for which a child is eligible at each visit, keeping in mind the minimum intervals between doses (**Table 5.1**).

The routine adult schedule, first published in its current form in 2002, is released in October of every year. The recommendations are now developed in conjunction with the AAFP, the American College of Obstetricians and Gynecologists, and the American College of Physicians. The schedule is given in two different formats—by age group (**Table 6.5**) and by underlying medical condition (**Table 6.6**).

TABLE 6.1 — Routine Immunization Schedule for Children 0 to 6 Years of Age, 2008

Vaccine (Route of Administration)	Birth	1	2	4	6	12	15	18	19-23	2-3	4-6
HepB (IM)[a]	Dose 1[b]	|--- Dose 2[c] ---|		Note[a]	|------------------------ Dose 3[c] ------------------------|						
Rotavirus (PO)[d]			Dose 1	Dose 2	(Dose 3)						
DTaP (IM)[e]			Dose 1	Dose 2	Dose 3		|------ Dose 4[f] ------|				Dose 5
Hib (IM)[g]			Dose 1	Dose 2	(Dose 3)[h]	|------ Dose 4 ------|					
PCV7 (IM)			Dose 1	Dose 2	Dose 3	|------ Dose 4 ------|					
IPV (IM or SC)[j]			Dose 1	Dose 2	|------------------ Dose 3 ------------------|						Dose 4
Influenza (IM or intranasal)					|------------------------ Annually[k] ------------------------|						
MMR (SC)[l]						|------ Dose 1 ------|				Dose 2[m]
Varicella (SC)[l]						|------ Dose 1 ------|				Dose 2[n]
HepA (IM)						Dose 1			|------ Dose 2 ------|	High-risk[o]	
MCV4 (IM)											High-risk[p]

High-risk conditions are discussed in Chapter 7, *Vaccination in Special Circumstances*, as well as individual vaccine sections.

[a] The following combination vaccines containing HepB are available: DTaP-HepB-IPV (Pediarix; 2, 4, 6 months); HepB-Hib (Comvax; 2, 4, 12 to 15 months). Use of these combination vaccines may mean that children will get an unnecessary dose of HepB at 4 months of age. Such extraimmunization is permissible and safe.

[b] Only monovalent vaccine can be used under 6 weeks of age. A birth dose should be given to all newborns before hospital discharge. For infants of HBsAg-negative mothers, the birth dose can be delayed only by an order from the provider and a copy of the mother's negative hepatitis B serology

laboratory report on the chart. Infants of HBsAg-positive mothers should receive both vaccine and hepatitis B immune globulin within 12 hours of birth and should be tested for HBsAg and HBsAb between 9 and 18 months of age (a few months after completion of the vaccine series). If the mother's status is unknown, vaccinate within 12 hours of birth and test the mother; hepatitis B immune globulin can still be given in the first week if the mother turns out to be HBsAg-positive.

c The second dose must be at least 4 weeks after the first dose; the third dose must be at least 16 weeks after the first dose and 8 weeks after the second dose; the last dose (third or fourth) should not be given before 24 weeks of age.

d Either HRV (2, 4 months) or PRV (2, 4, 6 months) may be used. Provisional recommendations released July 2008 state that the first dose should be given between 6 weeks and 14 weeks 6 days of age. All doses should be administered by 8 months 0 days of age. Vaccination should not be deferred if the product used for the previous dose is unavailable or not known. If any of the doses in the series is PRV, 3 total doses should be given.

e The following combination vaccines containing DTaP are available: DTaP-HepB-IPV (Pediarix; 2, 4, 6 months); DTaP-IPV/Hib (Pentacel; 2, 4, 6, 12 to 15 months); DTaP/Hib (TriHIBit; dose 4 only at 15 to 18 months); DTaP-IPV (KINRIX; dose 5 only at 4 to 6 years).

f The fourth dose may be given as early as 12 months of age, provided at least 6 months have elapsed since the third dose.

g The following combination vaccines containing Hib are available: HepB-Hib (Comvax; 2, 4, 12 to 15 months); DTaP-IPV/Hib (Pentacel; 2, 4, 6, 12 to 15 months); DTaP/Hib (TriHIBit; dose 4 only at 15 to 18 months).

h A dose at 6 months is not required if the first 2 doses were PRP-OMPC (PedvaxHIB or Comvax).

i One dose of PCV7 (Prevnar) should be given to all healthy children 24 to 59 months of age who have an incomplete schedule, including those who have never received PCV7. PPSV23 (Pneumovax 23) should be given to children ≥2 years of age with high-risk conditions.

j The following combination vaccines containing IPV are available: DTaP-HepB-IPV (Pediarix; 2, 4, 6 months); DTaP-IPV/Hib (Pentacel; 2, 4, 6, 12 to 15 months); DTaP-IPV (Kinrix; dose 5 only at 4 to 6 years).

k TIV (IM; multiple brands) may be used starting at 6 months of age and LAIV (intranasal; FluMist) starting at 2 years of age. All close contacts of children 0 to 59 months of age and close contacts of children with high-risk conditions also should be immunized. The dose of TIV between 6 and 35 months of age is 0.25 mL; beyond that it is 0.5 mL. Children <9 years of age who are receiving influenza vaccine for the first time, or who were vaccinated for the first time in the previous season and only received 1 dose, need 2 doses separated by 4 weeks. LAIV may be used for healthy children who do not have underlying conditions that predispose to complications of influenza.

l MMRV (ProQuad) may be used in place of MMR (M-M-R II) and varicella vaccine (Varivax). If used, the second dose may be given anytime ≥3 months after the first dose.

Continued

6

TABLE 6.1 — *Continued*

m For MMR, the second dose may be given anytime ≥4 weeks after the first dose.

n For monovalent varicella vaccine, the second dose may be given any time ≥3 months after the first dose. However, if the second dose is given ≥28 days after the first dose, this dose should be considered valid and should not be repeated.

o HepA (Havrix or Vaqta) is recommended for universal use in young children and for older children in certain high-risk groups. In some areas of the country, however, older children are routinely immunized.

p MCV4 (Menactra) should be given to children with high-risk conditions. MPSV4 (SC: Menomune–A/C/Y/W-135) is considered an acceptable alternative if MCV4 is not available. Children who received MPSV4 ≥3 years earlier and who remain at increased risk should receive MCV4.

Centers for Disease Control and Prevention. *MMWR.* 2008;57:Q1-Q4; Centers for Disease Control and Prevention. *MMWR Early Release.* 2008;57(July 17, 2008):1-60; ACIP provisional recommendations for the prevention of rotavirus gastroenteritis among infants and children. Centers for Disease Control and Prevention Web site. http://www.cdc.gov/vaccines/recs/provisional/downloads/roto-7-1-08-508.pdf. Accessed August 15, 2008.

TABLE 6.2 — Routine Immunization Schedule for Children 7 to 18 Years of Age, 2008

Vaccine (Route of Administration)	7-10 Years	11-12 Years	13-18 Years
Tdap (IM)		1 dose[a]	Catch-up[b]
HPV (IM; *females only*)		3 doses[c]	Catch-up
MCV4 (IM)	High-risk (1 dose)[d,e]	1 dose[e]	Catch-up[e]
PPSV23 (IM or SC)	------------------------ High-risk (1 dose)[f] ------------------------		
Influenza (IM or intranasal)	------------------------ Annually[g] ------------------------		
HepA (IM)	------------------------ High-risk (2 doses)[h] ------------------------		
HepB (IM)	------------------------ Catch-up (3 doses)[i] ------------------------		
IPV (IM or SC)	------------------------ Catch-up[j] ------------------------		
MMR (SC)	------------------------ Catch-up (2 doses)[k,l] ------------------------		
Varicella (SC)	------------------------ Catch-up (2 doses)[k,m] ------------------------		

High-risk conditions are discussed in Chapter 7, *Vaccination in Special Circumstances*, as well as individual vaccine sections.

[a] Boostrix may be given as early as 10 years of age. Adacel may be given starting at 11 years of age.

[b] Recommended for adolescents who missed the dose of Tdap at 11 to 12 years of age or who received Td instead of Tdap. In general, 5 years should elapse between the last dose of Td and a dose of Tdap, but shorter intervals are acceptable. Studies have demonstrated the safety of intervals as short as 2 years, but even shorter intervals can be used, particularly if the risk of pertussis exposure is high (in truth, there is no minimum interval between Td and Tdap).

[c] HPV4 (Gardasil) vaccine may be given as early as 9 years of age. The usual timing of doses is 0, 2, and 6 months.

[d] Children who received MPSV4 (SC; Menomune–A/C/Y/W-135) $\geq$3 years earlier and who remain at increased risk should receive a dose of MCV4 (Menactra).

[e] MPSV4 is considered an acceptable alternative if MCV4 is not available.

Continued

183

6

TABLE 6.2 — *Continued*

f   One-time revaccination in 3 to 5 years may be indicated.

g   All close contacts of children 0 to 59 months of age and close contacts of children with high-risk conditions also should be immunized. Children <9 years of age who are receiving influenza vaccine for the first time, or who were vaccinated for the first time in the previous season and only received 1 dose, need 2 doses separated by 4 weeks. LAIV (intranasal; FluMist) may be used for healthy nonpregnant individuals who do not have underlying conditions that predispose to complications of influenza.

h   In some areas of the country, older children are routinely immunized.

i   A 2-dose series of Recombivax HB is licensed for adolescents 11 to 15 years of age.

j   For children who received an all-IPV or all-OPV series, a fourth dose is not necessary if the third dose was given at ≥4 years of age. For children who received a mixed schedule, a total of 4 doses should be given regardless of age at vaccination.

k   MMRV (ProQuad) may be used in children 12 months to 12 years of age (the minimum interval between doses is 3 months).

l   The minimum interval between doses of MMR (M-M-R II) is 4 weeks.

m   For children <13 years of age, the minimum interval between doses of monovalent varicella vaccine (Varivax) is 3 months. However, if the second dose is given ≥28 days after the first dose, this dose should be considered valid and should not be repeated. For adolescents ≥13 years of age, the minimum interval is 4 weeks.

Centers for Disease Control and Prevention. *MMWR*. 2008;57:Q1-Q4; Centers for Disease Control and Prevention. *MMWR Early Release*. 2008;57(July 17):1-60.

TABLE 6.3 — Catch-Up Schedule for Children 4 Months to 6 Years of Age, 2008[a]

Vaccine	Minimum Age for First Dose	Dose 2	Dose 3	Dose 4	Dose 5
HepB[b]	Birth	4 weeks after dose 1	8 weeks after dose 2 and 16 weeks after dose 1 (4 weeks after dose 2)		
Rotavirus[c]	6 weeks	4 weeks after dose 1	4 weeks after dose 2		
DTaP	6 weeks	4 weeks after dose 1	4 weeks after dose 2	6 months after dose 3	6 months after dose 4[d]
Hib[e]	6 weeks	If dose 1 given at <12 months of age: 4 weeks after dose 1 If dose 1 given at 12 to 14 months of age: 8 weeks after dose 1 (final dose) If dose 1 given at ≥15 months of age: no further doses needed	If currently <12 months of age: 4 weeks after dose 2[f] If currently ≥12 months of age and dose 2 given at <15 months of age: 8 weeks after dose 2 (final dose)[f]	If currently 12 months to 5 years of age and received 3 doses at <12 months of age: 8 weeks after dose 3 (final dose)	
PCV7[g]	6 weeks	If dose 1 given at <12 months of age: 4 weeks after dose 1 If dose 1 given at ≥12 months of age or if current age is 24 to 59 months: 8 weeks after dose 1 (final dose) If dose 1 given at ≥24 months of age: no further doses needed	If currently <12 months of age: 4 weeks after dose 2 If currently ≥12 months of age: 8 weeks after dose 2 (final dose)	If currently 12 months to 5 years of age and received 3 doses at <12 months of age: 8 weeks after dose 3 (final dose)	
IPV	6 weeks	4 weeks after dose 1	4 weeks after dose 2	4 weeks after dose 3[h]	
MMR[i]	12 months	4 weeks after dose 1			

Continued

185

TABLE 6.3 — *Continued*

Vaccine	Minimum Age for First Dose	Dose 2	Dose 3	Dose 4	Dose 5
Varicella[i]	12 months	3 months after dose 1[j]			
HepA[k]	12 months	6 months after dose 1			

High-risk conditions are discussed in Chapter 7, *Vaccination in Special Circumstances*, as well as individual vaccine sections.

[a] This table should be used for children who start late or who are >1 month behind. The minimum interval between doses is shown. No routine vaccine series needs to be restarted, regardless of how much time has elapsed. Some combination vaccines can be used for catch-up.

[b] A 2-dose series of Recombivax HB is licensed for adolescents 11 to 15 years of age.

[c] Either HRV (2, 4 months) or PRV (2, 4, 6 months) may be used. Provisional recommendations released July 2008 state that the first dose should be given between 6 weeks and 14 weeks 6 days of age. All doses should be administered by 8 months 0 days of age. Vaccination should not be deferred if the product used for the previous dose is unavailable or not known. If any of the doses in the series is PRV, 3 total doses should be given.

[d] A fifth dose is not necessary if the fourth dose was given at ≥4 years of age. DTaP is not indicated for children ≥7 years of age.

[e] If first dose was given at 7 to 11 months of age, give 2 doses separated by 4 weeks plus a booster at 12 to 15 months of age.

[f] If the first 2 doses were PRP-OMPC (PedvaxHIB or Comvax), the third and final dose should be given at 12 to 15 months of age and at least 8 weeks after the second dose.

[g] One dose of PCV7 (Prevnar) should be given to all healthy children 24 to 59 months of age who have an incomplete schedule, including those who have never received PCV7. For children with high-risk conditions who have received <3 doses, give 2 doses at least 8 weeks apart. For children with high-risk conditions who have received 3 doses, give 1 dose.

[h] For children who received an all-IPV or all-OPV series, a fourth dose is not necessary if the third dose was given at ≥4 years of age. For children who received a mixed schedule, a total of 4 doses should be given regardless of age.

[i] MMRV (ProQuad) may be used in place of MMR (M-M-R II) and varicella vaccine (Varivax). If used, the second dose may be given any time ≥3 months after the first dose.

[j] If second dose of monovalent varicella vaccine is given ≥28 days after first dose, this dose should be considered valid and should not be repeated.

[k] In some areas of the country, older children are routinely immunized.

Centers for Disease Control and Prevention. *MMWR*. 2008;57:Q1-Q4.

TABLE 6.4 — Catch-Up Schedule for Children 7 to 18 Years of Age, 2008[a]

Vaccine	Minimum Age for First Dose	Dose 2	Dose 3	Dose 4
Td, Tdap[b]	7 years	4 weeks after dose 1	If dose 1 of a tetanus and diphtheria toxoid–containing vaccine given at <12 months of age: 4 weeks after dose 2 If dose 1 of a tetanus and diphtheria toxoid–containing vaccine given at <12 months of age: 6 months after dose 2	If dose 1 of a tetanus and diphtheria toxoid–containing vaccine given at <12 months of age: 6 months after dose 3[c]
HPV	9 years	4 weeks after dose 1	12 weeks after dose 2 and 24 weeks after dose 1	
HepA[d]	12 months	6 months after dose 1		
HepB[e]	Birth	4 weeks after dose 1	8 weeks after dose 2 and 16 weeks after dose 1	
IPV	6 weeks	4 weeks after dose 1	4 weeks after dose 2	4 weeks after dose 3[f]
MMR[g]	12 months	4 weeks after dose 1		
Varicella[g]	12 months	If dose 1 given at ≥13 years of age: 4 weeks after dose 1 If dose 1 given at <13 years of age: 3 months after dose 1[h]		

Continued

6

187

TABLE 6.4 — *Continued*

High-risk conditions are discussed in Chapter 7, *Vaccination in Special Circumstances*, as well as individual vaccine sections.

[a] This table should be used for children who start late or who are >1 month behind. The minimum interval between doses is shown. No routine vaccine series needs to be restarted, regardless of how much time has elapsed. Some combination vaccines can be used for catch-up.

[b] Tdap should be substituted for a single dose of Td in the primary catch-up series or as a booster if age-appropriate. In general, 5 years should elapse between the last dose of Td and a dose of Tdap, but shorter intervals are acceptable.

[c] A booster (fourth) dose of Td (or Tdap if appropriate) is needed if any of the previous doses of tetanus and diphtheria toxoid–containing vaccine were given at <12 months of age.

[d] In some areas of the country, older children are routinely immunized.

[e] A 2-dose series of Recombivax HB is licensed for adolescents 11 to 15 years of age.

[f] For children who received an all-IPV or all-OPV series, a fourth dose is not necessary if the third dose was given at ≥4 years of age. For children who received a mixed schedule, a total of 4 doses should be given regardless of age.

[g] MMRV may be used in place of MMR and varicella vaccine for children 12 months to 12 years of age. If used, the second dose may be given any time ≥3 months after the first dose.

[h] If the second dose of monovalent varicella vaccine is given ≥28 days after the first dose, this should be considered valid and should not be repeated.

Centers for Disease Control and Prevention. *MMWR*. 2008;57:Q1-Q4.

TABLE 6.5 — Routine Immunization Schedule for Adults by Age, 2007-2008

Vaccine (Route of Administration)	19-49 Years	50-64 Years	≥65 Years
Td, Tdap (IM)[a]	1 dose of Td every 10 y (substitute Tdap for Td once <65 years of age if not previously given)		
HPV (IM)[b]	3 doses for females ≤26 years of age		
MMR (SC)[c]	1 or 2 doses	|------------------ High-risk (1 dose) ------------------|	
Varicella (SC)[d]	|---------------------------- 2 doses if not immune ----------------------------|		
Influenza (IM or intranasal; annual)[e]	High-risk (1 dose)	|------------------------------ 1 dose ------------------------------	
PPSV23 (SC)[f]	|--------------- High-risk (1-2 doses) ---------------|-------------------------------| 1 dose		
HepA (IM)[g]	|------------------------------ High-risk (2 doses) ------------------------------|		
HepB (IM)[h]	|------------------------------ High-risk (3 doses) ------------------------------|		
MCV4 (IM), MPSV4 (SC)[i]	|------------------------------ High-risk (1-2 doses) ------------------------------|		
Zoster (SC)[j]			1 dose

High-risk conditions are discussed in Chapter 7, *Vaccination in Special Circumstances*, as well as individual vaccine sections.

[a] Only Adacel is licensed for adults. If vaccination history is uncertain, a primary series consisting of 2 doses of Td separated by 4 weeks with a booster dose 6 to 12 months later should be given; Tdap can be substituted for any one of the Td doses. In general, 5 years should elapse between the last dose of Td and a dose of Tdap, but shorter intervals are recommended for postpartum women, close contacts of infants <12 months of age, and health care workers (studies have demonstrated the safety of intervals as short as 2 years, but even shorter intervals are acceptable; in truth, there is no minimum interval between Td and Tdap). Td should be given to pregnant women in the second or third trimester if they have not been vaccinated in the past 10 years; however, in some circumstances Td can be deferred so that Tdap can be given postpartum, or Tdap may be given during pregnancy (see *Chapter 7*). If a pregnant woman received Td in the past 10 years, Tdap should be given postpartum. Td or Tdap also may be used in wound management.

[b] The usual timing of doses for HPV4 (Gardasil) is 0, 2, and 6 months. Women should be vaccinated regardless of history of HPV-induced disease and regardless of history of sexual activity.

Continued

6

TABLE 6.5 — *Continued*

c See **Table 9.12** for criteria for immunity to measles, mumps, and rubella.

d See **Table 9.19** for what constitutes evidence of immunity to varicella. The usual timing of doses is 0 and 4 to 8 weeks. Special consideration should be given to those who have close contact with individuals at high risk for varicella complications, exposure, or transmission. Pregnant women without evidence of immunity should receive a dose of varicella vaccine after delivery and before discharge from the hospital, with a second dose given 4 to 8 weeks later.

e LAIV (intranasal; FluMist) may be used for healthy nonpregnant adults ≤49 years of age who do not have underlying conditions that predispose to complications of influenza.

f One-time revaccination in 5 years is indicated for certain high-risk conditions and for individuals ≥65 years of age if they were previously vaccinated at <65 years of age.

g The usual timing of doses for Havrix is 0 and 6 to 12 months and for Vaqta 0 and 6 to 18 months. HepA-HepB (Twinrix) may be used on a 0-, 1-, and 6-month schedule or a 0-, 7-, 21-to-30–day, and 12-month schedule.

h The usual timing of doses is 0, 1 to 2, and 4 to 6 months. For patients on hemodialysis and for other immunocompromised adults, high-dose formulations are used (Recombivax HB 40 mcg/mL or 2 simultaneous doses of Engerix-B 20 mcg/mL).

i MCV4 (Menactra) is preferred at <56 years of age but MPSV4 (Menomune–A/C/Y/W-135) is an acceptable alternative. One-time revaccination with MPSV4 in 3 to 5 years may be indicated.

j Individuals should be vaccinated regardless of history of chickenpox or shingles.

Centers for Disease Control and Prevention. *MMWR.* 2007;56:Q1-Q4.

TABLE 6.6 — Routine Immunization Schedule for Adults by Medical Condition and Other Indications, 2007-2008

Vaccine	Pregnancy	Immunocompromised[a]	HIV Infection—CD4 <200/mcL	HIV Infection—CD4 ≥200/mcL	Chronic Medical Condition[b]	Asplenia or Terminal Complement Deficiency	Chronic Disease Liver	Chronic Disease Kidney	Health Care Personnel
Td, Tdap	Note[c]	----- Td every 10 years ----- Substitute Tdap for Td once <65 years of age if not previously given -----	------	------	------	------	------	------	------
HPV	Note[d]	------ Females ≤26 years of age ------	------	------	------	------	------	------	------
MMR	Contraindicated	Contraindicated	Contraindicated	------ If not immune[e] ------	------	------	------	------	If not immune[e]
Varicella	Contraindicated	Contraindicated	Contraindicated	------ If not immune[e] ------	------	------	------	------	If not immune[e]
Influenza (annual)	------	------ TIV ------	------	------	------	------	------	------	TIV or LAIV
PPSV23	Note[f]	------	------	------	------	------	------	------	Note[f]
HepA	------	------ If not immune[e] ------	------	------	------	------	If not immune[e,g]	------	Note[f]
HepB	------	------ Note[f] ------	------	------ If not immune[e] ------	------	------	------	If not immune[e]	Note[f]
MCV4, MPSV4	------	------ Note[f] ------	------	------	------	If not immune[e]	------	------	Note[f]
Zoster	Contraindicated	------ Contraindicated ------	------	Note[h]	------ If not immune and ≥60 years of age[e] ------	------	------	------	------

Continued

191

TABLE 6.6 — *Continued*

See **Table 6.5** and specific vaccine sections for details and dosing recommendations.

ᵃ Includes immunosuppression due to medication and radiation but does not include HIV infection. Live vaccines are generally contraindicated.

ᵇ Includes diabetes, heart disease, pulmonary disease, and alcoholism.

ᶜ Tdap may be indicated for pregnant women in certain circumstances (see Chapter 7, *Vaccination in Special Circumstances*).

ᵈ HPV vaccine should not routinely be given to pregnant women.

ᵉ Vaccinate individuals in this category who meet the age requirements and who lack documentation of vaccination or have no evidence of prior infection. Definitions for evidence of immunity can be found in some individual vaccine sections.

ᶠ Vaccinate if some other risk factor is present.

ᵍ Includes patients who receive clotting factor concentrates.

ʰ Zoster vaccine may be considered for HIV-infected individuals ≥60 years of age who are not immunosuppressed.

Centers for Disease Control and Prevention. *MMWR*. 2007;56:Q1-Q4.

Vaccination in Special Circumstances

General Considerations for Patients With Impaired Immunity

Vaccination of patients with impaired immunity requires special consideration for a number of reasons:

- *The balance between risks and benefits is complex*—Immuno-compromised individuals are at greater risk for complications and death from vaccine-preventable diseases. At the same time, they may be at increased risk for complications from live vaccines, and the response to all vaccines may be suboptimal. Decisions regarding vaccination are therefore more complicated than for healthy individuals and must take into account the prevalence of disease and probability of exposure, the nature and degree of immunodeficiency, the type of vaccine and the likelihood of adverse effects, the efficacy of the vaccine when immunity is impaired, and the confounding effects of other interventions. Unfortunately, in many situations there are few data available to provide guidance.

- *Immunocompromised states differ qualitatively*—Qualitative differences dictate not only which vaccines are indicated but which vaccines represent a danger to the patient. Congenital immunodeficiencies may affect humoral immunity, cell-mediated immunity, phagocyte function, or complement function in different and interconnected ways. Humoral immune defects place patients at higher risk for invasive infection with encapsulated bacteria, demanding special consideration for vaccination against *Haemophilus influenzae* type b, *Streptococcus pneumoniae*, and *Neisseria meningitidis*. Whereas isolated humoral defects do not increase the risk of serious varicella per se, they may predispose the patient to bacterial complications of varicella. Therefore, varicella vaccine is indicated in patients with isolated humoral defects—as long as they are not receiving immune globulin replacement, in which case varicella vaccine is contraindicated (antibodies in immune globulin will inactivate the vaccine virus). Similarly, phagocyte dysfunction per se does not substantially weaken defenses against influenza virus, but it does increase the risk of bacterial superinfection. Thus patients with chronic granulomatous disease, whose neutrophils fail to undergo oxidative burst, should receive influenza vaccine yearly in order to prevent bacterial pneumonia. Complement deficiencies put patients at risk for bacterial infections but carry no implications for the safety of live or inactivated vaccines.

Secondary immune deficiency states, such as those resulting from immunosuppressive medications, nephrotic syndrome, malnutrition, splenectomy, or bone marrow transplantation, also differ qualitatively from one another.

• *Immunocompromised states differ quantitatively*—In general, patients with cell-mediated immune defects should not receive live vaccines because of the risk of dissemination. However, cellular defects may range from mild to profound, and these differences affect the risk-benefit assessment for vaccination. For example, whereas varicella vaccine *should be avoided* in an HIV-infected individual with very low CD4 count, poor T-cell function, and a history of opportunistic infections, it *should be given* to a mildly symptomatic HIV-infected child whose CD4 percentages have been ≥15%. In the former situation, the risk of vaccination is too great; in the latter, the risk of vaccination is small and is outweighed by the potential consequences of natural disease. Similarly, MMR may be given to HIV-infected children without profound immunosuppression as determined by CD4 counts. DiGeorge syndrome, a quantitative T-cell deficiency resulting from thymic dysplasia, is quite variable in expression. Whereas those patients with low CD4 and CD8 counts and abnormal T-cell function should not receive live vaccines, live vaccines are probably safe in those patients with normal T-cell studies.

• *Immune responses may be suboptimal*—Data on the immunogenicity of many vaccines in immunocompromised individuals are lacking. Some patients would not be expected to respond at all. For example, there is no point in giving inactivated vaccines to patients with X-linked agammaglobulinemia because they do not make antibody. On the other hand, patients with common variable immunodeficiency may or may not respond, and such vaccines are worth giving with the hope of some benefit. Some patients who have normal concentrations of antibody may *still* not respond appropriately to certain vaccines. In fact, this constitutes an operational definition of antibody deficiency with normal immunoglobulins or antibody dysfunction syndrome, most often diagnosed by failure to respond to PPSV23. In some cases, more intensive immunization regimens are necessary to achieve protective immunity. The immune globulin replacement therapy received by some patients with humoral defects protects them from disease but also limits the usefulness of live vaccines, which can be inactivated by passively acquired antibodies.

• *Immunization of close contacts is important but may carry some risks*—Immunocompromised patients can be protected by ensuring that close contacts, especially other household members, are appropriately immunized. For example, AIDS patients may not respond well to influenza vaccine but can be protected from influenza by immunizing family members.

Likewise, HepA should be given to contacts of immunosuppressed persons if the family resides in a high-incidence area. Live vaccines carry the theoretic risk of transmission from vaccinees to immunocompromised contacts, in whom they could cause disease. A historical example of this is vaccine-associated poliomyelitis resulting from transmission of OPV within the home. However, the risk of transmission varies by vaccine, and some live vaccines carry no risk of transmission at all. Likewise, the consequences of transmission range from demonstrably serious (eg, smallpox vaccine) to only theoretic (eg, rotavirus vaccine). **Table 7.1** summarizes recommendations for use of live vaccines in household contacts of immunocompromised persons.

- *Official recommendations may differ from product labeling—* Many package inserts list immunodeficiency states as contraindications to vaccination. This labeling reflects allowable claims and mandated precautions that derive from data presented to the FDA at the time of licensure. Subsequent recommendations may be discordant with product labeling because of the availability of new data or reasoned re-evaluations of the pertinent risks and benefits. Practitioners should be aware of these discrepancies. For example, the package insert for

TABLE 7.1 — Use of Live Vaccines in Household Contacts of Immunocompromised Individuals

Vaccine	Recommendation
LAIV	Contraindicated if the household contact is profoundly immunosuppressed (eg, bone marrow transplant patient who requires specialized protective environment)
MMR	May be used
Rotavirus	May be used
	Use good hand hygiene
Smallpox	Contraindicated
Ty21a	May be used
	Use good hand hygiene
Varicella	May be used
	If vaccinee develops skin lesions, he or she should avoid contact with the immunocompromised person until the lesions resolve
YF	May be used
Zoster	May be used
	If vaccinee develops skin lesions, standard precautions should suffice to protect contacts

7

Varivax (varicella vaccine) cautions against vaccinating individuals who receive immunosuppressive therapy and those with cellular or humoral immunodeficiencies. The official recommendations, however, allow for vaccination of certain individuals with these conditions.

- *Passive immunoprophylaxis may be indicated*—Immunocompromised individuals who receive intravenous immune globulin on a monthly basis are probably protected against measles and varicella, although in the case of exposure, consideration should be given to shortening the interval to the next dose by 1 or 2 weeks. Other immunocompromised individuals at risk for serious measles should receive intramuscular immune globulin (0.5 mL/kg, maximum 15 mL) within 6 days of exposure. The AAP recommends immune globulin prophylaxis for *all* HIV-infected children and adolescents exposed to measles, regardless of vaccination status, degree of symptoms, and level of immune suppression (the dose for asymptomatic HIV-infected individuals is 0.25 mL/kg); the ACIP specifies prophylaxis only for *symptomatic* HIV infection.

Varicella zoster immune globulin (VariZIG) should be given within 96 hours of exposure to immunosuppressed individuals who are not immune to chickenpox (see Chapter 9, *Routine Vaccines*, for definition of immunity; individuals who had natural disease or are fully vaccinated and later become immunosuppressed are considered immune). The only product available in the United States is VariZIG, but this must be obtained under an investigational new-drug protocol (FFF Enterprises, phone number 800-843-7477). Intravenous immune globulin can be used if VariZIG is not available. Chemoprophylaxis with acyclovir (20 mg/kg/dose given 4 times per day, maximum dose 800 mg) is another option. If used, it should be given for 7 days beginning about a week after exposure—this is intended to limit the primary viremia. Susceptible HIV-infected individuals without evidence of immunosuppression do not need immunoprophylaxis.

Tetanus immune globulin should be administered to HIV-infected children with tetanus-prone wounds, regardless of their immunization status.

Specific Immune Deficiency States Other Than HIV Infection

Certain live vaccines, such as LAIV, MMRV, smallpox vaccine, typhoid Ty21a, and zoster vaccine are generally contraindicated in all patients with impaired immunity. Yellow fever vaccine should only be used in extraordinary, unavoidable circumstances. MMR and varicella vaccine can be used in certain defined immunodeficiency states, whereas the guidelines for rotavirus vaccine are permissive and dependent on the provider's assessment of the risks and benefits.

The following are general guidelines for use of common vaccines in persons with impaired immunity.

■ **Humoral Deficiencies**
- *Typical syndromes*: X-linked agammaglobulinemia, common variable immunodeficiency, IgA deficiency, IgG subclass deficiency, antibody deficiency with normal immunoglobulins (vaccine nonresponder state or antibody dysfunction syndrome), transient hypogammaglobulinemia of infancy
- *Safety issues*: Varicella vaccine may be given and MMR may be considered. Patients with selective IgA deficiency can probably receive all vaccines safely because they have adequate serum IgG responses.
- *Special considerations*: Inactivated vaccines are not effective in patients with severe deficiencies of immune globulin synthesis. Since many of these patients receive monthly immune globulin, live viral vaccines are unlikely to be effective as they are neutralized by passively acquired antibodies. Less severely affected individuals who are not receiving immune globulin may benefit from vaccination; in these cases, postimmunization antibody titers may be used to confirm responses.

■ **Defects of Cell-Mediated Immunity**
- *Typical syndromes*: severe combined immunodeficiency, DiGeorge syndrome, hyper-IgM syndrome (CD40 ligand deficiency), bare lymphocyte syndrome, autoimmune polyendocrinopathy candidiasis-ectodermal dystrophy (chronic mucocutaneous candidiasis), Wiskott-Aldrich syndrome, ataxia-telangiectasia (humoral immunity is affected in most of these syndromes as well)
- *Safety issues*: Live vaccines are generally contraindicated.
- *Special considerations*: Live vaccines can be considered in some situations—for example, varicella vaccine for DiGeorge syndrome patients with minimal T-cell dysfunction. Inactivated vaccines may be given, but effective responses are variable.

■ **Phagocyte Disorders**
- *Typical syndromes*: chronic granulomatous disease, leukocyte adhesion deficiency, Chédiak-Higashi syndrome, myeloperoxidase deficiency, hyper-IgE/recurrent infection syndrome (Job's syndrome), secondary granule deficiency
- *Safety issues*: Live bacterial vaccines are contraindicated.
- *Special considerations*: Effective responses to all routine vaccines probably occur. Influenza vaccine is indicated to reduce the risk of secondary bacterial infection.

■ **Complement Deficiencies**
- *Typical syndromes*: deficiency of individual early (C1-C4) or late (C5-C9) components, properdin deficiency, mannose-

7

binding lectin deficiency, factor I deficiency, secondary deficiency due to complement consumption
- *Safety issues*: All vaccines can be used.
- *Special considerations*: Patients with early component deficiencies are particularly susceptible to infection with gram-positive organisms, such *S pneumoniae,* and should probably receive both pneumococcal and meningococcal vaccines. Those with late component deficiencies are uniquely susceptible to infection with *N meningitidis* and should be vaccinated against this pathogen. Influenza vaccine is indicated to reduce the risk of secondary bacterial infection.

■ Steroids
- *Typical syndromes*: asthma, juvenile rheumatoid arthritis
- *Safety issues*: Live vaccines may be contraindicated in some patients.
- *Special considerations*: Because steroids may be immunosuppressive, they represent a potential problem in the use of live vaccines. Any patient receiving steroids in any form who has clinical or laboratory evidence of immunosuppression should not receive live vaccines. In addition, patients whose underlying disease itself is immunosuppressive should not receive live vaccines, except under special circumstances. The following guidelines are offered for live vaccines in other situations:
  - *Topical, inhaled, and compartmental depot injections*: Vaccination is acceptable.
  - *Physiologic replacement*: Vaccination is acceptable.
  - *Less than 2 mg/kg/day (<20 mg if >10 kg; daily or alternating days) of prednisone or equivalent*: Vaccination is acceptable.
  - *Greater than 2 mg/kg/day (>20 mg if >10 kg; daily or alternating days) of prednisone or equivalent for <14 days*: Vaccinate right after stopping steroid therapy. Do not vaccinate if steroid therapy will extend to 14 days or more.
  - *Greater than 2 mg/kg/day (>20 mg if >10 kg; daily or alternating days) of prednisone or equivalent for ≥14 days*: Vaccinate 1 month after stopping therapy.

■ Chemotherapy and Solid Organ Transplantation
- *Typical syndromes*: leukemia, lymphoma, severe autoimmune disorder, renal, heart, or liver transplant
- *Safety issues*: Live vaccines are generally contraindicated during active therapy, but may be considered before and after treatment.
- *Special considerations*: Live-virus vaccines are usually withheld for at least 3 months after immunosuppressive chemotherapy has been discontinued. This interval may vary with the type and intensity of immunosuppressive therapy, radiation therapy, underlying disease, and other factors. For children who are >12 months of age, previously immunized,

and are scheduled to undergo solid-organ transplantation, antibody titers against measles, mumps, rubella, and varicella should be obtained. Children who are susceptible should be given MMR, varicella vaccine, or both at least 1 month before transplantation (MMRV should not be used). Antibody titers to measles, mumps, rubella, and varicella should be measured in all patients 1 year after transplantation. Although live-virus vaccines are usually contraindicated in these patients because they are receiving chronic immunosuppressive medications, those who are seronegative are candidates for passive immunization if exposed to disease. Solid-organ transplant patients should receive TIV ≥6 months after transplantation and then annually for life. Routine Hib and PCV7 vaccination are only recommended in children and should be given prior to transplant. Meningococcal vaccine is not routinely indicated. Inactivated vaccines should be given about 1 year after transplantation to ensure immunogenicity.

■ **Anatomic and Functional Asplenia**
- *Typical syndromes*: congenital, traumatic, or surgical asplenia, sickle cell disease, polysplenia syndrome
- *Safety issues*: All vaccines can be used.
- *Special considerations*: Patients with asplenia, whether anatomic or functional, are at risk for life-threatening infection with encapsulated organisms, particularly *S pneumoniae*. The basis for this risk lies in impaired clearance of opsonized bacteria, coordination of lymphocyte responses, and synthesis of IgM and phagocytosis-enhancing factors. The following guidelines are offered:
  - *All asplenic individuals*: Yearly influenza vaccine should be given, beginning at 6 months of age, to prevent secondary bacterial infection. Family members should be immunized as well. Live vaccines may be given. Prophylactic antibiotics are indicated in certain individuals.
  - *Children who are anatomically or functionally asplenic from birth (including sickle cell disease) or are splenectomized in the first 2 years of life*: PCV7 and Hib should be given according to the routine schedule. At 2 years of age, MCV4 and PPSV23 should be given. A second dose of PPSV23 should be given 3 to 5 years later, and a dose of MPSV4 could be considered at that time.
  - *Elective splenectomy*: PCV7 (PPSV23 for adults), Hib, and MCV4 (if the patient is 2 to 55 years of age; beyond 55 years of age, MPSV4 should be used) should be given at least 2 weeks before surgery. Consider one-time revaccination 3 to 5 years later with PPSV23 and MPSV4.
  - *Traumatic splenectomy beyond 2 years of age*:
    - *Patient has already received the routine PCV7 and Hib series*: The patient should receive 1 dose of PPSV23, a booster dose of Hib, and MCV4 (if the patient is 2 to 55

years of age; beyond 55 years of age, MPSV4 should be used). Consider one-time revaccination 3 to 5 years later with PPSV23 and MPSV4.

- *Patient never received PCV7 or Hib (this includes adults)*: Children between 24 and 59 months of age should receive 2 doses of PCV7 followed by 1 dose of PPSV23, each separated by 2 months. They should also receive 2 doses of Hib 2 months apart. Children ≥5 years of age should receive 1 dose of Hib and 1 dose of PPSV23. MCV4 should be given if the patient is 2 to 55 years of age; beyond 55 years of age, MPSV4 should be used.

■ Chronic Disease

Individuals with chronic underlying disease may be unusually susceptible to infectious disease, whether they have immune deficiency in the classic sense. As a general rule, all routine vaccines should be given unless they are specifically contraindicated. Additional vaccines are indicated as well. There is no reason (other than a true contraindication) not to give yearly TIV to any patient ≥6 months of age who has a chronic underlying disease that might put them at risk for complications or secondary bacterial infection. This would include patients with chronic cardiac (eg, congenital heart disease), respiratory (eg, cystic fibrosis), allergic (eg, asthma), hematologic (eg, sickle cell disease), metabolic (eg, diabetes), neuromuscular (eg, muscular dystrophy), hepatic (eg, cirrhosis), and renal (eg, chronic renal failure) disorders. Patients who are particularly susceptible to pneumococcal infection, such as those with nephrotic syndrome, should receive pneumococcal vaccine as well; cochlear implants also represent a particular risk for pneumococcal disease. Patients with chronic liver disease are also at risk for severe hepatitis A and should receive HepA and HepB.

HIV Infection

Vaccine practice in HIV-infected individuals depends on the degree of immunosuppression:

- *Perinatally exposed infants whose HIV status is indeterminate*—These are infants who are born to HIV-infected mothers and are in the process of being evaluated for, but have no current evidence of, HIV infection. They should receive all routine vaccines, including rotavirus vaccine in infancy and MMR and varicella vaccine at 12 to 15 months of age (by this age HIV infection will have effectively been ruled out in most of them). Influenza vaccine should be given beginning at 6 months of age; LAIV may be used beginning at 2 years of age if the child is otherwise healthy and household contacts are not profoundly immunosuppressed. All household contacts, including the mother, should receive influenza vaccine as well.

- *Perinatally exposed infants who are not infected with HIV*—Guidelines released in February 2008 by the Working Group on Antiretroviral Therapy and Medical Management of HIV-Infected Children state that HIV infection is reasonably excluded in at-risk infants who have negative virologic tests (eg, PCR) at ≥14 days and ≥1 month of age, or one negative virologic test at ≥2 months of age, or one negative HIV antibody test at ≥6 months of age. These infants should receive all routine vaccines, as described.
- *HIV-infected infants and children*—Many children with HIV infection who receive highly active antiretroviral therapy or are natural long-term nonprogressors are relatively healthy and can be immunized according to the routine childhood schedule. The recommendations regarding rotavirus vaccine are permissive—they essentially say that the risks of giving this live vaccine should be weighed against the benefits. The risks would appear to be very low in HIV-infected infants who are not severely immunosuppressed. Special attention should be paid to influenza immunization, not only to protect the child but to prevent spread of influenza to HIV-infected household members. MMR and varicella vaccine should be given to HIV-infected children who do not have evidence of severe immunosuppression, regardless of whether symptoms are present. In children, levels of immunosuppression are defined by CD4 count or percentage (**Table 7.2**); for adolescents and adults, severe immunosuppression is defined by a CD4 count <200 cells/mcL. It is prudent to administer the 2 required doses of each vaccine as early as possible, as immune function may deteriorate before 4 to 6 years of age when the second doses are routinely administered. Given the minimum intervals of 1 month for MMR and 3 months for varicella vaccine, a simple approach would be to give both vaccines at 12 to 15 months of age and then again 3 months later. Remember, MMRV should not be used in HIV-infected individuals.

    HIV-infected children are at increased risk for invasive pneumococcal and meningococcal disease. The routine PCV7 schedule should be used, and 1 or 2 doses of PPSV23 after the first 2 years of life should be considered (**Table 9.17**). For children ≥5 years of age who never received a pneumococcal vaccine, it would be reasonable to administer 2 doses of PCV7 followed by a dose of PPSV23, each separated by 2 months; a second dose of PPSV23 could be given 3 to 5 years later. One dose of MCV4 would also be reasonable at 2 years of age.
- *HIV-infected adolescents and adults*—**Table 6.6** summarizes vaccination recommendations for older individuals with HIV infection. Note that if the CD4 count is ≥200 cells/mcL, the schedule is the same as for healthy adults, with three exceptions: 1) TIV should always be used instead of LAIV; 2) all nonimmune patients (not just high-risk patients) should be

TABLE 7.2 — Classification of HIV Infection in Children

Immunosuppression	Age <12 Months		Age 1-5 Years		Age 6-12 Years	
	CD4 Cells/mcL[a]	CD4%[a]	CD4 Cells/mcL	CD4%	CD4 Cells/mcL	CD4%
None	≥1500	≥25	≥1000	≥25	≥500	≥25
Moderate	750 to 1499	15 to 24	500 to 999	15 to 24	200 to 499	15 to 24
Severe	<750	<15	<500	<15	<200	<15

[a] Either the CD4 count or the CD4 percentage can be used to determine the immunologic category. If these indicate different categories, the more severe one should be used.

Centers for Disease Control and Prevention. *MMWR.* 1994;43(RR-12):1-10.

immunized with HepB; and 3) PPSV23 should be given soon after diagnosis (rather than waiting for routine vaccination at 65 years of age). For those with CD4 counts <200 cells/mcL, the same caveats hold true, but in addition MMR, varicella vaccine, and zoster vaccine are contraindicated. Meningococcal vaccination is indicated only if other risk factors are present.

Hematopoietic Stem Cell Transplantation (HSCT) and Leukemia

Allogeneic HSCT presents a complicated vaccination paradigm. The underlying disease itself may be immunosuppressive, the therapy used to prepare for transplantation ablates existing immunity, immunosuppressive therapy is given after the procedure (sometimes for life), and graft-versus-host disease may further compromise immune function. Moreover, the adopted immune system of the donor provides unreliable immunity of uncertain duration; fortunately, immune memory can be recalled by immunization after engraftment (it is not clear whether lasting benefits accrue from immunization of the donor prior to transplant). Although graft-versus-host disease is not an issue with autologous transplantation and the conditioning regimens may be less severe, studies show that vaccine-induced immunity may be lost after transplantation. **Table 7.3** provides a useful guide to revaccination of HSCT patients.

There are studies demonstrating loss of immunity to some vaccine antigens after successful treatment for acute leukemia. However, official guidelines for revaccination are hard to come by. Some centers favor testing for antibodies once chemotherapy is completed, with selective revaccination using those antigens for which the patient's antibody levels have fallen below protective levels. The problem is that seroprotection correlates are not known for all diseases. Another approach is to routinely revaccinate with some or all antigens.

Pregnancy and Breast-feeding

Whereas vaccination during pregnancy poses *theoretic* risks to the developing fetus, there is no evidence directly linking any routine vaccines, even live ones, to birth defects. Nevertheless, pregnant women should be vaccinated only when the risk for exposure to disease is high and the infection would pose a significant risk to the mother or fetus. Delaying vaccination until the second or third trimester, when possible, is reasonable in order to minimize concerns about teratogenicity, despite the evidence against this. An exception is TIV, which should be given regardless of trimester to women who are or will be pregnant during influenza season.

TABLE 7.3 — Revaccination of Hematopoietic Stem-Cell Transplant Recipients

Disease/Infectious Agent	Time After Transplant/Vaccine (Months)		
	12	14	24
Diphtheria, tetanus, pertussis:			
Age <7 years	DTaP	DTaP	DTaP
Age 7-9 years	Td	Td	Td[a]
Age ≥10 years	Tdap[b]	Td	Td
Hepatitis A	HepA (2 doses separated by 6 to 12 months) if 1 year of age or otherwise indicated[c] ---------		
Hepatitis B	HepB[d]	HepB[d]	HepB[d]
Haemophilus influenzae type b	Hib[e]	Hib[e]	Hib[e]
Human papillomavirus	HPV4 vaccine (3 doses at 0, 2, and 6 months for females 9 to 26 years of age) ---------		
Influenza	TIV yearly beginning before transplant and resuming ≥6 months after transplant[f] ---------		
Measles, mumps, rubella			MMR (2 doses separated by 6 to 12 months) if immunocompetent[g,h]
Neisseria meningitidis	MCV4 (one dose) if 11 to 18 years of age or otherwise indicated[i] ---------		
Rotavirus	Rotavirus vaccine cannot be initiated beyond infancy ---------		
Streptococcus pneumoniae	PCV7 (2 doses separated by 2 months) followed by PPSV23 (≥2 months after last dose of PCV7)[j] ---------		
Polio	IPV	IPV	IPV
Varicella	Varicella vaccine is contraindicated[h,k] ---------		
Zoster	Zoster vaccine is contraindicated ---------|Consider[l] ---------		

[a] Tdap should be substituted 1 time for Td if the patient is ≥10 years of age (in general, an interval of at least 2 years is recommended between Td and Tdap, but intervals of <2 years may be used if the risk of pertussis is high or if there is an infant under 1 year of age in the household).

b Boostrix is licensed for use in individuals 10 to 18 years of age; Adacel is licensed for individuals 11 to 64 years of age.

c HepA is recommended for all children in the second year of life, and catch-up immunization for older children has been routine in certain parts of the country. Transplant patients falling in these groups should be vaccinated. For example, a 2-year-old living anywhere in the United States who received a transplant at 6 months of age should be vaccinated. A 10-year-old living in California who was vaccinated at 5 years of age and received a transplant at 9 years of age should be revaccinated. HepA should also be considered for persons who have chronic liver disease or GVHD, persons living in endemic areas who otherwise would qualify for routine vaccination, and persons living in areas experiencing outbreaks. IGIM in addition to vaccine is preferred for travel.

d HepB is recommended for all individuals ≤18 years of age and for high-risk adults. Test for HBsAb 1 to 3 months after the third dose; if negative, repeat the 3-dose series one time.

e Hib should be given regardless of age.

f LAIV (FluMist; MedImmune) is contraindicated. Children 6 months to 9 years of age who are receiving influenza vaccine for the first time post-transplant, or who were vaccinated for the first time post-transplant in the previous season and only received 1 dose, need 2 doses separated by 4 weeks. Chemoprophylaxis should be considered for all patients regardless of vaccination status.

g A 4-week interval may be used in outbreak situations. MMRV (ProQuad; Merck) should not be used. Patients who are still considered immunocompromised or who have chronic GVHD should not receive MMF.

h Passive immunoprophylaxis should be given to all measles- and varicella-exposed patients regardless of personal history of disease or vaccination.

i HSCT recipients without GVHD are not at increased risk for invasive meningococcal disease per se. However, 1 dose of MCV4 (Menactra) is routinely recommended for all individuals 11 to 18 years of age. HSCT recipients with chronic GVHD should also be vaccinated or revaccinated with MCV4, and routine penicillin prophylaxis should be given (as if the patient were asplenic).

j One-time revaccination with PPSV23 (Pneumovax 23; Merck) in 3 to 5 years should be considered. Routine penicillin prophylaxis is recommended for patients with chronic GVHD (as if the patient were asplenic).

k Studies are looking at the safety and immunogenicity of varicella vaccine in HSCT patients >2 years out from transplantation who are presumed to be immunocompetent.

l Providers may consider immunizing HSCT recipients who are immunocompetent and who are ≥24 months post-transplant.

Adapted from: Centers for Disease Control and Prevention. *MMWR*. 2000;49(RR-10):1-128. Modifications are based on new recommendations and new vaccines licensed since 2000. Practice varies from one transplantation center to another.

7

205

In considering vaccines and pregnancy, clinicians should be aware of the following:

- Approximately 2% of all newborns have a major congenital malformation; it follows that some women who are vaccinated during pregnancy will have infants with birth defects. While a causal relationship with the vaccine may be lacking, there may be a tendency to attribute the birth defect to the vaccine. Pregnant women should be counseled about this before being vaccinated. Along the same lines, it stands that some children of women who receive thimerosal-containing vaccines (eg, some brands of TIV) during pregnancy will develop autism. Despite the overwhelming evidence against a causal association between thimerosal (which contains mercury) and autism (see Chapter 8, *Addressing Concerns About Vaccines*)—and despite the fact that there is no official preference for thimerosal-free TIV during pregnancy—it might be prudent to use thimerosal-free vaccine in pregnant women if it is available (some states actually require this).
- Very few vaccines have been tested for safety and efficacy in large numbers of pregnant women. For this reason, almost all vaccines are classified as Pregnancy Category C (defined as: animal studies show adverse effects and there are no adequate studies in pregnant women, *or* no animal studies have been done and there are no adequate studies in pregnant women) by the FDA. With this designation, the benefits in pregnant women may be acceptable despite the potential risks.
- Live vaccines are generally contraindicated during pregnancy, with the exceptions noted in **Table 7.4**. However, inadvertent receipt of live vaccines is not a reason to terminate the pregnancy because there is no definitive evidence of maternal-fetal transmission or fetal harm. In the case of varicella vaccine, if a pregnant woman is known to be susceptible to varicella and a close contact develops a rash after vaccination, exposure should be avoided until the vaccinee's lesions are crusted over. Some manufacturers maintain registries of women inadvertantly vaccinated during pregnancy in order to gather data on outcomes; the phone numbers for reporting are usually given in the package insert.
- The only live vaccine that is contraindicated in household contacts of pregnant women is the smallpox vaccine.
- Theoretical concerns include the possibilities that the immune response in pregnant women will be suboptimal; that transplacental antibodies might interfere with the infant's ability to respond to vaccines; and that in-utero antigen exposure could lead to immune tolerance in the baby.
- The rationale for some official recommendations is difficult to understand; for example:
  - HepB is recommended during pregnancy if indicated, despite its Pregnancy Category C designation. On the other

hand, HPV4, which is analogous to HepB in that it consists of a single recombinant-derived protein, is not recommended during pregnancy, despite its Pregnancy Category B designation (defined as: animal studies show no adverse effects but there are no adequate studies in pregnant women, *or* animal studies show adverse effects but adequate studies in pregnant women fail to demonstrate harm to the fetus) and despite the fact that inactivated vaccines have never been known to harm the fetus. Arguably, the risk of the average woman acquiring HPV during pregnancy is higher than the risk of her acquiring hepatitis B.

- MPSV4 and PPSV23 are very similar vaccines in that both consist of purified polysaccharide. Yet MPSV4 falls under the use-if-indicated column and PPSV23 falls under the special-language column, wherein no specific recommendation is actually made.

- HepA and IPV are very similar vaccines in that they consist of inactivated whole virions and both carry a Pregnancy Category C designation. Yet the language regarding use in pregnancy differs—for HepA, the recommendations state that "the theoretical risk to the developing fetus is expected to be low", whereas for IPV, they state that "vaccination of pregnant women should be avoided on theoretical grounds....". Why is the language different and how should this be interpreted in practice? In these situations, providers simply have to consider the risks and benefits and act accordingly.

- A tetanus toxoid booster is indicated for pregnant women who are unlikely to be immune to tetanus. See **Table 7.4** for a discussion of the criteria for immunity and when Tdap may be substituted for Td.

- There are no known risks of passive immunization during pregnancy. In fact, VariZIG is *recommended* for susceptible pregnant women who are exposed to varicella because the risk of complicated disease in the mother is high (it is not know whether passive immunization protects the fetus).

- Breast-feeding per se is not a contraindication to the use of any vaccines, including live ones, except for pre-event use of smallpox vaccine.

In April 2008, an ACIP working group offered guidance on the drafting of recommendations for vaccination during pregnancy and breastfeeding. Hopefully, this will lead to more uniformity in future statements.

Preterm and Low Birth Weight Infants

Preterm (<37 weeks' gestation) and low birth weight (<2500 g) infants are at particular risk for vaccine-preventable diseases

TABLE 7.4 — Vaccine Use During Pregnancy

Administer Because of Pregnancy	Administer if Indicated for Other Reasons[a]	Not Recommended or Contraindicated[b]	Special Language Contained in the Recommendation[c]	
TIV[d]	HepB	HPV4	Anthrax	Vaccinate only if the potential benefits outweigh the potential risks
Td or Tdap[e]	MPSV4	LAIV		
	Rabies vaccine	MMR	HepA	Theoretic risk is low
		Varicella vaccine		Consider for women at high risk of exposure
		Zoster vaccine	JE vaccine	Administer if travel to an endemic area is unavoidable and if there is increased risk for exposure
			IPV	Avoid on theoretic grounds
				Consider if risk of polio is increased and immediate protection is required
			MCV4	No data available in pregnant women
			PPSV23	Safety during first trimester not evaluated
			Smallpox vaccine	Administer only to pregnant women who have been exposed to smallpox
			Typhoid (TViPSV and Ty21a)	No data available in pregnant women
			YF vaccine	Administer if travel to an endemic area is unavoidable and if there is increased risk for exposure

[a] The recommendations for these vaccines are clear: give if indicated. Examples would include HepB for an unvaccinated pregnant injecting drug user; MPSV4 for an unvaccinated pregnant woman who has been diagnosed with a terminal complement component deficiency (MCV4 may be preferred

in this situation, depending on age, but the recommendations for use of MCV4 in pregnancy are less clear); and rabies vaccine for a pregnant woman who is bitten by a bat.

[b] Some of these vaccines, such as MMR, are contraindicated because they are live and there is the theoretic risk of harm to the fetus. Others, such as HPV, are inactivated and are unlikely to cause harm, but nevertheless are not recommended during pregnancy (see text). Inadvertent administration of MMR or varicella vaccine during pregnancy is not a reason to terminate the pregnancy. Pregnancy should be avoided for 1 month following MMR or varicella vaccine administration. Zoster vaccine is only indicated at ≥60 years of age and would therefore be unlikely to be used during pregnancy.

[c] The recommendations for these vaccines are less than clear-cut. Providers have to use their best judgment in balancing the risks and benefits.

[d] Pregnancy increases the risk of complicated influenza. Therefore, TIV should be given regardless of trimester to women who are or will be pregnant during influenza season.

[e] Babies born to mothers who are not immune to tetanus are at risk for neonatal tetanus. Previously vaccinated pregnant women who have not received a tetanus toxoid–containing vaccine in the past 10 years should receive a Td booster; Tdap may be substituted if the risk for pertussis is high. Previously unvaccinated women should receive 2 doses of Td separated by 4 weeks, followed by Tdap postpartum, at least 6 months after the second dose; alternatively, Tdap may be substituted for one of the earlier doses of Td. If there is sufficient evidence of tetanus immunity (any one of the following: antibody level ≥0.1 IU/mL; received primary series as an adolescent or adult), Td *can* be deferred during pregnancy in favor of giving Tdap postpartum (Tdap boosts immunity to pertussis, helping to protect the newborn by preventing pertussis in the mother). Tdap can be given during pregnancy (second or third trimester is preferred) if the risk of pertussis is elevated; this might be true, for example, for adolescents, health care workers, and child care providers. Whether given during pregnancy or postpartum, the recommended interval since the last Td is 2 years, but shorter intervals can be used if there is no history of moderate or severe reaction to tetanus toxoid. The following should be mentioned with regard to administration of Tdap during pregnancy:

- The AAP recommends Tdap for pregnant adolescents.
- There are no data on safety, immunogenicity, pregnancy outcomes, and protection of the infant against pertussis.
- Boosted pertussis antibodies in the mother may interfere with the "take" of pertussis vaccine in the infant.
- The second or third trimester is preferred.
- Td or Tdap can be used for wound management during pregnancy if it's been ≥5 years since the last tetanus shot.

Modified from: Guidelines for vaccinating pregnant women. Centers for Disease Control and Prevention. Centers for Disease Control and Prevention Web site. http://www.cdc.gov/vaccines/pubs /downloads/b_preg_guide.pdf. Accessed August 15, 2008; Centers for Disease Control and Prevention. *MMWR.* 2008;57(RR-4):1-51.

7

because of relatively immature immune systems. Comorbidities contribute to this risk and cause delays in immunization. These infants should be vaccinated according to the routine schedule, using the routine doses, at the appropriate chronologic age. The only vaccine for which weight is relevant is HepB. Infants weighing <2000 g at birth whose mothers are HBsAg-negative should receive the first dose of vaccine at 1 month of age (rather than at birth) or at hospital discharge. Infants weighing <2000 g at birth whose mothers are HBsAg-positive or HBsAg-unknown should receive the first dose of vaccine within 12 hours of birth and should also receive HBIG 0.5 mL intramuscularly at a separate site from the vaccine. In these cases, the birth dose of vaccine does not count toward completion of the HepB series; 3 additional doses should be given as follows:

- *Mother HBsAg-positive*: doses at 1, 2, and 6 months of age. Test for HBsAg and HBsAb at 9 to 18 months of age. If HBsAg is negative and HBsAb is <10 mIU/mL, repeat 3-dose vaccine series.
- *Mother HBsAg-unknown*: doses at 1, 2, and 6 months of age and test the mother; if she is HBsAg-positive, proceed as above.
- *Mother HBsAg-negative*: doses at 1, 2, and 6 to 18 months of age.

Rotavirus vaccine should be given to preterm infants who are being discharged from the nursery or who are already home, keeping in mind that the first dose should be given between 6 weeks and 14 weeks 6 days of age. The decision to give rotavirus vaccine to preterm infants (or other infants who have been hospitalized since birth) who will be staying in the hospital is complicated by the fact that vaccine virus can be shed in the stool and presents the theoretic risk of nosocomial transmission. However, shedding occurs in <10% of infants after the first dose of PRV and in 26% after the first dose of HRV. Horizontal transmission has not been documented for either vaccine; therefore, standard precautions should suffice to obviate concerns.

Preterm infants can experience cardiorespiratory events, such as apnea, bradycardia, and oxygen desaturation, following vaccination and should be closely observed for at least 48 hours.

International Adoptees, Refugees, and Immigrants

The Immigration and Nationality Act requires all immigrants entering the United States to show proof of having received all ACIP-recommended vaccines before a visa is granted. International adoptees <11 years of age are exempted from this requirement, but the adoptive parents must sign an affidavit indicating their intention to comply with immunization requirements after the child arrives. Refugees are also exempted from immunization requirements at the time of entry, but must show proof of immunization at the time they apply for permanent residency.

The following issues are germane to the immunization management of individuals from other countries, particularly international adoptees:

- Vaccination records are considered valid only if they are in written form and contain the vaccines, dates of administration, proper intervals between doses, and age at the time of immunization.
- Written records must be translated and interpreted correctly, and even then may be inaccurate or fraudulent.
- The immunization schedule in many countries differs from that in the United States. Some children will need additional vaccines to comply with the US schedule.
- Vaccines in some countries may have inadequate potency, especially because of handling issues.
- Serologic correlates of protection exist for some diseases but not for others. Testing may be expensive and the results require interpretation.
- There is no harm in revaccinating individuals who have already been vaccinated, although reactogenicity to DTaP and pneumococcal polysaccharide vaccines may increase if too many doses are given within a short time frame.

It is desirable for all individuals entering the United States permanently to receive all routinely recommended vaccines. For reasons mentioned, the simplest approach is to start over and revaccinate. An alternative, although somewhat less practical, approach is to test for antibodies to the major vaccine antigens and administer those vaccines to which the child has no immunity. Young infants can be vaccinated according to the routine childhood schedule (**Table 6.1**); older children can be vaccinated according to catch-up schedules (**Tables 6.3** and **6.4**), with attention paid to the minimum allowable intervals between doses (**Table 5.1**). For adults who immigrate to the United States, consideration should be given to vaccination with MMR, Tdap, HepB, and varicella vaccine. Individuals from hepatitis B–endemic areas should be screened for HBsAg; if positive, vaccination is not necessary.

Health Care Personnel (HCP)

HCP, as well as individuals who work in residential institutions, may be exposed to vaccine-preventable diseases and may transmit them to patients or residents, as well as their own families. Individuals who fit into this category include staff, physicians, nurses, students, and ancillary personnel; in essence, anyone who might have contact with patients. The risk of infection might be particularly high for people working in emergency departments or ambulatory care settings, especially if the facility serves underimmunized populations. The consequences of transmission to patients might be particularly high where ever there are vulnerable patients, such as intensive care units, newborn nurseries, obstetric wards, chronic care facilities, and oncology or transplant units. HCP should be up-to-date on all routinely recommended vaccines.

Hospitals and other facilities may develop policies that require documentation of immunization or immunity, and these should be part of a comprehensive occupational health program. Immunizations should be provided at no cost to the worker. Studies have shown that this preventative strategy is more cost-effective than treating patients and their contacts for vaccine-preventable diseases. The extent to which these recommendations are carried out varies considerably from institution to institution. Importantly, vaccination cannot be forced upon HCP who are reluctant to be vaccinated, although some institutions have developed strategies wherein individuals must sign a release form in order to opt out. In these situations, it should be emphasized that exposure to a vaccine-preventable disease could result in leave without pay during the period of potential communicability, and worker's compensation benefits would not apply unless the disease actually developed.

Diseases that deserve particular attention include the following:

- *Measles, mumps, and rubella*—Individuals born in or after 1957 are considered immune only if they meet the following criteria:
  - Measles and mumps: physician-diagnosed disease, or serologic evidence of immunity, or 2 doses of MMR (or equivalent monovalent vaccines) separated by at least 1 month and initiated on or after the first birthday
  - Rubella: serologic evidence of immunity (because so many rash illnesses can mimic rubella, a personal history of rubella is unreliable and should not be used to judge immune status), or at least one dose of a rubella-containing vaccine on or after the first birthday.

  Any health care worker who is not immune should receive 2 doses of MMR separated by at least 1 month. Even though individuals born before 1957 are considered immune to these diseases, regardless of whether they recall having had them, health care facilities should consider recommending one dose of MMR to unimmunized HCP born before 1957 who lack the above criteria for immunity.

- *Hepatitis B*—HepB is recommended for all HCP who are likely to be exposed to blood or blood-containing body fluids. In fact, the Bloodborne Pathogens Standard (see Chapter 3, *Standards, Principles, and Regulations*) mandates that vaccination be made available at no cost to all employees with potential blood contact. Personnel should be tested for HBsAb 1 to 2 months after the third dose, and those who test negative

(<10 mIU/mL) should receive another 3-dose series (one time only). If they remain seronegative after this, they should be tested for HBsAg, since chronic carriage could explain failure to respond to the vaccine. Persons who do not respond to a total of 6 properly administered doses should also be counseled about precautions to prevent hepatitis B infection and the need for HBIG if there is an exposure. Individuals who received the HepB series in the past need not be tested for HBsAb when they enter a health–care related job, but they should be tested at the time of an exposure and if they are seronegative, managed accordingly.

- *Varicella*—All HCP should be immune to varicella (the criteria for evidence of immunity are given in **Table 9.19**). Note that HCP born before 1980 are not assumed to be immune, as are other people, and that serologic screening in those with a questionable personal history of chickenpox is probably cost-effective. Those who are not immune should receive 2 doses of varicella vaccine separated by 4 to 8 weeks (postvaccination serology is not recommended because the vast majority of vaccinees seroconvert). Vaccinated individuals can return to work immediately, but if a rash develops (for example, vesicles at the inoculation site), the worker should not have contact with immunocompromised patients—he or she can continue to work with patients who are immunocompetent as long as the lesions are kept covered. Those who develop a generalized rash after vaccination should be furloughed until the rash resolves. Vaccinated personnel who are exposed to chickenpox or shingles should be observed carefully during days 10 through 21 postexposure; symptoms suggestive of varicella should prompt a medical leave, and if varicella develops, the worker should remain on leave until all the lesions are crusted or faded and there are no new lesions within a 24-hour period. Personnel who have had only one dose of varicella vaccine and are exposed to the virus should receive a second dose within 5 days of exposure (as long as it has been at least 4 weeks since the first dose) and should be observed carefully as above.

- *Influenza*—All HCP should be immunized to influenza in the fall of each year. Either TIV or LAIV (if age appropriate) can be used, except for HCP who are in close contact with severely immunosuppressed patients (the equivalent of HSCT patients who are in protective environments); if a health care worker receives LAIV, he or she should avoid contact with such patients for 7 days postvaccination. Nationally, less than half of HCP receive influenza vaccine every year. Responding to this dismal statistic, in 2007 the Joint Commission on Accreditation of Health Care Organizations approved a standard that requires accredited organizations to offer influenza vaccination to staff and even volunteers with close patient contact. Influenza vaccine coverage rates among HCP should be followed as an integral part of all health care–facility patient safety programs.

- *Tetanus, diphtheria, pertussis*—All HCP should have completed a primary series of tetanus and diphtheria vaccines and should receive a Td booster every 10 years. For those <65 years of age, one dose of Tdap should be given as soon as possible (a minimum interval of 2 years between the last Td and Tdap is safe, and shorter intervals may be used). The dose of Tdap "resets the clock" for subsequent 10-year Td boosters.

Travel

Travelers going to Canada, Western Europe, Australia, and New Zealand are probably at no higher risk for illness than those traveling within the United States. For other destinations, however, consideration may need to be given to specialized vaccines or to accelerated schedules for routine vaccines, depending to some extent on what circumstances the traveler will encounter. Travel to certain areas may require other measures, including malaria chemoprophylaxis, insect avoidance, food hygiene, and the availability of emergency medical services. Moreover, certain individuals may be at higher risk than others for particular diseases.

Travel medicine clinics, which may be available at local health departments, academic medical centers, or in private practice settings, maintain up-to-date information and provide vaccination services for travelers. Primary care physicians who choose to provide travel vaccines to their patients should be aware of the following:

- *Planning*—Consultation should take place *at least* 4 to 6 weeks before departure in order to allow for the development of protective immunity after vaccination. More time may be required if certain vaccines will need to be ordered.
- *Itinerary*—It is not enough to know where the person will be traveling. The duration of stay and the particular activities in which the person will be engaged can help determine risk. For example, a 2-day stay in a sophisticated urban hotel carries different risks than extended field work in rural areas.
- *Routine vaccines*—All travelers should be up-to-date on routinely recommended vaccines. Some special considerations are listed below:
  - *Childhood vaccination schedule*: The routine childhood schedules (**Tables 6.1** and **6.2**) provide some flexibility in the timing of doses. For example, the third dose of HepB and IPV can be given as early as 6 months of age and the fourth dose of Hib and PCV7 as early as 12 months of age. The fourth dose of DTaP can be given as early as 12 months

214

of age provided that at least 6 months have elapsed since the third dose. Varicella vaccine and HepA can be given as early as 12 months of age. The first dose of MMR should be given to all infants 6 to 12 months of age who will be traveling outside the United States (reimmunization with 2 doses after the first birthday is necessary). For children in the second year of life, the second dose of MMR can be given as early as 4 weeks after the first dose, and a second dose of varicella vaccine as early as 3 months after the first dose. Physicians should be aware of flexibility in the schedule and administer all eligible vaccines before the anticipated date of travel.

– *HepA*: For most travelers to endemic areas, vaccination is now preferred over administration of immune globulin and should be initiated as soon as travel is considered. One dose of HepA at any time before departure is likely to provide protection for most healthy people (only monovalent HepA should be used for this purpose). For older adults, immunocompromised individuals, and persons with chronic liver disease or other chronic medical conditions, immune globulin (0.02 mL/kg) should be given (at a separate site) in addition to vaccine *if* there are <2 weeks before departure. Immune globulin alone should be given to infants <12 months of age and to individuals who cannot be or do not want to be vaccinated.

– *HepB*: For those travelers who might have missed universal immunization, HepB should be given if the person might be exposed to blood, have sexual contact with the local population, stay >6 months, or be exposed through medical treatment.

– *Influenza*: Influenza vaccine may be given to anyone ≥6 months of age who will be traveling to areas with influenza activity. This should be a priority for individuals at risk for complicated influenza, including children 6 to 23 months of age, adults ≥50 years of age, and those with medical risk factors (see *Chapter 9*).

– *Polio*: Previously immunized adults traveling to endemic areas should receive one dose of IPV (this does not need to be given again for subsequent travel). If travel of an infant to an endemic area is imminent, 3 doses of IPV can be given at 4-week intervals.

– *PPSV23*: All adults ≥65 years of age should be immunized.

– *Td*: Although boosters are recommended only every 10 years in adults, consideration should be given to a dose if >5 years have elapsed and the person will be working in situations where dirty wounds might be incurred or traveling to regions where diphtheria outbreaks have occurred. If the person has not yet received a dose of Tdap, this can be substituted for Td.

- *Mandatory vaccines*—The only vaccine covered by international health regulations at the present time is yellow fever vaccine, for which travelers to certain countries must have a valid International Certificate of Vaccination or Prophylaxis (see Chapter 10, *Specialized Vaccines*). However, some countries have their own regulations. For example, Saudi Arabia requires meningococcal vaccine for pilgrims visiting Mecca for the Hajj, and some countries may require the vaccine for individuals returning from the Hajj.
- *Recommended vaccines*—**Table 7.5** gives some general guidelines regarding vaccines for travel to certain parts of the world. Specific information about the vaccines is contained in the referenced sections of this book. Since disease outbreaks are always occurring and guidelines frequently change, the best advice is to check updated resources before traveling. The following web sites are useful for this purpose (Accessed August 15, 2008):
  - *Centers for Disease Control and Prevention: Travelers' Health*: http://wwwn.cdc.gov/travel/default.aspx
  - *World Health Organization: International Travel and Health*: http://www.who.int/ith/en
  - *International Society of Travel Medicine*: http://www.istm.org
  - *MDtravelhealth.com*: http://www.mdtravelhealth.com
  - *Travel Medicine, Inc.*: http://www.travmed.com

Other Special Circumstances

Table 7.6 covers other situations and groups that deserve special attention for certain vaccines.

ADDITIONAL READING

Impaired Immunity

Pirofski LA, Casadevall A. Use of licensed vaccines for active immunization of the immunocompromised host. *Clin Microbiol Rev*. 1998;11:1-26.

Recommendations of the Advisory Committee on Immunization Practices (ACIP): use of vaccines and immune globulins for persons with altered immunocompetence. *MMWR Recomm Rep*. 1993;42(RR-4):1-18.

HIV Infection

Measles immunization in HIV-infected children. American Academy of Pediatrics. Committee on Infectious Diseases and Committee on Pediatric AIDS. *Pediatrics*. 1999;103:1057-1060.

HSCT and Leukemia

Centers for Disease Control and Prevention; Infectious Diseases Society of America; American Society of Blood and Marrow Transplantation. Guidelines for preventing opportunistic infections among hematopoietic stem cell transplant recipients. *Biol Blood Marrow Transplant.* 2000;6:659-713.

Patel SR, Ortin M, Cohen BJ, et al. Revaccination of children after completion of standard chemotherapy for acute leukemia. *Clin Infect Dis.* 2007;44:635-642.

Singhal S, Mehta J. Reimmunization after blood or marrow stem cell transplantation. *Bone Marrow Transplant.* 1999;23:637-646.

Pregnancy

Advisory Committee on Immunization Practices Workgroup on the Use of Vaccines During Pregnancy and Breastfeeding. Guiding principles for development of ACIP recommendations for vaccination during pregnancy and breastfeeding. Centers for Disease Control and Prevention Web site. http://www.cdc.gov/vaccines/recs/acip/downloads/preg-principles05-01-08.pdf. Accessed August 15, 2008.

Preterm Infants

Saari TN; American Academy of Pediatrics Committee on Infectious Diseases. Immunization of preterm and low birth weight infants. American Academy of Pediatrics Committee on Infectious Diseases. *Pediatrics.* 2003;112:193-198.

Foreign Born

Cohen AL, Veenstra D. Economic analysis of prevaccination serotesting compared with presumptive immunization for polio, diphtheria, and tetanus in internationally adopted and immigrant infants. *Pediatrics.* 2006;117:1650-1655.

Greenaway C, Dongier P, Boivin JF, Tapiero D, Miller M, Schwartzman K. Susceptibility to measles, mumps, and rubella in newly arrived adult immigrants and refugees. *Ann Intern Med.* 2007;146:20-24.

Health Care Personnel

Immunization of health-care workers: recommendations of the Advisory Committee on Immunization Practices (ACIP) and the Hospital Infection Control Practices Advisory Committee (HICPAC). *MMWR Recomm Rep.* 1997;46(RR-18):1-42.

Pearson ML, Bridges CB, Harper SA; Healthcare Infection Control Practices Advisory Committee (HICPAC); Advisory Committee on Immunization Practices (ACIP). Influenza vaccination of health-care personnel: recommendations of the Healthcare Infection Control Practices Advisory Committee (HICPAC) and the Advisory Committee on Immunization Practices (ACIP). *MMWR Recomm Rep.* 2006;55(RR-2):1-16.

Travel

Arguin PM, Kozarsky PE, Reed C. *CDC Health Information for International Travel 2008.* Atlanta, GA: US Department of Health and Human Services, Public Health Service, Centers for Disease Control and Prevention, National Center for Preparedness, Detection and Control of Infectious Diseases, Division of Global Migration and Quarantine; 2007.

TABLE 7.5 — Particular Vaccine-Preventable Diseases by Region[a]

Region	Hepatitis A[b]	Japanese Encephalitis[c]	Meningococcus[d]	Polio[e]	Typhoid[f]	Yellow Fever[g]
Caribbean	✓				✓	✓
Central Africa	✓		✓	✓	✓	✓
East Africa	✓[h]		✓	✓	✓	✓
East Asia	✓	✓			✓	
Eastern Europe and Northern Asia	✓				✓	
Indian Ocean Islands	✓				✓	
Mexico and Central America	✓				✓	✓[i]
Middle East	✓		✓[j]	✓	✓	
North Africa	✓			✓	✓	
North America						
South Asia	✓	✓		✓	✓	
Southeast Asia	✓	✓		✓	✓	
Southern Africa	✓[k]			✓	✓	
Southern and Western Pacific	✓	✓[l]		✓[m]	✓	

South America			
Temperate	✓	✓	✓[n]
Tropical	✓	✓	✓
West Africa	✓	✓	✓
Western Europe	✓[o]	✓	✓

[a] Vaccination might not be indicated for every country in the region. Specific recommendations can be found at http://wwwn.cdc.gov/travel/regionList.aspx. Accessed August 15, 2008. Two diseases are not listed but deserve special comment:

Hepatitis B: HepB is recommended for all unvaccinated individuals traveling to or working in countries with intermediate to high levels of endemic transmission, which includes much of the world. Since exposure to blood or body fluids (through, for example, sexual contact or emergency medical treatment) may not be predictable, immunization should be strongly considered for all travelers.

Rabies: Rabies vaccine should be considered in most parts of the world if exposure to animals is expected. At particular risk are travelers spending a lot of time outdoors, or who are involved in activities such as bicycling, camping, hiking, or outdoor work. Children are considered at higher risk because they tend to play with animals and may not report bites. Spelunkers are also at risk because of potential exposure to bats.

[b] Risk increases with duration of travel and is highest for those who live in or visit rural settings, trek in back-country areas, or frequently eat or drink in areas with poor sanitation.

[c] The risk to short-term travelers and those staying in urban centers is very low. Risk increases with prolonged visits to rural settings, and with extensive outdoor, evening, and nighttime exposures such as bicycling, camping, working outdoors, or sleeping in unscreened structures without bed nets.

[d] Risk is increased for travelers to sub-Saharan Africa (the "meningitis belt") during the dry season, especially if there is prolonged contact with local populations. Saudi Arabia requires that Hajj and Umrah visitors have a certificate of meningococcal vaccination before entering.

[e] Adult travelers to endemic or epidemic areas who have had a primary immunization series in the past should receive a dose of IPV before departure. Saudi Arabia requires polio vaccination for those attending the Hajj.

[f] Risk is higher for those visiting relatives or friends and those who will not have access to cooked foods and safe beverages.

Continued

7

TABLE 7.5 — *Continued*

g Vaccination must occur at a certified center and vaccinees must receive an *International Certificate of Vaccination or Prophylaxis* that carries a Uniform Stamp. Some countries require a certificate from travelers arriving from infected areas, even if they are just in transit. Other countries require vaccination of all entering travelers, and still others may waive the requirements for travelers coming from noninfected areas and staying <2 weeks. Vaccination is also recommended for travel to countries that lie in the yellow fever–endemic zone but do not officially report the disease.

h Except Japan.

i Panama only.

j Saudi Arabia only.

k Except Australia and New Zealand.

l Torres Strait, far northern Australia, Papua New Guinea, Philippines.

m Philippines only.

n Northern and northeastern forested areas of Argentina only.

o Greenland only.

TABLE 7.6 — Vaccination in Other Special Circumstances[a]

Condition or Circumstance	Particular Risks and Considerations
Animal workers and veterinarians	Anthrax and rabies vaccines may be indicated
Bleeding diathesis	Use IM vaccines with caution
	Patients who receive clotting factors should be immunized against hepatitis A and hepatitis B
Children and adolescents on long-term aspirin therapy	At risk for Reye syndrome if they get influenza or varicella
	Do not give varicella or LAIV while on aspirin because of theoretic risk of Reye syndrome
College students living in dormitories	Should be immunized against meningococcus and influenza
Foreign field personnel	Should be immunized against travel-related diseases
Food handlers	HepA not routinely recommended, but could be considered on a local basis
Foresters	Rabies vaccine may be indicated
Injecting illegal drug users	Should be immunized against hepatitis A and hepatitis B
Laboratory workers	Should be immunized against laboratory pathogens for which vaccines are available (eg, *Neisseria meningitidis*)
Men who have sex with men	Should be immunized against hepatitis A and hepatitis B
Military personnel	Special immunizations may include meningococcus, influenza, anthrax, smallpox, and travel vaccines
Morticians	Should be immunized against hepatitis B
Native Americans and Alaskans	Special attention to timely immunization against pneumococcus and *Haemophilus influenzae* type b

Continued

7

TABLE 7.6 — *Continued*

Condition or Circumstance	Particular Risks and Considerations
Patients with cochlear implants or CSF leaks	Should be immunized against pneumococcus
Providers of essential community services	Should be immunized against influenza
Public safety workers	Should be immunized against hepatitis B
Residents of long-term–care facilities	Should be immunized against influenza
Sewage workers	Not at increased risk for typhoid or hepatitis A in the United States
Spelunkers	Rabies vaccine may be indicated
Staff of correctional facilities	Should be immunized against influenza and hepatitis B
Staff of day care centers	Should be immunized against influenza
Staff of institutions for developmentally disabled	Should be immunized against influenza and hepatitis B

^a This table assumes that all routinely recommended vaccine series and boosters have been given.

8

Addressing Concerns About Vaccines

Vaccines have saved more lives than virtually any other public health intervention, and they are safer now than ever before. Despite this, providers face the daily challenge of convincing parents and patients that vaccines are safe, effective, and necessary. It is true that good things have come from public concern about vaccines—the drive, for example, to replace DTwP with the less reactogenic DTaP. However, many of the sensational claims made about the dangers of vaccination by antivaccination activists, celebrities, and rogue scientists have not held up to scientific scrutiny. Despite this, these ideas have been popularized in the lay press and have made their way to the Internet. As a result, well-meaning parents, influenced by the negative things they hear and read, are refusing to have their children vaccinated. This has translated directly into personal and public harm, and many fear an impending public health crisis. This chapter provides some background on popular theories about vaccines, as well as tips on communicating the true risks and benefits with parents and patients.

Communicating Risks and Benefits

What do we mean when we say that vaccines are *safe*? One definition of the word safe is *harmless*. This definition would imply that any negative consequence of vaccines would make them unsafe. But we know that all vaccines have side effects. For example, parenterally administered vaccines can cause pain, redness, swelling, and tenderness at the site of injection. Some vaccines cause more severe side effects. For example, pertussis vaccine can very rarely cause persistent, inconsolable crying, high fever, hypotonic-hyporesponsive syndrome, and seizures with or without fever. While none of these severe symptoms result in permanent damage, they can be frightening. There are historical examples of serious side effects as well; for example, the oral polio vaccine caused paralytic polio, but only one case for every 2.3 million doses distributed. The recommendation to change to IPV in the year 2000 was based on recognition of this extremely rare side effect, which had by then become more of a risk than natural polio itself in the United States.

Few things in life meet the definition of harmless. Even everyday activities contain hidden dangers. For example, each year in the United States, 350 people are killed in bath- or shower-related accidents and 200 people are killed when food lodges in their trachea. Just being outdoors can be dangerous—100 people are killed each year by lightning. By the harmless criterion, even routine daily activities could be considered unsafe.

Another definition of the word safe is *having been preserved from a real danger*. Using this definition, the danger (*the disease*) must be significantly greater than the means of protecting against the danger (*the vaccine*). To put it another way, a vaccine's benefits must clearly and definitively outweigh its risks. For all routinely recommended vaccines, the benefits clearly outweigh the risks.

Scientists, public health officials, and providers tend to think (subconsciously, if not consciously) about vaccines in terms of probability and expected utility. The health value of getting a vaccine, and presumably the basis for decision making, can simplistically be seen as the difference between two things, shown in **Figure 8.1**: 1) the probability of avoiding the disease times the utility, or value, of avoiding the disease; and 2) the probability of a vaccine side effect times the disutility of that side effect. For example, the probability of avoiding measles through vaccination is nearly 100%, and the utility of avoiding measles for any given individual is very high (because 1 in 100 patients develop pneumonia and 1 in 1000 die). Thus the first part of the equation has a high value. On the other hand, the probability of getting fever and rash from MMR is low, say 5%, and the disutility of fever and rash is low, since it is self-limited. Thus the value of the second part of the equation is low and does not detract appreciably from

FIGURE 8.1 — Schematic Diagram of Probabilistic Thinking

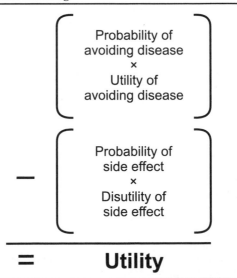

224

the value of the first part. In other words, the overall mental model overwhelmingly favors vaccination.

Lay people, however, think differently. At the societal level, the value of vaccines paradoxically decreases as their effectiveness increases; when disease is eliminated, the public perceives no benefit from vaccines. Another way to look at this is that when vaccines work, *nothing* (as opposed to *disease*) happens. This fact, combined with widespread attention given to rare adverse events, leads to the perception that vaccines do more harm than good. At the individual level, several thought processes might be operative in a parent's reluctance to have his or her child vaccinated. Some of these are heuristics, shortcut ways of thinking or rules of thumb that people use (subconsciously or consciously) to simplify complex decision making. In order to communicate effectively, physicians should understand these thought processes and be prepared to address them, armed with the information that is presented in this chapter. The goal of communication is not to convince doubtful parents to accept vaccination, but rather to listen to their concerns, provide accurate information, and facilitate their informed decision-making.

Here are some examples of heuristic thinking, along with some suggested responses:

- **Availability**—The ease with which a person remembers something correlates with the perceived probability that it will occur.
  - *Example*: A vivid, frightening news story about a child who has a serious anaphylactic reaction to a vaccine might make a parent think that anaphylaxis is more common than it really is.
  - *Response*: Factual information about side effects can be offered. For example, parents should know that the risk of anaphylaxis is estimated to be around 1 in a million.
- **Avoidance of ambiguity**—A known risk is more acceptable than an unknown risk.
  - *Example*: The serious sequelae of chickenpox (a disease with which the parent is familiar) seem more acceptable than the potential risks of the vaccine (with which the parent is not familiar).
  - *Response*: Explain to the parent that they may *think* they know chickenpox, but there is a side to it (eg, hemorrhagic varicella, necrotizing fasciitis, encephalitis, etc) that they have not seen—but you have. Convert the unknown risk of the vaccine to a known one by reviewing the safety data (Chapter 9, *Routine Vaccines*) and describing the rigorous pre- and postlicensure evaluation process that ensures safety (Chapter 2, *Vaccine Infrastructure in the United States*).
- **Do no harm**—A bad outcome is more tolerable if it occurs from inaction rather than action.

- *Example*: Hospitalization with influenza (something that just *happens*) is more tolerable than side effects of the vaccine (something that the parent has *caused* by choice).
- *Response*: Help the parent understand that nothing in medicine (or life for that matter) has zero risk, and that not taking a vaccine is actually an action to accept vulnerability to the disease.
- **Framing**—The context in which a decision is made affects the decision.
  - *Example*: A parent may be reluctant to take on the risks of vaccination because it involves making a decision on behalf of the child.
  - *Response*: Reframe the vaccination discussion around the viewpoint of the child, who would likely choose protection from disease if given the chance. In fact, there are studies showing that school-aged children who have had chickenpox would rather have had the shot.
- **Freeloading**—Herd immunity protects unvaccinated children.
  - *Example*: Since other children get the MMR, my child will not get measles and there is no reason for him or her to take the risk of the vaccine.
  - *Response*: The risk of measles is actually 35-fold higher in exemptors, even in communities where >90% of children are immunized. In truth, freeloaders *are* protected—that is, until enough people in a population are also freeloading. Then everyone is unprotected, and all it takes is a case of measles to arrive on an international flight for there to be an outbreak of disease.
- **Maintaining the status quo**—There is an aversion to taking on one risk to reduce another.
  - *Example*: I'm more comfortable just taking the risk of the disease since that's how things are now and so far my child has been fine.
  - *Response*: The status quo, ie, susceptibility to disease, is not the optimal position to be in because protection from disease is available.
- **Representativeness**—The probability that something will occur correlates with similarity of circumstances.
  - *Example*: A vaccine side effect is likely because it happened to a child just like mine who lives in the same community.
  - *Response*: Again, this is where the cold hard facts on adverse events can be helpful.

People will not undertake a risk-control measure like vaccination unless they believe they can effectively control the risk. In other words, they need to understand that the vaccine really does prevent the disease. In addition, the risk should be personally relevant and serious. While there are thought processes that tend to favor vaccination, such as *bandwagoning* (the tendency for individuals to choose the decision of the majority as what might be wise for themselves) and *altruism* (a willingness to take on personal risks if it is for the benefit of others), nothing substitutes for a straightforward discussion with patients and parents about risks and benefits.

There is a disconnect between what physicians do and what parents want. For example, parents want personal verbal communication from their physicians that conveys a sense of trust and respect. Time-motion studies, however, show that physicians spend <2 minutes discussing vaccines with their patients. Physicians are sometimes reluctant to mention risks for fear of "opening a can of worms," but parents are interested in relevant, practical information that can be easily understood. Here are some tips on getting to the point of what parents want to know:

- Describe which vaccines the child will receive today.
- Give the pertinent Vaccine Information Statements (VISs) to the parent (see Chapter 3, *Standards, Principles, and Regulations*)
- Explain why these vaccines are important.
- Review contraindications to each vaccine.
- Give a detailed account of the common, mild side effects and how to manage them.
- Give a brief account of any severe risks.
- Place today's vaccinations in the context of the overall schedule.

In addition, here are some suggestions regarding risk-communication in the office setting:

- *Begin the discussion early*—One of the advantages of the birth dose of HepB is that it opens the door to discussing vaccines immediately after parenthood has begun. In those initial discussions before hospital discharge, vaccines should be portrayed as part of the routine care the child will receive as he or she grows up. Parents who express doubt or concern should be targeted for further discussion and should receive printed materials and other resources well before the 2-month visit.
- *Use a team approach*—Communication should be a coordinated effort between doctors, nurses, and other office personnel. Even the receptionist can provide an introduction to the vaccination visit, give VISs, and direct the parent or guardian to informational materials in the waiting room. Office nurses (who are often trained in risk-benefit communication) are accessible, highly invested in immunization, and can have a great impact on parents. Each member of the team should be empowered and should know his or her function during the vaccination visit.
- *Organize the visit effectively*—Face-to-face time with the doctor can be increased by building efficiencies into the

227

visit, beginning with a preparatory phone call to remind the parent or guardian to bring the child's shot record and perhaps introducing the vaccines that are scheduled for the visit. Use of a screening questionnaire for contraindications (**Table 4.4**) can be helpful. Development of simple, direct messages and easy-to-understand printed materials can eliminate some questions and help focus the discussion. Ultimately, the use of newer combination vaccines may increase office efficiency and allow more time for communication.

- *Understand individual backgrounds*—Many factors affect risk perception, including educational, emotional, religious, psychological, spiritual, philosophical, and intuitive foundations. Families differ in their orientation toward the medical establishment—some are traditional and trusting, others are cautious, challenging, and oriented toward alternative practices (**Table 8.1**). Vaccine messages should be delivered with these differences in mind.

- *Layer information appropriately*—Information should be presented with sensitivity to individual needs. Providers should be aware of the patient's cognitive foundation and begin with information appropriate to that level. Parents who want to know more will ask.

- *Engage patients in a decision-making partnership*—Research repeatedly shows that parents trust their physicians more than anyone else for accurate, honest information. Building on this trust, the approach should be nonjudgmental, empathetic, and mutually respectful.

- *Remove barriers*—Insufficient time is the most important barrier to effective communication. Consider scheduling vaccination visits at off-peak hours.

- *Be aware of pitfalls*—Avoid the tendency to extrapolate from limited data and to fit equivocal data into preconceived notions. Risk comparisons (eg, "The chances of a severe reaction are the same as being struck by lightening") can backfire (eg, "We know two people who have been struck by lightening!"). Consciously avoid being paternalistic and belittling.

- *Check for understanding*—Make sure parents understand what you have told them and ask if they have any questions.

Vaccine Refusal

More and more parents are requesting alternative schedules, agreeing to only selected formulations and antigens, or refusing to have their children vaccinated at all—despite the best efforts of providers and public health agencies to communicate the scientific evidence that would allay their concerns. Surveys show that the majority of pediatricians and family practitioners have had at least one family in their practice that has refused vaccination. Overall,

TABLE 8.1 — Parent Phenotypes With Respect to Vaccination

Parent Type	Percentage	Characteristics	Implications
Relaxed	34	"Hands off" parenting style Less active in seeking information Less likely to implement safeguards for children	Provider may need to initiate discussion
Believer	33	Convinced of benefits of vaccination Respect and trust provider Support government requirements	Little reassurance needed
Cautious	23	Avidly seek information Very involved emotionally with children	May need extra time to address concerns
Unconvinced	10	Do not consider vaccination important, necessary, or safe Less trust in traditional sources of information, such as government and institutions	May respond to discussion based on personal experiences

Keane MT, et al. *Vaccine.* 2005;23:2486-2493.

8

approximately 15% of underimmunization in the United States can be attributed to parental concerns about safety. Ironically, *unvaccinated* children are more likely to come from backgrounds with ready access to health care—they have white, married, college-educated mothers and their household income is >\$75,000 (2001 dollars). In contrast, *undervaccinated* children—those who might be vaccinated if they had ready access to care—tend to be black, have single mothers without college educations and live near the poverty level in the inner city.

How should vaccine refusal be handled? First, listen to what the parent is saying. Providers may mistake the need for information or reassurance for flat-out refusal. Some parents may be refusing a single vaccine; others may be refusing all the vaccines that are due at a single visit. Few parents refuse all vaccines at all visits. Second, it must be recognized that whereas the decision not to vaccinate goes against the best medical advice, it rarely puts a child directly in harm's way. Ironically, this is due to the success of vaccination programs. The truth is that polio vaccine has eliminated indigenous polio from the Western Hemisphere; therefore, any given unvaccinated child in the United States is, on the whole, unlikely to get polio. In this context, refusing to allow a child to receive the polio vaccine can hardly be interpreted as actionable medical neglect. On the other hand, there are some situations where vaccine refusal could bring immediate harm to a child—during an epidemic, for example, or after a tetanus-prone injury. In such situations, it would be appropriate to involve governmental agencies or the courts to force action in the child's best interest. While states may be reluctant to act unless there is immediate and substantial danger, it is notable that the courts have repeatedly upheld compulsory immunization laws as a reasonable exercise of the state's power, even in the absence of an epidemic.

Third, parents need to understand that the decision not to immunize their children places other children at risk. Outbreaks are spread by unvaccinated individuals, and even vaccinated children whose parents have diligently tried to protect them can still get the disease—this is due to the (fortunately unusual) phenomenon of primary vaccine failure. In addition, some children cannot be immunized for medical reasons and can therefore only be protected by herd immunity. Thus, immunization can be construed as a civic duty, and failure to immunize can be seen as indirectly bringing the possibility of harm to others. If they understood the scientific facts about the safety of vaccines—and that is a big "if"—it is hard to imagine that most parents would not agree to having their children immunized on the basis of altruism alone. Many parents, however, fear things that have not been, and may not ever be, studied—side effects that could appear decades down the road, for example.

Yet there are still parents who will not agree to vaccination. For these situations, the American Academy of Pediatrics has developed a *Refusal to Vaccinate* form (available at http://www.cispimmunize.org, Accessed August 15, 2008) that can be signed by the parent. The form is not intended to be a legal document and it is not clear what legal protection it would afford the practitioner in the case of a bad outcome from a vaccine-preventable disease (nevertheless, it should be placed in the permanent medical record). Its main purpose is to encourage parents to rethink the issue and to document the provider's efforts to communicate the true risks and benefits of immunization. By signing the form, the parent acknowledges that he or she understands the purpose of the vaccine, why it is recommended, what the risks of vaccination are, and what the consequences of infection may be, including disease, death, permanent impairment, transmission to others, and exclusion from school during outbreaks. Some providers place an expiration date on the form in order to encourage readdressing the issue in the future.

Some parents want a modified schedule for their children, one that spreads the shots out over time, minimizing what they perceive to be a bolus of "toxins" and an assault on the child's immune system. Whereas the end of negotiation in this case—namely that the child receives all recommended vaccines—might justify the means, it also places a burden on the provider to prioritize the immunizations. If the parent will only allow two shots on a given day, which ones should be given and which ones deferred? The decision should be made based on the epidemiology and potential consequences of infection. So, for example, given the above discussion about polio, it might make sense to defer IPV in favor of DTaP, since pertussis is still prevalent and the consequences of infection include a high probability of hospitalization and the possibility of death. Deferral prolongs the period of vulnerability to disease, which in the case of polio may not be consequential; however, it also increases the likelihood that the vaccine series will not be completed.

The AAP takes the position that negotiation is in the best interest of the child. However, there is no law that says a provider must acquiesce to a parent's wishes. Some providers may not be willing to accept the potential exposure to liability that is inherent in negotiating a modified schedule. Others may feel that negotiation is a slippery slope—what if the next request is for half doses, or worse yet homeopathic ones? Still other providers may feel that drawing a hard line behind the recommended schedule is the best way to send the message that vaccinations—at the proper time, in the proper doses, and according to the proper schedule—is a critical component of preventive medicine; this alone might be enough to change some parents' minds. Unfortunately, there are no controlled trials comparing "hard-line" and "soft-line" approaches, and the provider is left to his or her best judgment in terms of how to proceed.

Ultimately, failure to come to terms about immunization may be symptomatic of other issues, such as a lack of mutual trust and inability to communicate, that could affect the care of the child. The American Medical Association Code of Ethics, Section E-8.115 (http://www.ama-assn.org/ama/pub/category/2498.html, Accessed August 15, 2008), states that physicians have the option of withdrawing from a case, so long as notice is given far enough in advance as to permit another medical provider to be secured. Ultimately, physicians need to decide whether to retain patients in their practice who refuse all immunizations. Bear in mind that despite the risks, retention allows continued opportunities to break down barriers and protects the child from seeking care from chiropractors and alternative medicine practitioners.

Many studies suggest that the most trusted person in this whole debate is you—the provider. Personally advocating for vaccination, tempered by compassionate engagement and recognition of a shared, firm commitment to the child's well-being, underpinned by unequivocal scientific data, is the most important thing you can do to ensure the protection of children. Parents should be part of the decision-making process, but many parents will want to know what you have done or would do with your own children.

The Costs of Public Concern

There is no controversy about this fact—public fear of vaccination leads to public harm. The best example is what happened in the United Kingdom in the late 1970s. Anecdotal case series claiming that the whole-cell pertussis vaccine caused encephalopathy, popularized in the lay press, led to widespread fear of the vaccine and to a wholesale drop-off in immunization rates. The result was a tragic increase in pertussis cases and many infant deaths. Not surprisingly, the same scenario played out in other countries that had successful antivaccination movements, but was not seen in countries that had sustained vaccine use. Similarly, claims that MMR vaccine causes autism led to dramatic declines in MMR uptake in the United Kingdom in the late 1990s—predictably resulting in outbreaks of measles. Studies in the United States during the 1980s and 1990s showed that people living in communities with high exemption rates were at higher risk for pertussis, and that individual children with nonmedical exemptions were anywhere from 22 to 35 times more likely to get measles. More recent studies have shown alarming increases in the rates of philosophical or personal-belief exemptions. States granting such exemptions have higher rates of pertussis, and the incidence of pertussis correlates directly with the ease with which such exemptions are obtained.

To understand the impact of vaccine refusal, one need go no further than Indiana, where in 2005 an unvaccinated teenager returned from a church mission trip to Romania, unknowingly incubating measles. The next day she attended a gathering of approximately 500 church members, and the result was 33 cases of measles among church members and 1 case in a hospital phlebotomist (who was not a church member). Three people were hospitalized and one spent 6 days on a ventilator. The vast majority of cases occurred in unvaccinated individuals. Several important things can be gleaned from the Indiana outbreak. First, fear of adverse events was the main reason people refused vaccination. In testament to the prevalence of misinformation, some families feared MMR because of the preservative thimerosal, which has never been part of the vaccine. Second, the church was largely white, middle class, and well educated, reflecting the demographic of unvaccinated children mentioned earlier. Third, the church itself had no official position on immunization—vaccine refusal was a subcultural phenomenon (20 of the 28 affected children were home-schooled, suggesting that there are other sociodemographic correlates of vaccine refusal). Fourth, even though the attack rate was much higher in unvaccinated individuals, some vaccinated individuals still got measles. This illustrates the real issue of primary vaccine failure and the fact that unvaccinated people place vaccinated people at risk (as discussed above). Fifth, the outbreak was almost entirely confined to church members—vaccination-coverage rates in the surrounding community were high enough to prevent spread. Finally, the case could not be made more clearly that diseases such as measles are only a plane flight away, and that all it takes to ignite an outbreak is for the virus to land in a community with enough susceptible individuals.

Vaccine Protest Organizations

A simple Internet search using terms such as vaccines or immunization yields a multitude of web sites that contain non-peer–reviewed data, frightening anecdotes, and pseudoscientific arguments intermingled with legitimate concerns for adverse events such as fever, redness, and swelling. Parents may have trouble separating the information from the misinformation. Many of these web sites are sponsored by organizations that claim authority, credibility, and scientific rigor. They offer strong emotive or political appeals, make explicit claims about vaccines that are unsupported or even contradicted by published data, and they call parents to action in opposing vaccine policy. **Figure 8.2** shows some of the explicit claims made by antivaccination organizations, and **Table 8.2** summarizes some of the rhetorical appeals used to reach parents.

Table 8.3 lists some web sites that have a vaccine-protest orientation. Providers should remain informed about the content of these sites in order to be better prepared to address issues that parents may raise.

234

FIGURE 8.2 — Content Attributes of Antivaccination Web Sites

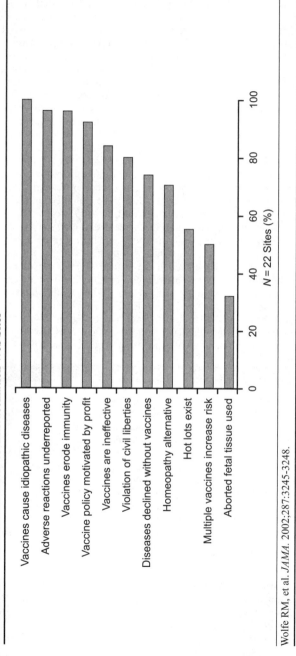

Wolfe RM, et al. *JAMA*. 2002;287:3245-3248.

TABLE 8.2 — Rhetorical Appeals Made by Vaccine-Protest Organizations on the Internet

Authoritative and Scientific
- Present their organization as a legitimate, official body with scientific credibility
- Reference self-published works and alternative medicine literature
- Use indiscriminate citations (eg, letters to newspapers, television interviews)
- Draw alternative conclusions from peer-reviewed studies
- Claim to present "both sides"
- Provide links to provaccine sites

Emotive Appeals
- Paint an "us" (the organization, concerned parents) vs "them" (the medical establishment, government, pharmaceutical industry) picture
- Describe physicians as willing conspirators or manipulated pawns
- Pit parents' love and compassion against cold, analytical science
- Feature anecdotal accounts of purported vaccine injury
- Suggest that responsible parenting means refusing vaccination
- Urge parents to resist coercion
- Warn the public about conspiracy
- Characterize vaccines as "unnatural" and suggest that a natural lifestyle will prevent disease

Search for Truth
- Depict their struggle as a search for truth against a backdrop of cover-up
- Highlight excavated "facts" that were hitherto neglected
- Portray rank-breaking doctors as enlightened heroes

Davies P, et al. *Arch Dis Child*. 2002;87:22-25.

Specific Concerns

What follows is a list of specific questions about vaccines that are on the minds of parents and patients. The answers lie in the science, and it is hoped that the information provided herein will serve as a foundation for effective communication of the true risks and benefits. Some of these issues were addressed by the Institute of Medicine (IOM) Immunization Safety Review Committee (**Table 2.2**).

■ Are Vaccines Still Necessary?
There is no question that vaccine-preventable diseases are less prevalent now than they were before vaccines were introduced (see **Table 1.5**). However, the myth still circulates that these

TABLE 8.3 — Web Sites With a Vaccine-Protest Orientation

URL	Sponsor
http://avn.org.au	Australian Vaccination Network
http://www.ctanet.fr/vaccination-information	French National League for Liberty in Vaccination
http://www.gval.com	Global Vaccine Awareness League
http://www.ias.org.nz/process.php?page=splash	Immunization Awareness Society of New Zealand
http://www.know-vaccines.org	KNOW Vaccines
http://members.aol.com/_ht_a/mccfhc	Missouri Citizens Coalition for Freedom in Health Care
http://www.909shot.com	National Vaccine Information Center
http://nyvic.org/nyvic	New Yorkers for Vaccination Information and Choice
http://vaccineinfo.net	Parents Requesting Open Vaccine Education (PROVE)
http://www.vaccines.bizland.com	People Advocating Vaccine Education (PAVE)
http://thinktwice.com/global.htm	Thinktwice Global Vaccine Institute
http://www.vaccinationnews.com	Vaccination News
http://www.vran.org	Vaccination Risk Awareness Network (VRAN)
http://home.san.rr.com/via	Vaccine Information & Awareness
http://www.vaccination.inoz.com	Vaccine Information Service
http://www.vaclib.org	Vaccination Liberation
http://whale.to/vaccines.html	Vaccine Website
http://www.vaccine-info.com	Vaccine-Info.com

Accessed August 15, 2008.

diseases were disappearing before we had the vaccines. Nothing could be farther from the truth, as anyone whose medical career has spanned the demise of *H influenzae* type b can testify to. In the early 1980s, 1 in 200 children per year, year in and year out, were affected by invasive *Haemophilus* disease. Call nights in the hospital were replete with cases of bacteremia, meningitis, periorbital cellulitis, and the like. Today's pediatric residents have never seen a case; the change occurred in the early 1990s, after licensure and universal use of Hib in infants. Incontrovertible associations between the introduction of a new vaccine and the beginning of the end of a disease have been seen many other times in recent history, including varicella, hepatitis A, and *S pneumoniae*.

Now that many of these diseases are rare, it is hard for parents and patients to understand why vaccines are still important. Here are a few reasons.

- *Some diseases are still prevalent*—Despite our successes, many vaccine-preventable diseases are still around. The choice not to vaccinate against pertussis, for example, is a choice to take a significant risk of getting the disease. The same is true for *S pneumoniae*. Newer vaccines have not yet had a chance to impact disease due to rotavirus and HPV. Influenza still kills 36,000 people every year in the United States.

- *Diseases could easily re-emerge*—Some diseases continue to circulate at very low levels. If immunization rates decrease, outbreaks are likely to occur. This is exactly what happened between 1989 and 1991 in the United States, when 55,622 cases of measles and 123 deaths from the disease were reported. The single most important contributing factor was low vaccine coverage, especially among preschoolers in inner cities. By 2003, after renewed efforts to achieve universal vaccination and the implementation of a 2-dose schedule, measles was no longer endemic in the United States. This means that there is enough population immunity to prevent sustained transmission. The situation could change dramatically if coverage rates fall. The outbreak of >6000 cases of mumps in the Midwest in 2006 is further evidence that diseases can re-emerge.

- *Infections can easily be imported from other parts of the world*—Diseases such as polio and diphtheria still occur in other countries. Tourism, immigration, and international business travel contribute to the ease with which these diseases can be imported into the United States. The outbreaks of measles that occurred in the United States in 2008 were probably due to importation from Europe.

- *Some diseases cannot be eradicated or extinguished*—Tetanus is a good example.

■ Is Natural Infection Better at Inducing Immunity?

It is true that natural infection may induce stronger and longer-lasting immunity than vaccines. Whereas immunity from disease often follows a single natural infection, immunity from vaccines usually occurs only after several doses and, in some cases, can wane with time. A notable example of waning immunity occurs with the pertussis vaccine—by the time children are teenagers, they have lost the protective immunity imparted by the childhood DTaP series (it is important to understand that even natural immunity to pertussis also wanes with time). As a result, teenagers account for a large proportion of reported cases and serve as a reservoir for transmission of the disease in the community. Fortunately, there are now vaccines that can boost immunity in adolescents and adults.

There are some diseases for which vaccines are actually better at inducing immunity than natural infection. Infants who are infected with *H influenzae* do not develop effective antibody responses due to an inherent maturational defect in recognizing polysaccharide antigens (see Chapter 1, *Introduction to Vaccinology*). Hib vaccines, on the other hand, are very effective in young infants because, in coupling the polysaccharide to proteins, they are capable of enlisting T-cell help in driving antibody production by B-cells.

The difference between vaccination and natural infection is the price paid for immunity. For chickenpox, the price paid for natural immunity might be pneumonitis, respiratory failure, encephalitis, or necrotizing fasciitis. For *S pneumoniae*, it might be mental retardation from meningitis—and that would only buy you immunity to the one serotype that caused the infection. Likewise, for HPV the price might be cervical dysplasia—and if you are lucky enough to resolve the infection and dysplasia without progression to cancer, you are left with immunity to only one HPV type (HPV4 protects against four serotypes). The price of immunity to shingles is a case of shingles, and, in some cases, postherpetic neuralgia. The cost of vaccine-induced protection against shingles is the cost of the vaccine, plus minor reactogenicity.

■ Can Multiple Vaccines Overload the Immune System?

One hundred years ago, children received one vaccine (smallpox). Forty years ago, children routinely received five vaccines (diphtheria, whole-cell pertussis, tetanus, polio, and smallpox) and as many as eight shots by 2 years of age. The routine childhood immunization schedule in 2007 called for as many as 34 separate vaccine doses (31 for boys), not including the yearly flu shot. The good news is that delivery of this long list of antigens prevents 16 different diseases. The bad news is that some people wonder if it is just too much.

The possibility of immune overload must be put into perspective. Every day, people are bombarded by antigens to which their immune systems must respond. This includes viruses and bacteria from the external environment as well as organisms from within, particularly those in the mouth, nasopharynx, and gut. Most people are not sick most of the time—this speaks to the robustness of the immune system's ability to meet these challenges. Even the most vulnerable people—neonates—seem to do just fine. Within a matter of hours of birth, the initially sterile GI tract becomes heavily colonized with a wide variety of bacteria, some of which are potentially harmful. Yet the specific secretory IgA responses that are engendered by colonization are, by and large, adequate to prevent invasion.

Even though children receive more vaccines today than they did 40 years ago, the number of separate immunologic challenges (ie, bacterial and viral proteins and bacterial polysaccharides) represented by the routine childhood schedule has actually decreased dramatically (**Table 8.4**). The main reason for this is the elimination of smallpox vaccine, which contained about 200 proteins, and the whole-cell pertussis vaccine, which contained about 3000 antigens. In this context, the vaccine schedule is "purer" than it used to be.

People fear that vaccines might weaken the immune system and thereby increase susceptibility to infectious agents not contained

8

TABLE 8.4 — Number of Separate Antigens Contained in Vaccines Routinely Recommended for Children and Adolescents

Vaccine	1960	1980	2000	2007
Smallpox	200			
Diphtheria	1	1	1	1
Tetanus	1	1	1	1
Pertussis	~3000[a]	~3000[a]	5[b]	5[b]
Polio	15	15	15	15
Measles		10	10	10
Mumps		9	9	9
Rubella		5	5	5
Hib			2	2
Varicella			69	69
PCV7			8	8
HepB			1	1
HepA				4
HPV4				4[c]
Rotavirus				5
MCV4				5
Influenza				12
Total	~3217	~3041	126	156

[a] Estimate of the number of proteins contained in whole-cell pertussis vaccine.
[b] Acellular pertussis vaccines contain anywhere from two to five separate antigens.
[c] Only recommended for girls.

Adapted from: Offit PA, et al. *Pediatrics*. 2002;109:124-129.

in the vaccines (so-called *heterologous infections*). Vaccines may cause temporary suppression of delayed-type hypersensitivity skin reactions or alter certain lymphocyte function tests in vitro. In addition, the measles vaccine may decrease immunogenicity of the varicella vaccine if the latter is administered within 30 days (and not given on the same day). However, the short-lived immunosuppression caused by certain vaccines does not result in an increased risk of heterologous infections. A huge study was done in Denmark that included 805,206 children, 2,900,463 person-years of follow-up, and 84,317 hospitalizations. No causal association was found between any of the childhood vaccines and hospitalization for any of seven different diagnoses unrelated to the vaccine-preventable diseases (acute upper respiratory tract infection, viral pneumonia, bacterial pneumonia, septicemia, viral central nervous system infection, bacterial meningitis, and diarrhea). Moreover, a study from Germany found that children who received the diphtheria, pertussis, tetanus, Hib, and polio vaccines in the first 3 months of life actually had *fewer* infections with vaccine-related as well as vaccine-unrelated pathogens.

Bacterial and viral infections, on the other hand, often *do* predispose children and adults to severe, invasive infections with other pathogens. For example, influenza infection clearly predisposes patients to pneumococcal and staphylococcal pneumonia. Similarly, varicella infection increases susceptibility to group A beta-hemolytic streptococcal infections including necrotizing fasciitis, toxic shock syndrome, and bacteremia. Thus if susceptibility to heterologous infection is the concern, vaccination makes more sense than no vaccination.

■ Does MMR Cause Autism?

In 1993, Wakefield and colleagues in London suggested that inflammatory bowel disease (IBD) might be caused by persistence of measles virus in intestinal tissue. In 1998, the group described 12 children with a form of chronic enterocolitis and regressive developmental disorders. Ten of these children had autism, and in eight, the onset of regression was temporally linked by the child's parent or physician to receipt of MMR. The authors suggested that a unique disease process, characterized by intestinal inflammation and regressive autism, was caused by replication of the three vaccine viruses in gut tissues.

Since a control group that was never exposed to the vaccine was not included in the study, a causal relationship between MMR and autism could not be established. Moreover, many questions about the integrity of the work were raised, spurred by the discovery that Wakefield had been commissioned by a group of lawyers to investigate the relationship between MMR and autism. At the very least, this raised the possibility that some of the patients in the 1998 study made their way to Wakefield *because* of his interest in this purported clinical entity—in other words, the study population might have been biased toward patients who already thought their symptoms were brought on by the vaccine. These and other concerns prompted 10 of the 12 original authors, in a 2004 statement, to retract their previous interpretation of the study. Seldom, however, has an imperfect study like this one had such a dramatic negative impact on public health (the closest thing was the pertussis-vaccine-causes-encephalopathy scare of the 1970s). The notion that MMR causes autism fed directly into the public's natural tendency to assume causality when two events are temporally associated—children get MMR at 1 year of age and the signs of autism become apparent right around the same time.

The evidence against an association between MMR and autism, summarized below, is overwhelming:

- *Persistent measles virus infection has not been found in IBD or autism*—Studies range from attempts to find the viral genome in bowel tissues using molecular amplification techniques to rigorous case-control studies. One such study done through the Vaccine Safety DataLink (VSD; see *Chapter 2*) showed no more exposure to MMR among 142 cases with IBD compared with 432 controls without IBD. A 2006 study found no differences in antimeasles antibody titers between 54 autistic children (51 had received MMR) and 34 controls (31 had received MMR), and no study subjects had detectable measles virus DNA sequences in their peripheral blood mononuclear cells.

- *Ecologic studies have shown no relationship between MMR uptake and increased incidence of autism*—Most studies show that autism cases are increasing dramatically, but many epidemiologists believe this is a reflection of expanded case definitions, diagnostic substitution for other neurodevelopmental conditions, and more public awareness rather than a true increase in incidence. In any event, studies done in very different settings—the United Kingdom, California, and Montréal, to name a few—consistently show that the incidence of autism over time does not parallel the uptake of MMR, as it would if MMR caused autism. **Figure 8.3** shows the data from the Montréal study. Another study from the United Kingdom showed no increase in cases of autism after introduction of MMR, which occurred in 1988. In addition, there was no clustering of cases of autism at various intervals up to 1 year after receipt of MMR vaccine. A second study by the same group expanded these observations to include 1 and 2 doses of MMR and longer intervals after receipt of vaccine, again finding no evidence for a causal association.

- *Retrospective studies show no new form of autism and no bowel symptoms associated with the introduction of MMR*—One study in the United Kingdom found that the proportion of children with developmental regression or bowel symptoms did not change significantly between 1979 and 1998, a period that included introduction of MMR. Similarly, a study of 262

FIGURE 8.3 — Birth Cohort Study in Montréal, Quebec: MMR

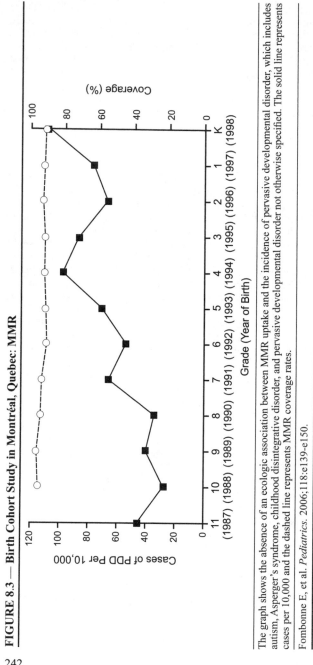

The graph shows the absence of an ecologic association between MMR uptake and the incidence of pervasive developmental disorder, which includes autism, Asperger's syndrome, childhood disintegrative disorder, and pervasive developmental disorder not otherwise specified. The solid line represents cases per 10,000 and the dashed line represents MMR coverage rates.

Fombonne E, et al. *Pediatrics.* 2006;118:e139-e150.

patients with autism found no evidence for the emergence of a new form of the disease that included intestinal symptoms following widespread use of MMR.

- *Case-control studies do not support an association*—One study done in the United Kingdom found that 78.1% of 1010 cases had received MMR before being diagnosed with autism, as compared with 82.1% of 3671 controls without autism, for an adjusted odds ratio of 0.86 (95% CI 0.68, 1.09). This means that the odds of being diagnosed with autism among individuals who had received MMR were essentially the same as those who had not received MMR. Another study, done in Atlanta, showed there was no difference in the proportion of children vaccinated with MMR before 18 or before 24 months of age among 624 case children and 1824 matched controls.

- *Cohort studies provide strong evidence against an association*—Cohort studies are among the most rigorous epidemiologic investigations. The methodology is simple—a cohort of subjects are assembled, exposure or nonexposure to the risk factor is determined, and the subsequent development of the outcome is ascertained. The rate of the outcome is then compared between exposed and nonexposed individuals; the ratio of the two is called the relative risk (RR), and an RR of 1 means there is no association between the exposure and the outcome. The beauty of retrospective cohort studies, wherein the cohort is identified in the past and followed to the present, is that the exposure and outcomes have already taken place, so that measurement of the exposure (in this case, receipt of MMR) cannot be biased by knowledge of the outcome (autism), and robust inferences can be made. **Figure 8**.4 shows the results of the Danish Cohort Study, which involved 537,303 children. The outcomes of autism or autistic-spectrum disorder were no more common in 1,647,504 person-years of exposure to MMR than they were in 482,360 person-years of nonexposure. The study further showed no association with age at vaccination, interval since vaccination, or the date of vaccination. This study provided very strong evidence against MMR as a cause of autism.

The science is clear—MMR does not cause autism. Moreover, there is no scientific rationale for giving the monovalent components in lieu of the combination. In fact, there is a significant downside—because one must allow for the minimum intervals between live vaccines not given on the same day (see Chapter 5, *General Recommendations*), breaking up the MMR prolongs the period of susceptibility to disease and increases the risk of not being immunized to all three.

FIGURE 8.4 — Danish Cohort Study of MMR and Autism

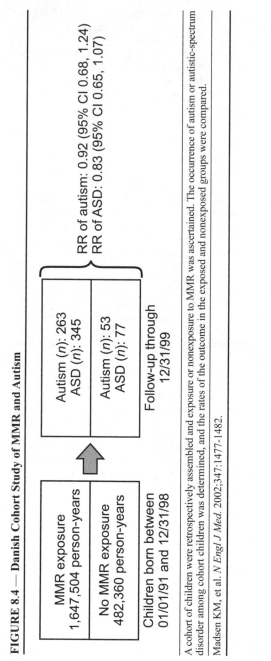

A cohort of children were retrospectively assembled and exposure or nonexposure to MMR was ascertained. The occurrence of autism or autistic-spectrum disorder among cohort children was determined, and the rates of the outcome in the exposed and nonexposed groups were compared.

Madsen KM, et al. *N Engl J Med.* 2002;347:1477-1482.

■ Did the Thimerosal Used as a Preservative in Vaccines Cause Autism?

High levels of mercury are known to damage the nervous system and kidneys. In addition, studies in the Faroe Islands, the Seychelles, and Iraq showed that fetuses can be harmed when pregnant women ingest large quantities of mercury. For these reasons, the FDA Modernization Act of 1997 required the FDA to compile a list of drugs and foods that contain mercury. At that time (and really since the beginning of the modern vaccine era), some vaccines used thimerosal, which contains *ethylmercury* as a preservative so these vaccines were included in the FDA list. Preservatives were necessary in multidose vials to prevent contamination with bacteria or fungi.

The cumulative level of mercury represented by the routine vaccine schedule for infants was within the acceptable range published by the FDA, the Agency for Toxic Substance and Disease Registry, and the WHO. However, it slightly exceeded the level considered to be safe by the Environmental Protection Agency (EPA). To determine safe levels of mercury, the EPA evaluated a study performed in Iraq where pregnant women were accidentally exposed to large quantities of *methylmercury* (a more toxic organic compound than ethylmercury) that had been used to disinfect grain. The EPA then estimated the lowest dose of mercury that was found to cause neurodevelopmental delay in infants as a result of fetal exposure. From this, the lowest dose of methylmercury that could possibly harm an unborn child was calculated and then divided by ten, yielding a very conservative estimate of the lowest acceptable dose of mercury.

There are many problems with using the study in Iraq to determine levels of thimerosal in vaccines that would be safe in children. Among them is the fact that the mercury contained in thimerosal is in the form of *ethylmercury*, which behaves in the body much differently that *methylmercury*. In addition, vaccines are administered to children after, not before, they are born, when the nervous system is more mature and, therefore, much less likely to be susceptible to harmful effects.

Nevertheless, the Public Health Service and the AAP issued a joint statement on July 9, 1999, calling for manufacturers to eliminate thimerosal from vaccines as a precautionary measure, stating the following: "The current levels of thimerosal will not hurt children, but reducing those levels will make safe vaccines even safer." One might wonder how safe vaccines can be made safer, particularly by removing a component that had not been shown to be harmful in the first place. The consequences of this statement ranged from confusion on the part of providers, dismantling of the machinery that had been put in place to deliver the birth dose of HepB, failure to give HepB to many high-risk infants, an onslaught of litigation, and a loss of public confidence. The effects were still evident in 2008, with a barrage of celebrities on television talk shows claiming that thimerosal is responsible for the "epidemic" of autism, op-ed pieces in newspapers, and nearly 5000 thimerosal injury claims pending under the National Vaccine Injury Compensation Program (VICP; see *Chapter 3*). The issue climaxed in early 2008, when a special court for the VICP ruled that multiple vaccinations received in a single day had aggravated an underlying mitochondrial disorder in a child, ultimately manifesting as regressive encephalopathy with features of autistic spectrum disorder. This reignited the controversy, even though the ruling was strictly applicable only to this case of a child with a previously undiagnosed and very rare metabolic defect.

The evidence against an association between thimerosal and autism, or any other neurodevelopmental problem, is overwhelming.

- *Biologic studies do not show toxic levels of mercury in infants receiving thimerosal-containing vaccines*—In a pilot study published in 2002, 40 full-term infants ≤6 months of age were given vaccines containing thimerosal and 21 were given thimerosal-free vaccines. No infants had blood mercury concentrations exceeding 29 parts per billion, the level thought to be safe in cord blood. Stool concentrations were high, suggesting elimination through the GI tract. A follow-up study looking at 216 infants and conducted in Argentina was published in 2008. The blood half-life of mercury after administration of thimerosal-containing vaccines was 3.7 days. The highest levels of mercury were seen in the first 24 hours after vaccination, and all were ≤8 ng/mL (some infants received as much as 57.5 mcg of mercury at one time through the vaccinations). Inorganic mercury was detected in stools within days. The results suggest rapid elimination of ethylmercury from the body after vaccination with thimerosal-containing vaccines.

- *Ecologic studies show continued increases in autism cases well after thimerosal was removed from vaccines*—Whether one looks in Denmark and Sweden, where thimerosal was removed from vaccines in 1992, or Canada, where no vaccines contained thimerosal after 1996, the data are remarkably consistent—continued increases in reported cases of autism (data from the Canadian study are shown in **Figure 8.5**). A study from California published in 2008 showed no decrease in autism prevalence by age or birth cohort several years after the last lots of thimerosal-containing vaccines would have expired. As discussed earlier, epidemiologists do not uniformly agree that there is a *true* increase in the incidence of autism. However, there *are* many cases being diagnosed, and while the causes remain elusive, the ecologic data argue very strongly against thimerosal being one of them.

- *Cohort studies provide strong evidence against an association*—**Figure 8.6** shows the results of the Danish Cohort

FIGURE 8.5 — Birth Cohort Study in Montréal, Quebec: Thimerosal

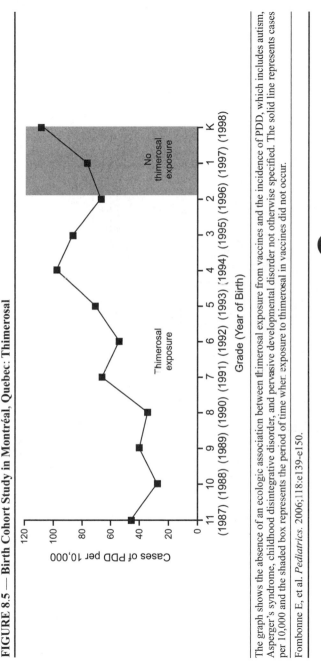

The graph shows the absence of an ecologic association between thimerosal exposure from vaccines and the incidence of PDD, which includes autism, Asperger's syndrome, childhood disintegrative disorder, and pervasive developmental disorder not otherwise specified. The solid line represents cases per 10,000 and the shaded box represents the period of time when exposure to thimerosal in vaccines did not occur.

Fombonne E, et al. *Pediatrics.* 2006;118:e139-e150.

FIGURE 8.6 — Danish Cohort Study of Thimerosal and Autism

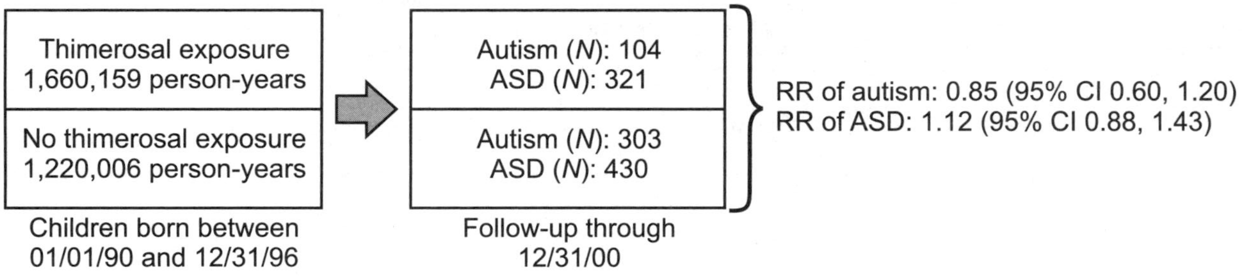

A cohort of children were retrospectively assembled and exposure or nonexposure to thimerosal in vaccines was ascertained. The occurrence of autism or ASD among cohort children was determined, and the rates of the outcome in the exposed and nonexposed groups were compared.

Hviid A., et al. *JAMA*. 2003;290:1763-1766.

Study, which involved 467,450 children. The outcomes of autism or autistic-spectrum disorder were no more common in 1,660,159 person-years of exposure to thimerosal than they were in 1,220,006 person-years of nonexposure. The study further showed no evidence of a dose-response relationship between cumulative amounts of ethylmercury exposure and autism, thus providing very strong evidence against thimerosal as a cause. A prospective cohort study in the United Kingdom (children were enrolled at birth and behavioral data were collected regularly thereafter) involving over 14,000 children showed that poor prosocial behavior at 47 months of age was correlated with ethylmercury exposure by 3 months of age. However, the same study showed that ethylmercury exposure was associated with *better* outcomes in eight other areas, including conduct, fine motor development, reported tics, and the need for special education. A 2-phased retrospective cohort study in the United States involving over 100,000 children also found no consistent associations with neurodevelopmental outcomes. Finally, in a 2007 study, 1047 children were given a 3-hour assessment involving 42 different neuropsychologic test; no consistent associations were seen between exposure to thimerosal-containing vaccines and the test results.

Authoritative bodies involved in vaccine practice and policy are virtually unanimous in rejecting the purported link between thimerosal and autism (**Table 8.5**). As of 2008, the only childhood vaccines that still contain thimerosal as a preservative are two brands of TIV (although a preservative-free formulation for children is available). Thimerosal activists argue, however, that vaccines labeled *preservative-free* are still not safe because they contain trace amounts of thimerosal, levels that are essentially below the limit of detection. Since a product cannot be labeled *thimerosal-free* if thimerosal is used anywhere in the manufacturing process, companies have either dropped out of the market or scrambled to revise their protocols and package their products in single-dose vials or prefilled syringes. The public has paid the price in dollars as well as in availability. All of this without a shred of scientific evidence that thimerosal was a problem to begin with.

■ **Does Pertussis Vaccine Cause Brain Damage?**

In 1974, Kulenkampff and coworkers published an uncontrolled case series of children who allegedly developed mental retardation and epilepsy following receipt of the whole-cell pertussis vaccine. Over the next several years, fear of the pertussis vaccine generated by media coverage of this report caused a decrease in pertussis immunization rates in British children from 81% to 31%; the decrease in vaccine use resulted in >100,000 cases and 36

TABLE 8.5 — Organizations Opposed to Antithimerosal Legislation[a]

- Ambulatory Pediatric Association
- American Academy of Family Physicians
- American Academy of Physician Assistants
- American College of Allergy, Asthma, and Immunology
- American College of Preventive Medicine
- American Liver Foundation
- American Medical Directors Association
- American Pharmacists Association
- Association of Immunization Program Managers
- Children's Hospital of Philadelphia Vaccine Education Center
- Council of State and Territorial Epidemiologists
- Every Child by Two
- Hepatitis B Foundation
- Hepatitis Foundation International
- Immunization Action Coalition
- Infectious Diseases Society of America
- National Coalition for Adult Immunization
- National Foundation for Infectious Diseases
- Parents of Kids With Infectious Diseases
- Pediatric Infectious Diseases Society
- Society for Adolescent Medicine
- Society of Teachers of Family Medicine

[a] Signatories on a letter to Congress dated April 3, 2006. The letter stated that there was no scientific evidence that thimerosal in vaccines posed any health risk. It also raised concerns that antithimerosal legislation would compound ongoing vaccine shortages, hamper the influenza vaccination program, increase costs, add complexity to the vaccine delivery system, and affect global immunization programs. Available at http://www.immunize.org/thimerosal/official.asp. Accessed August 15, 2008.

deaths from pertussis. Decreased immunization rates and increased pertussis deaths also were seen in Japan, Sweden, and Wales.

The National Childhood Encephalopathy Study (NCES), conducted in the United Kingdom from 1976 to 1979, suggested the possibility of a relationship between the vaccine and encephalopathy, although methodologic problems with this study were quickly highlighted. For example, the study included only a small number of cases that had been exposed to the vaccine. The IOM independently analyzed the NCES data in 1991 and concluded that there was a rare but causal relationship with encephalopathy in the immediate postvaccination period, even though there was no evidence that permanent brain damage occurred. A reanalysis by the IOM in 1994 reached a different conclusion—whole-cell pertussis vaccine did not cause encephalopathy.

In a study published in 2006, the records of four large US health maintenance organizations were used to address this issue once again. A total of 452 children with encephalopathy diagnosed between 1981 and 1995 were compared with matched controls without encephalopathy. Exposure to pertussis vaccine in any postvaccination time period was no more common among cases than controls. The maximum possible all-cause incidence of encephalopathy after pertussis immunization was 1 in 370,000, which is no different from the background rate of encephalopathy in young children.

Despite the data and despite the fact that acellular pertussis vaccines have replaced whole-cell vaccines, encephalopathy remains an injury that can be compensated through the Vaccine Injury Table under the VICP (see *Chapter 3*).

■ Do Vaccines Cause Guillain-Barré Syndrome (GBS)?

GBS is an acute, immune-mediated, demyelinating peripheral neuropathy characterized by progressive symmetric weakness. Most cases occur after an infectious event, including *Campylobacter jejuni* enteritis. GBS came to the forefront during the 1976-1977 flu season, when an association with swine flu vaccination was found. The mechanism is unclear, but may involve molecular mimicry, whereby an epitope on the vaccine triggers an immune response to a self antigen, which in this case is on neurons. Alternatively, autoimmunity may have been triggered by a bystander effect, wherein self-reactive T- and B-cells, normally held in check, are stimulated by the vaccine. In any event, recent studies have failed to show a consistent relationship between subsequent versions of the influenza vaccine and GBS. One study looked at two influenza seasons in the United States in the early 1990s and found an RR of 1.7 (95% CI 1.0, 2.8), corresponding to approximately one additional case of GBS per million people vaccinated (the background rate of GBS is about 10 to 20 cases per 1,000,000). Another study in the United Kingdom spanning the years 1992 to 2000 found 228 incident cases of GBS; seven cases occurred within 42 days of any immunization (three were after influenza immunization) and 221 were not associated with immunization, for an RR of 1.03 (95% CI 0.48, 2.18). Finally, a study from Canada published in 2006 demonstrated no seasonality of GBS and no increase in hospital admission for GBS after the introduction of a universal influenza immunization program. If influenza vaccine does cause GBS, it is extremely rarely and barely above background. A personal history of GBS within 6 weeks of influenza vaccination is listed as a precaution to further doses (**Table 5.3**).

By September 2006, 17 cases of GBS associated with MCV4 administration had been reported to VAERS (the vaccine was licensed in January 2005). Most of the cases occurred within 2 weeks of vaccination, a time frame that would fit with a causal relationship. The rate of GBS among immunized teenagers, calculated based on doses distributed, was estimated to be about 0.20 per 100,000 person-months. This rate was similar to the background rate of GBS calculated from the VSD database, but it was slightly higher than that seen in the Healthcare Cost and Utilization Project, a multistate hospital discharge database. It was estimated that if GBS is truly caused by MCV4, there would be 1 extra case for every 800,000 teenagers vaccinated. Universal adolescent vaccination continues to be recommended, although a personal history of GBS is listed as a precaution (**Table 5.3**).

■ Do Vaccines Cause Multiple Sclerosis (MS)?

The hypothesis that vaccines might cause MS was fueled by anecdotal reports of MS following HepB administration and two case-control studies showing an increase in the incidence of MS in vaccinated individuals that was not statistically significant. However, two large case-control studies evaluated whether HepB causes MS or whether HepB, tetanus, or influenza vaccines exacerbate symptoms of MS. The first study in a cohort of nurses identified 192 women with MS and 645 matched controls. The RR of multiple sclerosis associated with exposure to HepB was 0.9 and the RR within 2 years before the onset of disease was 0.7. There also was no association between the number of doses of HepB and the risk of MS. The second study included 643 patients in Europe with MS relapse occurring between 1993 and 1997. Exposure to vaccination in the 2-month period before relapse was compared with the four previous 2-month control periods. The RR of relapse associated with the use of any vaccine was 0.71, and with HepB, tetanus, and influenza vaccines it was 0.67, 0.75, and 1.08, respectively.

Other well-controlled studies also found that influenza vaccine did not exacerbate symptoms of MS. In a retrospective study of 180 patients with relapsing MS, *infection* with influenza virus was more likely than *immunization* with influenza vaccine to cause an exacerbation of symptoms, suggesting that influenza vaccine is actually likely to prevent exacerbations of MS.

■ Are Vaccines Made From Fetal Tissue?

Rubella, HepA, rabies, and varicella vaccines are grown in cultured human embryo fibroblasts (MRC-5 or WI-38) because these are the only cells that replicate the viruses in high enough titer for mass production. Each cell line was first obtained from an aborted fetus in the early 1960s. These very same embryonic cells have been passaged in tissue culture in the laboratory since then, and no new fetal material has ever been involved. Nevertheless, this situation represents a moral dilemma for some individuals. In helping patients work through this, it may be worth emphasizing that the original abortion was not done specifically with the intent to produce vaccines, that it occurred in the distant past, that the vaccine producers never intended for fetuses to be aborted, and that the moral imperative to save lives through vaccination might outweigh their objection to what they consider to be a singular, distant moral transgression. Many religious organizations, including the United States Conference of Catholic Bishops, have used these arguments to support vaccination, despite their opposition to abortion.

■ Do Vaccines Cause Allergies and Autoimmune Disease?

Developed countries have seen an increase in the incidence of allergic diseases during the same time that many new vaccines have been introduced, leading some to believe there is a relationship. The theoretical basis for this belief has to do with the *hygiene hypothesis* which holds that "clean living" brought on in part by the elimination of vaccine-preventable diseases creates an immunologic environment during ontogeny that is replete with type 2 helper T cells and deficient in T regulator cells (see *Chapter 1*), an environment that promotes allergy and autoimmunity. However, several large epidemiologic studies favor rejection of this hypothesis. One well-controlled study identified 18,407 children with asthma who were born between 1991 and 1997 and compared them with a control group without asthma. Relative risks of asthma in vaccinated compared to unvaccinated children were 0.92 for DTwP, 1.09 for the oral polio vaccine, and 0.97 for the MMR vaccine. In children who had at least two medical encounters during their first year of life, the RR for asthma following receipt of Hib was 1.07, and for HepB it was 1.09.

Another large well-controlled study of 669 children prospectively evaluated the risk of allergies following receipt of the pertussis vaccine. Infants were randomized to receive a 2-component DTaP vaccine, a 5-component DTaP, DTwP, or DT beginning at 2 months of age. Children were followed for >2 years and the risk of allergies was determined by parent questionnaires and examination of medical records. Allergic disorders studied included asthma, atopic dermatitis, allergic rhinoconjunctivitis, urticaria, and food allergies. No difference in the incidence of allergic diseases was observed in children who did or did not receive pertussis vaccine. Of interest, children with natural pertussis infections were more likely to develop allergic diseases than children not infected with pertussis.

A cohort study from Tasmania published in 2007 showed small and inconsistent associations between receipt of diphtheria toxoid and asthma, eczema, and food allergies. The authors, however, acknowledged the problems with this and other similar studies: the possibility of recall bias (wherein parents of children with allergies may falsely recall immunizations that were not actually given), difficulty ascertaining the timing of vaccination and types of vaccines that were given, inaccurate reporting of allergies by parents, and health care–seeking behavior on the part of parents (certain parents may seek both immunizations and diagnoses of allergy). Many of these factors could have led to an increased association between immunizations and atopic conditions.

In addition, the hypothesis in many studies of vaccines and allergies is that unimmunized children have the "benefit" of exposure to the actual infections that the vaccines are designed to prevent. Few, if any, studies offer evidence of this. In addition, remember that for live vaccines, vaccination *is* infection. Taken together, the data argue strongly that vaccines do not cause allergies and asthma.

Several uncontrolled observational studies claimed that the introduction of vaccines, particularly Hib, into certain populations caused an increase in the incidence of type 1 diabetes. The purported link is vaccine-induced enhancement of preexisting subclinical islet cell autoimmunity. Once again, the data do not support an association. One study from the VSD compared 252 cases of type 1 diabetes with 768 matched controls without diabetes. The odds ratio was 0.28 for the association between diabetes and DTwP, 1.36 for MMR, 1.14 for Hib, 0.81 for HepB, 1.16 for varicella vaccine, and 0.92 for DTaP. For children vaccinated at birth with HepB, the odds ratio for diabetes was 0.51 and for those vaccinated at 2 months of age or later was 0.86. In another study, 21,421 children who received Hib between 1988 and 1990 in the United States were followed for 10 years and the risk of type 1 diabetes was 0.78 when compared with a group of 22,557 children who did not receive the vaccine. Several other well-controlled retrospective studies also found that immunizations are not associated with an increased risk of developing type 1 diabetes.

Figure 8.7 shows a representative result from the Danish Cohort Study of childhood vaccination and type 1 diabetes. A total of 739,694 children were included and there were 4,720,517 person-years of follow-up. Not surprisingly, the risk of diabetes was much higher in children who had at least one sibling with diabetes. None of the childhood vaccines, however, in any number of doses, was associated with diabetes.

■ Can Vaccines Transmit Mad Cow Disease (MCD)?

By July of 2000 approximately 175,000 cows in the United Kingdom had developed bovine spongiform encephalopathy, more commonly referred to as MCD, a progressive deterioration of the nervous system. At the same time, >70 people in the United Kingdom had developed a progressive neurologic condition termed *variant Creutzfeldt-Jakob disease* (vCJD) that likely resulted from eating meat prepared from cows with MCD. Both MCD and vCJD are caused by prions, which are proteinaceous, self-replicating infectious particles. In July 2000, the FDA convened a meeting to discuss the possibility that some vaccines were made using serum or gelatin derived from cows in countries that had MCD, including England. Although the risk of transmission of vCJD to humans from such vaccines was considered theoretic and remote, the recommendation was made that vaccines use bovine materials originating from countries without endogenous

FIGURE 8.7 — Danish Cohort Study of Vaccines and Diabetes

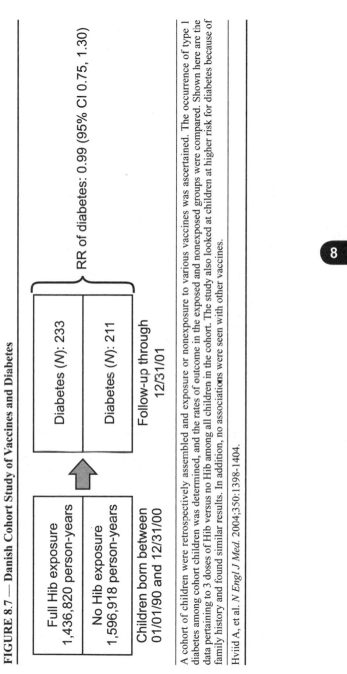

RR of diabetes: 0.99 (95% CI 0.75, 1.30)

Full Hib exposure
1,436,820 person-years

Diabetes (N): 233

No Hib exposure
1,596,918 person-years

Diabetes (N): 211

Children born between
01/01/90 and 12/31/00

Follow-up through
12/31/01

A cohort of children were retrospectively assembled and exposure or nonexposure to various vaccines was ascertained. The occurrence of type 1 diabetes among cohort children was determined, and the rates of outcome in the exposed and nonexposed groups were compared. Shown here are the data pertaining to 3 doses of Hib versus no Hib among all children in the cohort. The study also looked at children at higher risk for diabetes because of family history and found similar results. In addition, no associations were seen with other vaccines.

Hviid A, et al. *N Engl J Med.* 2004;350:1398-1404.

MCD. This recommendation was published in the *MMWR* on December 22, 2000, and was followed by a New York Times article published on February 8, 2001 entitled *Five Drug Makers Use Material With Possible Mad Cow Link*.

Prions are found in the brains of cows with MCD and in the brains of humans with vCJD. They can also be found in the spinal cord and retina. However, blood from infected animals and from infected people has never been shown to be a source of infection to humans. The likely source of prions for people in England was hamburger, not steak, and hamburger may be prepared in a manner that includes the spinal cord. Steak, on the other hand, represents only the muscles of cows and, therefore, does not contain prions.

Vaccines may contain trace amounts of animal products used during the manufacturing process. For example, vaccines are grown in laboratory cells that require many growth factors for maintenance. An excellent source of these growth factors is fetal bovine serum, which is naturally filtered by the 6-layered bovine placenta. Many proteins are excluded from the bovine fetal circulation by these layers (for example, bovine fetal blood contains 1/500th of the antibodies found in bovine maternal blood). Maternal-fetal transmission of prions has never been documented in animals and fetal blood is not known to contain prions. Moreover, the fetal bovine serum used in vaccine manufacture is highly diluted and eventually removed from cells during purification of vaccine viruses. It should be pointed out as well that prions propagate in mammalian brain but not in cell culture.

Another product from cows and pigs that may be used in vaccines is gelatin, a protein formed by boiling skin or connective tissue such as hooves. Gelatin is used to stabilize vaccines so that they remain effective after distribution. Since prions are not detected in the skin or connective tissue of animals, gelatin does not represent a risk to patients.

Final reassurance comes from the fact that transmission of prions occurs from eating the brains of infected animals or from directly inoculating preparations of brains of infected animals into the brains of experimental animals. Transmission of prions has not been documented after inoculation into the muscles or under the skin, which are the routes used for vaccination. Taken together, the chances that currently licensed vaccines contain prions and represent a risk to humans is essentially zero.

■ Can Vaccines Cause Cancer?

The polio vaccine used in the late 1950s and early 1960s was contaminated with a monkey virus called simian virus 40 (SV40), present in the monkey kidney cells used to grow the vaccine. Investigators found SV40 DNA in biopsy specimens obtained from patients with mesothelioma, osteosarcoma, and non-Hodgkin's lymphoma. Interestingly, SV40 DNA was present in the cancers of people who had received the polio vaccine that was contaminated with SV40, but it was also present in those who had not. SV40 DNA was even found in the cancers of people born after 1963, a time when the vaccine no longer contained SV40. A study published in 2004 shed some light on this. Some of the primers that were being employed in the PCR reactions used to amplify DNA sequences of SV40 were directed at a region of the T antigen. As it turns out, these sequences are also present in common laboratory plasmids. How did they get there? They were engineered into the plasmids during the first attempts to create expression vectors for eukaryotic cells, but this happened so long ago that their presence was not well known. When alternative T-antigen primers were used, only a few cancers were positive. Moreover, this study found no evidence of T-antigen RNA transcript production and no T-antigen protein expression in the tumors.

Finally, epidemiologic studies do not show an increased risk of cancers in those who received polio vaccine between 1955 and 1963.

■ **Did the Polio Vaccine Cause the AIDS Pandemic?**

In 1999, Edward Hooper published a book entitled *The River: A Journey to the Source of HIV and AIDS*. The central hypothesis was that the origin of AIDS could be traced to poliovirus vaccines that were administered orally in the Belgian Congo between 1957 and 1960. This assertion was based on the following assumptions: 1) all poliovirus vaccines were grown in monkey kidney cells; 2) those cells were contaminated with simian immunodeficiency virus (SIV), which is closely related to HIV; and 3) people were inadvertently infected with SIV that then mutated to HIV and caused the AIDS epidemic.

The following facts, however, exonerate polio vaccines as a cause of AIDS:

- SIV is found in chimpanzees, not monkeys, and chimpanzee cells were never used to grow polio vaccine.
- SIV and HIV are not very close genetically and mutation from SIV to HIV would have required centuries, not years.
- Both SIV and HIV are enveloped viruses that are easily disrupted by extremes of pH. If given by mouth (as was oral polio vaccine), both of these viruses would likely be destroyed in the acid environment of the stomach.
- Original lots of the polio vaccine (including those used in Africa for the polio vaccine trials) did not contain HIV, SIV, or chimpanzee genetic sequences when analyzed by molecular amplification techniques.

Unfortunately, fears of polio vaccine based on this unfounded theory might have adversely affected vaccine use where it is need most—in the developing world where the last vestiges of wild type poliovirus reside.

■ Can Vaccines Cause SIDS?

In 1999, the ABC news program *20/20* aired a story claiming that HepB caused sudden infant death syndrome (SIDS). The story included a picture of a 1-month-old girl who died of SIDS only 16 hours after receiving the second dose of HepB. In 1991, before routine use of the HepB was fully implemented for all infants, about 5000 children died every year from SIDS. Within 10 years of that recommendation, vaccine uptake had increased to about 90% and the incidence of SIDS had decreased dramatically to about 1600 cases per year. This decrease was due to the introduction of the "Back to Sleep" program, in which parents were encouraged to place their infants on their backs or sides when going to sleep. The lack of an ecologic correlation between SIDS and HepB was supported by VAERS data showing very few neonatal deaths following HepB after approximately 86 million doses were given. Several studies actually show *lower* SIDS rates among infants who receive vaccines when compared with those who do not. While this may reflect biases wherein healthier or better-cared-for infants are the ones who are immunized, the data clearly do not indicate vaccines as a risk factor for SIDS. Temporal associations arise because some vaccines happen to be given just at the time of the peak-age incidence of SIDS.

A study published in 2004 looked at a cohort of 361,696 infants between 1993 and 1998. A total of 1363 infants in the cohort died in the first 29 days of life; only 5% of them had been vaccinated with HepB, whereas 66% of those who survived the first month of life had been immunized. Moreover, there was no difference in the proportion of vaccinated and unvaccinated infants who died of unexpected causes, and the SIDS death rate was the same (3.3 per 100,000) for vaccinated and unvaccinated infants.

Communication

Ball LK, Evans G, Bostrom A. Risky business: challenges in vaccine risk communication. *Pediatrics.* 1998;101:453-458.

Davis TC, Fredrickson DD, Arnold CL, et al. Childhood vaccine risk/benefit communication in private practice office settings: a national survey. *Pediatrics.* 2001;107:e17.

Davis TC, Fredrickson DD, Bocchini C, et al. Improving vaccine risk/benefit communication with an immunization education package: a pilot study. *Ambul Pediatr.* 2002;2:193-200.

Evans G, Bostrom A, Johnston RB, Fisher BL, Stoto MA. *Risk Communication and Vaccination: Summary of a Workshop.* Washington, DC: National Academy Press; 1997.

Fredrickson DD, Davis TC, Bocchini JA Jr. Explaining the risks and benefits of vaccines to parents. *Pediatr Ann.* 2001;30:400-406.

Vaccine Refusal

American Medical Association. Council on Ethical and Judicial Affairs. Termination of the physician-patient relationship. In: *Code of Medical Ethics: Current Opinions.* 2002–2003 ed. Chicago, IL: American Medical Association; 2002:110.

Diekema DS; American Academy of Pediatrics Committee on Bioethics. Responding to parental refusals of immunization of children. *Pediatrics.* 2005;115:1428-1431.

Flanagan-Klygis EA, Sharp L, Frader JE. Dismissing the family who refuses vaccines: a study of pediatrician attitudes. *Arch Pediatr Adolesc Med.* 2005;159:929-934.

Freed GL, Clark SJ, Hibbs BF, Santoli JM. Parental vaccine safety concerns. The experiences of pediatricians and family physicians. *Am J Prev Med.* 2004;26:11-14.

Gust DA, Strine TW, Maurice E, et al. Underimmunization among children: effects of vaccine safety concerns on immunization status. *Pediatrics.* 2004;114:e16-e22.

Salmon DA, Moulton LH, Omer SB, DeHart MP, Stokley S, Halsey NA. Factors associated with refusal of childhood vaccines among parents of school-aged children: a case-control study. *Arch Pediatr Adolesc Med.* 2005;159:470-476.

Smith PJ, Chu SY, Barker LE. Children who have received no vaccines: who are they and where do they live? *Pediatrics.* 2004;114:187-195.

Costs of Public Concern

Feikin DR, Lezotte DC, Hamman RF, Salmon DA, Chen RT, Hoffman RE. Individual and community risks of measles and pertussis associated with personal exemptions to immunization. *JAMA.* 2000;284:3145-3150.

Gangarosa EJ, Galazka AM, Wolfe CR, et al. Impact of anti-vaccine movements on pertussis control: the untold story. *Lancet.* 1998;351:356-361.

Jansen VA, Stollenwerk N, Jensen HJ, Ramsay ME, Edmunds WJ, Rhodes CJ. Measles outbreaks in a population with declining vaccine uptake. *Science.* 2003;301:804.

Omer SB, Pan WK, Halsey NA, et al. Nonmedical exemptions to school immunization requirements: secular trends and association of state policies with pertussis incidence. *JAMA.* 2006;296:1757-1763.

Parker AA, Staggs W, Dayan GH, et al. Implications of a 2005 measles outbreak in Indiana for sustained elimination of measles in the United States. *N Engl J Med.* 2006;355:447-455.

Salmon DA, Haber M, Gangarosa EJ, Phillips L, Smith NJ, Chen RT. Health consequences of religious and philosophical exemptions from immunization laws: individual and societal risk of measles. *JAMA.* 1999;282:47-53.

Vaccine Protest Organizations

Poland GA, Jacobson RM. Understanding those who do not understand: a brief review of the anti-vaccine movement. *Vaccine.* 2001;19:2440-2445.

Blume S. Anti-vaccination movements and their interpretations. *Soc Sci Med.* 2006;62:628-642.

Immune Overload

Black SB, Cherry JD, Shinefield HR, Fireman B, Christenson P, Lampert D. Apparent decreased risk of invasive bacterial disease after heterologous childhood immunization. *Am J Dis Child.* 1991;145:746-749.

Davidson M, Letson GW, Ward JI, et al. DTP immunization and susceptibility to infectious diseases. Is there a relationship? *Am J Dis Child.* 1991;145:750-754.

Hviid A, Wohlfahrt J, Stellfeld M, Melbye M. Childhood vaccination and nontargeted infectious disease hospitalization. *JAMA.* 2005;294:699-705.

Offit PA, Quarles J, Gerber MA, et al. Addressing parents' concerns: do multiple vaccines overwhelm or weaken the infant's immune system? *Pediatrics.* 2002;109:124-129.

Otto S, Mahner B, Kadow I, Beck JF, Wiersbitzky SK, Bruns R. General non-specific morbidity is reduced after vaccination within the third month of life—the Greifswald study. *J Infect.* 2000;41:172-175.

Storsaeter J, Olin P, Renemar B, et al. Mortality and morbidity from invasive bacterial infections during a clinical trial of acellular pertussis vaccines in Sweden. *Pediatr Infect Dis J.* 1988;7:637-645.

MMR and Autism

Afzal MA, Minor PD, Begley J, et al. Absence of measles-virus genome in inflammatory bowel disease. *Lancet.* 1998;351:646-647.

D'Souza Y, Fombonne E, Ward BJ. No evidence of persisting measles virus in peripheral blood mononuclear cells from children with autism spectrum disorder. *Pediatrics.* 2006;118:1664-1675.

Dales L, Hammer SJ, Smith NJ. Time trends in autism and in MMR immunization coverage in California. *JAMA.* 2001;285:1183-1185.

Davis RL, Kramarz P, Bohlke K, et al; Vaccine Safety Datalink Team. Measles-mumps-rubella and other measles-containing vaccines do not increase the risk for inflammatory bowel disease: a case-control study from the Vaccine Safety Datalink project. *Arch Pediatr Adolesc Med.* 2001;155:354-359.

DeStefano F, Bhasin TK, Thompson WW, Yeargin-Allsopp M, Boyle C. Age at first measles-mumps-rubella vaccination in children with autism and school-matched control subjects: a population-based study in metropolitan Atlanta. *Pediatrics.* 2004;113:259-266.

Farrington CP, Miller E, Taylor B. MMR and autism: further evidence against a causal association. *Vaccine.* 2001;19:3632-3635.

Fombonne E, Chakrabarti S. No evidence for a new variant of measles-mumps-rubella-induced autism. *Pediatrics.* 2001;108:e58.

Kaye JA, del Mar Melero-Montes M, Jick H. Mumps, measles, and rubella vaccine and the incidence of autism recorded by general practitioners: a time trend analysis. *BMJ.* 2001;322:460-463.

Shattuck PT. The contribution of diagnostic substitution to the growing admninistrative prevalence of autism in US special education. *Pediatrics.* 2006;117:1028-1037.

Smeeth L, Cook C, Fombonne E, et al. MMR vaccination and pervasive developmental disorders: a case-control study. *Lancet.* 2004;364:963-969.

Taylor B, Miller E, Farrington CP, et al. Autism and measles, mumps, and rubella vaccine: no epidemiological evidence for a causal association. *Lancet.* 1999;353:2026-2029.

Taylor B, Miller E, Lingam R, Andrews N, Simmons A, Stowe J. Measles, mumps, and rubella vaccination and bowel problems or developmental regression in children with autism: population study. *BMJ.* 2002;324:393-396.

Wakefield AJ, Murch SH, Anthony A, et al. Ileal-lymphoid-nodular hyperplasia, non-specific colitis, and pervasive developmental disorder in children. *Lancet.* 1998;351:637-641.

Thimerosal and Autism

Andrews N, Miller E, Grant A, Stowe J, Osborne V, Taylor B. Thimerosal exposure in infants and developmental disorders: a retrospective cohort study in the United Kingdom does not support a causal association. *Pediatrics.* 2004;114:584-591.

Centers for Disease Control and Prevention (CDC). Thimerosal in vaccines: a joint statement of the American Academy of Pediatrics and the Public Health Service. *MMWR Morb Mortal Wkly Rep.* 1999;48:563-565.

Freed GL, Andreae MC, Cowan AE, Katz SL. The process of public policy formulation: the case of thimerosal in vaccines. *Pediatrics.* 2002;109:1153-1159.

Heron J, Golding J; ALSPAC Study Team. Thimerosal exposure in infants and developmental disorders: a prospective cohort study in the United Kingdom does not support a causal association. *Pediatrics.* 2004;114:577-583.

Luman ET, Fiore AE, Strine TW, Barker LE. Impact of thimerosal-related changes in hepatitis B vaccine birth-dose recommendations on childhood vaccination coverage. *JAMA.* 2004;291:2351-2358.

Madsen KM, Lauritsen MB, Pedersen CB, et al. Thimerosal and the occurrence of autism: negative ecological evidence from Danish population-based data. *Pediatrics.* 2003;112:604-606.

Offit PA, Jew RK. Addressing parents' concerns: do vaccines contain harmful preservatives, adjuvants, additives, or residuals? *Pediatrics.* 2003;112:1394-1397.

Pichichero ME, Gentile A, Giglio N, et al. Mercury levels in newborns and infants after receipt of thimerosal-containing vaccines. *Pediatrics.* 2008;121:e208-e214.

Stehr-Green P, Tull P, Stellfeld M, Mortenson PB, Simpson D. Autism and thimerosal-containing vaccines: lack of consistent evidence for an association. *Am J Prev Med.* 2003;25:101-106.

Thompson WW, Price C, Goodson B, et al; Vaccine Safety Datalink Team. Early thimerosal exposure and neuropsychological outcomes at 7 to 10 years. *N Engl J Med.* 2007;357:1281-1292.

Verstraeten T, Davis RL, DeStefano F, et al; Vaccine Safety Datalink Team. Safety of thimerosal-containing vaccines: a two-phased study of computerized health maintenance organization databases. *Pediatrics.* 2003;112:1039-1048.

Pertussis Vaccine and Encephalopathy

Gale JL, Thapa PB, Wassilak SG, Bobo JK, Mendelman PM, Foy HM. Risk of serious acute neurological illness after immunization with diphtheria-tetanus-pertussis vaccine. A population-based case-control study. *JAMA.* 1994;271:37-41.

Golden GS. Pertussis vaccine and injury to the brain. *J Pediatr.* 1990;116:854-861.

Griffin MR, Ray WA, Mortimer EA, Fenichel GM, Schaffner W. Risk of seizures and encephalopathy after immunization with the diphtheria-tetanus-pertussis vaccine. *JAMA.* 1990;263:1641-1645.

Howson CP, Howe CJ, Fineberg HV, eds. *Adverse Effects of Vaccines: A Report of the Committee to Review the Adverse Consequences of Pertussis and Rubella Vaccines.* Washington, DC: National Academy Press; 1991.

Kulenkampff M, Schwartzman JS, Wilson J. Neurological complications of pertussis inoculation. *Arch Dis Child.* 1974;49:46-49.

Miller D, Madge N, Diamond J, Wadsworth J, Ross E. Pertussis immunisation and serious acute neurological illnesses in children. *BMJ.* 1993;307:1171-1176.

Pollock TM, Morris J. A 7-year survey of disorders attributed to vaccination in North West Thames region. *Lancet.* 1983;1:753-757.

Ray P, Hayward J, Michelson D, et al; Vaccine Safety Datalink Group. Encephalopathy after whole-cell pertussis or measles vaccination: lack of evidence for a causal association in a retrospective case-control study. *Pediatr Infect Dis J.* 2006;25:768-773.

Shields WD, Nielsen C, Buch D, et al. Relationship of pertussis immunization to the onset of neurologic disorders: a retrospective epidemiologic study. *J Pediatr.* 1988;113:801-805.

Stratton KR, Howe CJ, Johnston RB, eds. *DPT Vaccine and Chronic Nervous System Dysfunction: A New Analysis.* Washington, DC: National Academy Press; 1994.

Influenza Vaccine and Guillain-Barré Syndrome

Centers for Disease Control and Prevention (CDC). Update: Guillain-Barré syndrome among recipients of Menactra meningococcal conjugate vaccine—United States, June 2005-September 2006. *MMWR Morb Mortal Wkly Rep.* 2006;55:1120-1124.

Haber P, DeStefano F, Angulo FJ, et al. Guillain-Barré syndrome following influenza vaccination. *JAMA.* 2004;292:2478-2481.

Hughes RA, Charlton J, Latinovic R, Gulliford MC. No association between immunization and Guillain-Barré syndrome in the United Kingdom, 1992 to 2000. *Arch Intern Med.* 2006;166:1301-1304.

Juurlink DN, Stukel TA, Kwong J, et al. Guillain-Barré syndrome after influenza vaccination in adults: a population-based study. *Arch Intern Med.* 2006;166:2217-2221.

Lasky T, Terracciano GJ, Magder L, et al. The Guillain-Barré syndrome and the 1992-1993 and 1993-1994 influenza vaccines. *N Engl J Med.* 1998;339:1797-1802.

HepB and Multiple Sclerosis

Ascherio A, Zhang SM, Hernán MA, et al. Hepatitis B vaccination and the risk of multiple sclerosis. *N Engl J Med.* 2001;344:327-332.

Confavreux C, Suissa S, Saddier P, Bourdès V, Vukusic S; Vaccines in Multiple Sclerosis Study Group. Vaccinations and the risk of relapse in multiple sclerosis. *N Engl J Med.* 2001;344:319-326.

De Keyser J, Zwanikken C, Boon M. Effects of influenza vaccination and influenza illness on exacerbations in multiple sclerosis. *J Neurol Sci.* 1998;159:51-53.

Fourrier A, Touze E, Alperovitch A, Begaud B. Association between hepatitis B vaccine and multiple sclerosis: a case-control study. *Pharmacoepidemiol Drug Saf.* 1999;8:S140-S141.

Hall A, Kane M, Roure C, Meheus A. Multiple sclerosis and hepatitis B vaccine? *Vaccine.* 1999;17:2473-2475.

Miller AE, Morgante LA, Buchwald LY, et al. A multicenter, randomized, double-blind, placebo-controlled trial of influenza immunization in multiple sclerosis. *Neurology.* 1997;48:312-314.

Sturkenboom MCJM, Abenhaim L, Wolfson C, Roulet E, Heinzelf O, Gout O. Vaccinations, demyelination, and multiple sclerosis study (VDAMS). *Pharmacoepidemiol Drug Saf.* 1999;8:S170-S171.

Fetal Cell Lines

Grabenstein JD. On the moral acceptability of certain viral vaccines. *Catholic Pharmacist.* 1996;29:2-4.

Hayflick L. The limited in vitro lifetime of human diploid cell strains. *Exp Cell Res.* 1965;37:614-636.

United States Conference of Catholic Bishops. Fact Sheet: Embryonic stem cell research and vaccines using fetal tissue. USCCB Web site. http://www.usccb.org/prolife/issues/bioethic/vaccfac2.shtml. Accessed August 15, 2008.

Zimmerman RK. Ethical analyses of vaccines grown in human cell strains derived from abortion: arguments and Internet search. *Vaccine* 2004;22:4238-4244.

Allergies and Autoimmune Diseases

Anderson HR, Poloniecki JD, Strachan DP, Beasley R, Björkstén B, Asher MI; ISAAC Phase 1 Study Group. Immunization and symptoms of atopic disease in children: results from the International Study of Asthma and Allergies in Childhood. *Am J Public Health.* 2001;91:1126-1129.

Black SB, Lewis E, Shinefield HR, et al. Lack of association between receipt of conjugate *Haemophilus influenzae* type b vaccine (HbOC) in infancy and risk of type 1 (juvenile onset) diabetes: long term follow-up of the HbOC efficacy trial cohort. *Pediatr Infect Dis J.* 2002;21:568-569.

DeStefano F, Gu D, Kramarz P, et al; Vaccine Safety Datalink Research Group. Childhood vaccinations and risk of asthma. *Pediatr Infect Dis J.* 2002;21:498-504.

DeStefano F, Mullooly JP, Okoro CA, et al; Vaccine Safety Datalink Team. Childhood vaccinations, vaccination timing, and risk of type 1 diabetes mellitus. *Pediatrics.* 2001;108:e112.

Graves PM, Barriga KJ, Norris JM, et al. Lack of association between early childhood immunizations and beta-cell autoimmunity. *Diabetes Care.* 1999;22:1694-1697.

Heijbel H, Chen RT, Dahlquist G. Cumulative incidence of childhood-onset IDDM is unaffected by pertussis immunization. *Diabetes Care.* 1997;20:173-175.

Hummel M, Füchtenbusch M, Schenker M, Ziegler AG. No major association of breast-feeding, vaccinations, and childhood viral diseases with early islet autoimmunity in the German BABYDIAB Study. *Diabetes Care.* 2000;23:969-974.

Kramarz P, DeStefano F, Gargiullo PM, et al. Does influenza vaccination exacerbate asthma? Analysis of a large cohort of children with asthma. Vaccine Safety Datalink Team. *Arch Fam Med.* 2000;9:617-623.

Nakajima K, Dharmage SC, Carlin JB, et al. Is childhood immunisation associated with atopic disease from age 7 to 32 years? *Thorax.* 2007;62:270-275.

Nicholson KG, Nguyen-Van-Tam JS, Ahmed AH, et al. Randomised placebo-controlled crossover trial on effect of inactivated influenza vaccine on pulmonary function in asthma. *Lancet.* 1998;351:326-331.

Nilsson L, Kjellman NI, Björkstén B. A randomized controlled trial of the effect of pertussis vaccines on atopic disease. *Arch Pediatr Adolesc Med.* 1998;152:734-738.

Offit PA, Hackett CJ. Addressing parents' concerns: do vaccines cause allergic or autoimmune diseases? *Pediatrics.* 2003;111:653-659.

Reid DW, Bromly CL, Stenton SC, Hendrick DJ, Bourke SJ. A double-blind placebo-controlled study of the effect of influenza vaccination on airway responsiveness in asthma. *Respir Med.* 1998;92:1010-1011.

Schaub B, Lauener R, von Mutius E. The many faces of the hygiene hypothesis. *J Allergy Clin Immunol.* 2006;117:969-977.

Wickens K, Crane J, Kemp T, et al. A case-control study of risk factors for asthma in New Zealand children. *Aust N Z J Public Health.* 2001;25:44-49.

Mad Cow Disease

Centers for Disease Control and Prevention (CDC). Public health service recommendations for the use of vaccines manufactured with bovine derived materials. *MMWR Morb Mortal Wkly Rep.* 2000;49:1137-1138.

Minor PD, Will RG, Salisbury D. Vaccines and variant CJD. *Vaccine.* 2000;19:409-410.

Transcripts of 27 July, 2000, Joint Meeting of the Transmissible Spongiform Encephalopathy and Vaccines and Related Biologicals Products Advisory Committees. The Food and Drug Administration Web site. http://www.fda.gov/cber/bse/bse.htm#tran. Accessed August 15, 2008.

Vaccines and Cancer

Ferber D. Virology. Monkey virus link to cancer grows stronger. *Science.* 2002;296:1012-1015.

López-Ríos F, Illei PB, Rusch V, Ladanyi M. Evidence against a role for SV40 infection in human mesotheliomas and high risk of false-positive PCR results owing to presence of SV40 sequences in common laboratory plasmids. *Lancet.* 2004;364:1157-1166.

Vaccines and AIDS

Berry N, Davis C, Jenkins A, et al. Vaccine safety. Analysis of oral polio vaccine CHAT stocks. *Nature.* 2001;410:1046-1047.

Korber B, Muldoon M, Theiler J, et al. Timing the ancestor of the HIV-1 pandemic strains. *Science.* 2000;288:1789-1796.

Plotkin SA. CHAT oral polio vaccine was not the source of human immunodeficiency virus type 1 group M for humans. *Clin Infect Dis.* 2001;32:1068-1084.

Poinar H, Kuch M, Pääbo S. Molecular analyses of oral polio vaccine samples. *Science.* 2001;292:743-744.

Vaccines and SIDS

Eriksen EM, Perlman JA, Miller A, et al. Lack of association between hepatitis B birth immunization and neonatal death: a population-based study from the vaccine safety datalink project. *Pediatr Infect Dis J.* 2004;23:656-662.

Fleming PJ, Blair PS, Platt MW, Tripp J, Smith IJ, Golding J. The UK accelerated immunisation programme and sudden unexpected death in infancy: case-control study. *BMJ.* 2001;322:822.

Griffin MR, Ray WA, Livengood JR, Schaffner W. Risk of sudden infant death syndrome after immunization with the diphtheria-tetanus-pertussis vaccine. *N Engl J Med.* 1988;319:618-623.

Niu MT, Salive ME, Ellenberg SS. Neonatal deaths after hepatitis B vaccine: the vaccine adverse event reporting system, 1991-1998. *Arch Pediatr Adolesc Med.* 1999;153:1279-1282.

9
Routine Vaccines

This chapter contains key information about vaccines that are routinely given in the United States and the diseases they prevent. Specifics about vaccine formulation, labeling, and general use are provided. See other chapters for discussion of concomitant use with other vaccines (Chapter 5, *General Recommendations*), catch-up schedules (Chapter 6, *Schedules*), use in special populations (Chapter 7, *Vaccination in Special Circumstances*), and public concerns (Chapter 8, *Addressing Concerns About Vaccines*).

Diphtheria, Tetanus, Pertussis

■ The Pathogens

Diphtheria

Corynebacterium diphtheriae is an aerobic, nonencapsulated, non–spore-forming, pleomorphic gram-positive bacillus that has a club-like appearance on Gram stain. Infection occurs on mucous membranes of the upper respiratory tract or in the skin, where the organism elaborates a potent exotoxin that works by inactivating tRNA transferase, preventing amino acids from being added to nascent polypeptide chains during protein synthesis. On respiratory surfaces like the throat, necrotic cells, inflammatory exudate, bacteria, and fibrin coalesce into adherent *pseudomembranes*. Local effects of the toxin include paralysis of the palate and hypopharynx; distant effects can be seen in the kidneys, liver, heart, and nervous system.

Tetanus

Clostridium tetani is a nonencapsulated, gram-positive, obligately anaerobic bacillus that has a drumstick or tennis racket appearance on Gram stain because of terminally located spores. Initial infection usually takes place in a deep, penetrating wound, where the organism elaborates *tetanospasmin*, a potent neurotoxin. The toxin spreads via the bloodstream and lymphatics to distant sites, where it is taken up into nerves through the neuromuscular junction and transported to the CNS. There it prevents the release of neurotransmitters at inhibitory synapses, causing unopposed lower motor-neuron activity, with resultant spasms and rigidity.

Pertussis

Bordetella pertussis is a tiny, aerobic, gram-negative coccobacillus that is tropic for ciliated respiratory epithelium. Attachment is mediated by several proteins, including *filamentous hemagglutinin* (FHA), *fimbriae* (FIM), and *pertactin* (PRN). The major virulence factor is *pertussis toxin* (PT), a complex molecule that causes increased intracellular levels of cAMP and disruption of cellular function. PT also facilitates adherence, promotes lymphocytosis, inhibits phagocytosis, increases insulin production (causing hypoglycemia) and increases sensitivity to histamine (causing vascular permeability and hypotension). PT and other toxins, including *tracheal cytotoxin* and *adenylate cyclase toxin*, are involved in the genesis of protracted cough.

■ Clinical Features

Diphtheria

The disease most often presents as *membranous nasopharyngitis* or *obstructive laryngotracheitis* associated with low-grade fever. Less commonly, cutaneous, vaginal, conjunctival, or otic infection can occur. Serious complications include upper airway obstruction caused by extensive membrane formation, myocarditis, and peripheral neuropathy. The case fatality rate is as high as 10% but is higher in young children and adults >40 years of age. Treatment includes antibiotics as well as equine antitoxin (available through the CDC), which neutralizes circulating toxin and prevents disease progression.

Tetanus

Most cases occur within 14 days of injury. Shorter incubation periods have been associated with more heavily contaminated wounds, more severe disease, and worse prognosis. *Generalized tetanus* (lockjaw) initially manifests with trismus, followed within a week by neck stiffness, dysphagia, rigidity of the abdominal muscles, and generalized muscle spasms. Severe spasms, often aggravated by external stimuli, persist for 3 to 4 weeks, and complete recovery may take months. *Neonatal tetanus* results from contamination of the umbilical stump. *Localized tetanus* manifests as muscle spasms in areas contiguous with an infected wound. *Cephalic tetanus* refers to cranial nerve dysfunction associated with infected wounds on the head and neck. Both localized and cephalic tetanus may precede generalized tetanus. Treatment includes tetanus immune globulin (BayTet; Bayer), which neutralizes unbound toxin. The case fatality rate is about 10%.

Pertussis

Classic *whooping cough* begins with mild upper respiratory tract symptoms (*catarrhal stage*) that last for 1 to 2 weeks. This progresses to severe paroxysms of cough (*paroxysmal stage*), often followed by a characteristic inspiratory whoop, that last for 4 to 6 weeks. Post-tussive emesis is common and the cough can be forceful enough to cause injury—rib fractures and even carotid artery dissections have been reported. Fever is minimal or absent and symptoms wane gradually (*convalescent stage*) over 6 to 10 weeks, giving rise to the colloquial term *the hundred-day cough*. Complications include seizures, pneumonia, and encephalopathy.

Pertussis is most severe during the first year of life. During 2000 to 2004, approximately 2500 cases were reported in infants <12 months of age—63% were hospitalized for a median duration of 5 days. Almost all deaths occur in young infants; of the 100 pertussis-related deaths reported from 2000 to 2004, 90 were among infants <4 months of age. Disease in infants <6 months of age may be atypical, with prominent apnea and absent whoop. Older children and adults may also have atypical disease, manifest solely as persistent cough, making recognition and treatment difficult. Infection in immunized children and older persons is often mild.

■ Epidemiology and Transmission

Diphtheria

Humans are the only known reservoir of *C diphtheriae*. Patients excrete the organism for 2 to 6 weeks in nasal discharge, from the throat, or from eye or skin lesions. Antibiotic treatment shortens the period of communicability. Transmission results from intimate contact, and illness is more common in crowded living situations. Although *infection* can still occur in immunized persons, *disease* generally does not because any elaborated toxin is neutralized by antibody. Respiratory diphtheria is seen in winter and spring; summer epidemics can occur in warm, moist climates where skin infections are prevalent. Despite dramatic declines in diphtheria in the United States since the 1940s (at the present time, an average of two to three annual cases are reported), toxigenic *C diphtheriae* can still be found in some populations. Diphtheria continues to be a significant cause of morbidity and mortality in developing countries.

Tetanus

Tetanus is not transmissible from person to person. Spores of *C tetani* are ubiquitous in the environment, especially where there is soil contaminated with excreta. Wounds, recognized or unrecognized, are where the organism multiplies and elaborates toxin. Contaminated wounds, those that result from deep puncture, and those with devitalized tissue are at greatest risk. Disease occurs worldwide but is more frequent in warmer climates and during warmer months, in part because contaminated wounds are more common. In 2003, the number of reported cases in the United States reached a low of 20. Neonatal tetanus is rare in the United States (two cases reported since 1989) but common in developing countries, where pregnant women may not be fully immunized and nonsterile umbilical cord–care practices are followed.

Pertussis

Humans are the only known hosts for *B pertussis*. Transmission occurs through respiratory droplets and direct contact with respiratory secretions, and acquisition rates approach 80% in susceptible household contacts. Patients are most contagious during the catarrhal stage, before the onset of paroxysms; communicability then diminishes rapidly but may persist for ≥3 weeks after onset of cough. Antibiotic therapy decreases infectivity and may limit spread. Asymptomatic infection has been demonstrated but may not be a significant factor in transmission.

Studies show that the prevalence of pertussis among adolescents and adults who have prolonged-cough illness may be as high as 50%. Many of these cases go unrecognized and untreated, and chemoprophylaxis of contacts does not take place, facilitating persistence and spread through communities. In fact, older individuals in the environment—parents, older siblings, non-household adults— are the most important source of transmission to young infants. Nearly 26,000 cases of pertussis were reported in 2004, but it is estimated that >1 million annual cases actually occur. The incidence of disease—approximately 100 cases per 100,000—is highest among infants <6 months of age. However, the greatest number of reported cases occurs among adolescents and young adults. School-based outbreaks are common.

■ Background on Immunization Program

Diphtheria

Introduction of diphtheria toxoid vaccines in the United States in the 1940s led to a dramatic reduction in disease incidence. High levels of vaccination have made diphtheria rare in the United States, and most cases today occur in unvaccinated or inadequately vaccinated persons. However, immunization does not completely eliminate the potential for transmission because it does not prevent carriage of the organism in the nasopharynx or on the skin. The consequences of inadequate immunization at the population level were demonstrated in Russia and other former Soviet countries in the 1990s, when over 150,000 cases and 5000 deaths occurred.

Tetanus

Following the introduction of tetanus toxoid vaccines in the United States, the incidence of tetanus declined from 0.4 per 100,000 in 1947 to 0.05 per 100,000 since the mid 1970s. Currently, the majority of tetanus cases occur in persons who have not completed a 3-dose primary series or who have uncertain vaccination histories. From 1998 to 2000, only one death is known to have occurred in an individual who had completed a primary immunization series; in this case, however, the last dose of tetanus toxoid was 11 years before the onset of illness. In contrast, 19 deaths occurred in individuals who had not completed a primary series or who had unknown vaccination histories. Because naturally acquired immunity to tetanus toxin does not occur, universal primary vaccination with appropriately timed boosters is the only way to protect persons in all age groups.

Pertussis

In the early 1940s, there were an average of 175,000 reported cases per year in the United States, for an incidence of 150 per 100,000. At the peak of activity in the prevaccine era, there were 265,000 cases of pertussis and 7500 deaths per year. After the introduction of universal infant immunization in the 1940s, the number of cases dramatically declined, dipping below 2000 around 1980 (for an incidence of approximately 1 per 100,000). Between 1980 and 2005, however, there was a dramatic *increase* in cases, making pertussis the only disease preventable by a routinely recommended vaccine that was on the rise. During this time, from 1991 to 1996, the whole-cell pertussis vaccine was gradually replaced by acellular vaccines, which were more effective and less reactogenic.

Some of the resurgence in reported pertussis cases was due to better diagnostic testing (eg, the use of PCR) and increased case-finding, but an important factor also was *waning immunity*. Protection from childhood immunization—and even from natural infection, for that matter—wanes after about 5 to 10 years. With the approval of Tdap vaccines for adolescents and adults in 2005, booster immunization became a possibility and, along with that, the opportunity to reduce disease in that age group as well as to impact a reservoir of pertussis in the community. The experience in Canada validated this approach—adolescent booster immunization was started there in 2000, and overall cases of pertussis steadily declined. In 2006, Tdap was recommended for all adolescents and adults in the United States.

9

■ Available Vaccines

Characteristics of the diphtheria, tetanus, and pertussis vaccines licensed in the United States are given in **Tables 9.1** and **9.2**.

■ Efficacy and/or Immunogenicity

Essentially 100% of individuals who receive any of the available diphtheria or tetanus toxoid-containing vaccines achieve protective antibody levels. The acellular pertussis vaccines have not been compared directly in head-to-head clinical trials, but efficacy estimates overlap enough so as to consider the products equivalent in terms of protection.

Tripedia was studied in trials in Sweden and Germany. In the Swedish trial involving 1389 infants who received 2 doses, efficacy was estimated at 81% for culture-confirmed cases with coughing spasms ≥21 days. In a German case-control study involving 16,780 children, 75% of whom had received Tripedia, efficacy of 3 doses was estimated at 80%; in this study, pertussis was defined as ≥21 days of cough plus a positive culture or a household contact with a positive culture.

In an Italian trial sponsored by the NIH that enrolled 15,601 infants, 4481 of whom received 3 doses of Infanrix, efficacy against typical pertussis (≥21 days of cough plus culture or

TABLE 9.1 — Diphtheria, Tetanus, and Pertussis Vaccines

	Adacel	Boostrix	Daptacel[a]	Infanrix[b]	Tripedia[c]
Trade name					
Abbreviation	Tdap	Tdap	DTaP	DTaP	DTaP
Manufacturer/distributor	Sanofi Pasteur	GlaxoSmithKline	Sanofi Pasteur	GlaxoSmithKline	Sanofi Pasteur
Type of vaccine:	Inactivated, purified subunits and toxoids	Inactivated, purified subunits and toxoids	Inactivated, purified subunits and toxoids	Inactivated, purified subunits and toxoids	Inactivated, purified subunits and toxoids
Composition:					
Diphtheria toxoid	2 Lf units	2.5 Lf units	15 Lf units	25 Lf units	6.7 Lf units
Tetanus toxoid	5 Lf units	5 Lf units	5 Lf units	10 Lf units	5 Lf units
Inactivated pertussis toxin	2.5 mcg	8 mcg	10 mcg	25 mcg	23.4 mcg
Filamentous hemagglutinin	5 mcg	8 mcg	5 mcg	25 mcg	23.4 mcg
Pertactin	3 mcg	2.5 mcg	3 mcg	8 mcg	—
Fimbriae types 2 and 3	5 mcg	—	5 mcg	—	—
Adjuvant	Aluminum phosphate (0.33 mg aluminum)	Aluminum hydroxide (≤0.39 mg aluminum)	Aluminum phosphate (0.33 mg aluminum)	Aluminum hydroxide (≤0.625 mg aluminum)	Aluminum potassium sulphate (≤0.17 mg aluminum)
Preservative	None	None	None	None	None
Excipients and contaminants:					
Formaldehyde	≤5 mcg	≤100 mcg	≤5 mcg	≤100 mcg	≤100 mcg

Glutaraldehyde	$\leq$50 ng	—	$\leq$50 ng	—	—
2-phenoxyethanol	3.3 mg	—	3.3 mg	—	—
Polysorbate 80	—	$\leq$100 mcg	—	$\leq$100 mcg	Unspecified amount
Thimerosal	—	—	—	—	$\leq$0.3 mcg mercury
Gelatin	—	—	—	—	Unspecified amount
Latex	None	Tip cap and plunger of prefilled syringe contain dry natural rubber	Vial stopper contains dry natural rubber	Tip cap and plunger of prefilled syringe contain dry natural rubber	Vial stopper contains dry natural rubber
Labeled indications	Active booster immunization	Active booster immunization	Active immunization	Active immunization	Active immunization
Labeled ages	11 to 64 years	10 to 18 years	6 weeks to 6 years	6 weeks to 6 years	6 weeks to 6 years
Dose	0.5 mL	0.5 mL	0.5 mL	0.5 mL	0.5 mL
Route of administration	Intramuscular	Intramuscular	Intramuscular	Intramuscular	Intramuscular
Usual schedule	1 dose	1 dose	2, 4, 6, 15 to 20 months, 4 to 6 years of age	2, 4, 6, 15 to 20 months, 4 to 6 years of age	2, 4, 6, 15 to 18 months, 4 to 6 years of age
How supplied (number in package):					
1-dose vial	(5, 10)	(10)	(1, 5, 10)	(10)	(10)
Prefilled syringe	(5)	(5)	—	(5)	—

9

Continued

TABLE 9.1 — *Continued*

Trade name	Adacel	Boostrix	Daptacel[a]	Infanrix[b]	Tripedia[c]
Storage	Refrigerate	Refrigerate	Refrigerate	Refrigerate	Refrigerate
	Do not freeze	Do not freeze	Do not freeze	Do not freeze	Do not freeze
Reference package insert	January 2006	June 2007	March 2008	August 2007	December 2003

[a] A DTaP vaccine similar to Daptacel is also available in combination with Hib and IPV (Pentacel; Sanofi Pasteur); in this case, ActHIB is reconstituted with liquid DTaP-IPV that is packaged with the product. Pentacel is indicated at 2, 4, 6, and 15 to 18 months of age.

[b] Infanrix is available in combination with HepB and IPV (Pediarix; GlaxoSmithKline). Pediarix is indicated at 2, 4, and 6 months of age. Infanrix is also available in combination with IPV (Kinrix; GlaxoSmithKline). Kinrix is indicated for the booster dose at 4 to 6 years of age.

[c] Tripedia is also available in combination with Hib (TriHIBit; Sanofi Pasteur); in this case the Hib (ActHIB) is supplied lyophilized in 1-dose vials and the liquid Tripedia that is packaged with the Hib is used for reconstitution. TriHIBit is indicated only for the fourth dose of DTaP.

serologic confirmation) was 84%. Efficacy against milder disease, defined as >7 days of cough, was 71%. Protection against typical pertussis was sustained to 6 years of age. In a German household-contact study involving 22,000 children, Infanrix was 89% effective against typical pertussis and 81% effective against disease with ≥7 days of paroxysmal cough.

In a Swedish trial involving 9829 infants, 2587 of whom received 3 doses of Daptacel, efficacy against typical pertussis was 85%. Efficacy against milder disease, defined as ≥1 day of cough, was 78%. Protection was sustained during the 2-year follow-up period.

Both Tdap vaccines, Boostrix and Adacel, were licensed on the basis of immunogenicity rather than efficacy. In each case, the antibody response to pertussis antigens after a single dose was noninferior to the analogous infant DTaP vaccines, for which efficacy had been previously demonstrated.

■ **Safety**

Local pain, swelling, and erythema are common after DTaP administration, reported in up to 40% of vaccinees during the primary series. The rate of local reactions is higher with dose 4 and dose 5, and swelling of the entire limb, sometimes accompanied by fever, has been reported. Such reactions are self-limited, resolve without sequelae, and are *not* contraindications to further doses. Clinically significant fever is reported in <5% of DTaP recipients.

Tdap appears to be slightly more painful than Td, with local pain and/or tenderness in up to 75% of vaccinees (60% to 70% for Td); swelling and erythema occur in around 20% of recipients of either Tdap or Td. Fever occurs in <5%.

• *Contraindications for DTaP*
  – Allergic reaction to previous dose of vaccine or any vaccine component (risk of recurrent allergic reaction)
  – Encephalopathy within 7 days of receiving a pertussis-containing vaccine (risk of recurrent encephalopathy [causality not established] and difficulty distinguishing illness from vaccine reaction)
  – Progressive neurologic disorder (risk of neurologic deterioration [causality not established] and difficulty distinguishing illness from vaccine reaction)
• *Contraindications for Tdap*
  – Allergic reaction to previous dose of vaccine or any vaccine component (risk of recurrent allergic reaction)
  – Encephalopathy within 7 days of receiving a pertussis-containing vaccine (risk of recurrent encephalopathy [causality not established] and difficulty distinguishing illness from vaccine reaction)
• *Contraindications for DT, Td, and TT*
  – Allergic reaction to previous dose of vaccine or any vaccine component (risk of recurrent allergic reaction)

TABLE 9.2 — Diphtheria and Tetanus Vaccines[a]

	Decavac	Diphtheria and Tetanus Toxoids Adsorbed USP (for Pediatric Use)	Tetanus Toxoid Adsorbed
Trade name			
Abbreviation	Td	DT	TT
Manufacturer/distributor	Sanofi Pasteur	Sanofi Pasteur	Sanofi Pasteur
Type of vaccine	Inactivated, toxoids	Inactivated, toxoids	Inactivated, toxoids
Composition	Diphtheria toxoid (2 Lf units) Tetanus toxoid (5 Lf units)	Diphtheria toxoid (6.7 Lf units) Tetanus toxoid (5 Lf units)	Tetanus toxoid (5 Lf units)
Adjuvant	Aluminum potassium sulfate (≤0.28 mg aluminum)	Aluminum potassium sulfate (≤0.17 mg aluminum)	Aluminum potassium sulfate (≤0.25 mg aluminum)
Preservative	None	None	None
Excipients and contaminants	Formaldehyde (≤0.02%) Thimerosal (≤0.3 mcg mercury)	Formaldehyde (≤0.02%) Thimerosal (≤0.3 mcg mercury)	Formaldehyde (≤0.02%) Thimerosal (≤0.3 mcg mercury)
Latex	None	Vial stopper contains dry natural rubber	None
Labeled indications	Active immunization against diphtheria and tetanus	Active immunization against diphtheria and tetanus	Active immunization against tetanus
Labeled ages	≥7 years	6 weeks to 6 years	≥7 years
Dose	0.5 mL	0.5 mL	0.5 mL
Route of administration	Intramuscular	Intramuscular	Intramuscular

Usual schedule	2 doses 4 to 8 weeks apart; reinforcing dose 6 to 12 months after dose 2; booster dose	3 doses 4 to 8 weeks apart; reinforcing dose 6 to 12 months after dose 3; booster dose	2 doses 4 to 8 weeks apart; reinforcing dose 6 to 12 months after dose 2; booster dose
How supplied (number in package)	1-dose vial (10) Prefilled syringe (10)	1-dose vial (10)	1-dose vial (10)
Storage	Refrigerate Do not freeze	Refrigerate Do not freeze	Refrigerate Do not freeze
Reference package insert	December 2005	October 2001	December 2005

[a] Tetanus and Diphtheria Toxoids Adsorbed for Adult Use made by the Massachusetts Public Health Biologic Laboratories is no longer available. Tenivac, manufactured by Sanofi Pasteur, is licensed in the United States but not distributed.

- *Precautions for DTaP*
  - Moderate or severe acute illness (difficulty distinguishing illness from vaccine reaction)
  - Any of these conditions after receiving a DTaP vaccine
    - Otherwise unexplained fever ≥105°F (40.5°C) within 48 hours (risk of recurrent fever)
    - Collapse or shock-like state (hypotonic hyporesponsive episode) within 48 hours (risk of recurrent reaction)
    - Persistent, inconsolable crying lasting ≥3 hours within 48 hours (risk of recurrent reaction)
    - Seizure with or without fever occurring within 72 hours (risk of recurrent seizure)
  - Guillain-Barré syndrome within 6 weeks of receiving a tetanus toxoid–containing vaccine (risk of recurrent Guillain-Barré syndrome)
- *Precautions for Tdap*
  - Moderate or severe acute illness (difficulty distinguishing illness from vaccine reaction)
  - Progressive neurologic disorder (risk of neurologic deterioration [causality not established] and difficulty distinguishing illness from vaccine reaction)
  - Guillain-Barré syndrome within 6 weeks of receiving a tetanus toxoid–containing vaccine (risk of recurrent Guillain-Barré syndrome)
  - Severe local (Arthus-type) reaction to previous dose of tetanus and/or diphtheria toxoid–containing vaccine in the last 10 years (risk of recurrent reaction)
- *Precautions for DT, Td, and TT*
  - Moderate or severe acute illness (difficulty distinguishing illness from vaccine reaction)
  - Guillain-Barré syndrome within 6 weeks of receiving a tetanus toxoid–containing vaccine (risk of recurrent Guillain-Barré syndrome)
  - Severe local (Arthus-type) reaction to previous dose of tetanus and/or diphtheria toxoid–containing vaccine in the last 10 years (risk of recurrent reaction)

■ Recommendations for General Use

All individuals should be vaccinated against diphtheria, tetanus, and pertussis, and immunity should be maintained through booster immunization. The primary series of DTaP consists of doses at 2, 4, 6, and 15 to 18 months of age; dose 4 may be given at 12 to 14 months of age if ≥6 months have elapsed since dose 3 and the child is unlikely to return at 15 to 18 months of age. A booster dose of DTaP is given at 4 to 6 years of age (this is optional if dose 4 was given at ≥4 years of age), and while there is a preference to use the same brand of DTaP for all 5 doses, any brand may be used if this is not feasible. An additional booster in the form of Tdap is given at 11 to 12 years of age. If contraindications to pertussis immunization exist, DT may be used for children and Td may be used for adolescents. However, if pertussis vaccination is deferred during the first year of life because of the possibility of an evolving neurologic condition, DT should not be given because the risk of diphtheria or tetanus is very low. By 1 year of age, if the neurologic condition is deemed to be nonprogressive, the DTaP series may be initiated; if the condition *is* progressive, the series should be given as DT.

Children who have had well-documented pertussis (ie, laboratory confirmed or linked to a confirmed case) may not need further pertussis immunization until they reach adolescence and become eligible for the booster dose of Tdap. However, since the duration of protection from natural disease is unknown and there is no harm in continuing the vaccine series, it makes practical sense do so unless there are contraindications. Patients who have had diphtheria or tetanus should still be immunized because natural infection does not confer immunity (the amount of toxin is too small to induce effective immune responses).

All individuals 11 to 64 years of age who have never had a dose of Tdap should have one. As a matter of routine, the dose should be given at 11 to 12 years of age, in place of the historically recommended dose of Td. Tdap may be given at the same time as MCV4 and (for girls) HPV vaccine. The AAP recommends a minimum interval of 1 month between MCV4 and Tdap if they are not given on the same day; the ACIP does not recommend a minimum interval.

If not given at 11 to 12 years of age, Tdap should be given at the next available opportunity, provided enough time has elapsed since the last tetanus toxoid–containing vaccine (the risk of local reactions increases when too many doses of tetanus toxoid are given too close together). The manufacturers of Tdap recommend a minimum interval of 5 years between the last dose of a tetanus toxoid–containing vaccine and a dose of Tdap. However, there are data supporting the safety of intervals as short as 2 years, and in truth there is no absolute minimum interval—Tdap may be given regardless of when the last tetanus toxoid–containing vaccine was received. Giving it earlier than 5 years should be considered when the risk of pertussis or its complications (in the individual or his or her contacts) is elevated (eg, outbreak situations, household exposure, chronic pulmonary and neurologic conditions, individuals who have close contact with infants <12 months of age, health care workers, women who may become pregnant).

As a matter of routine, Tdap should replace the next scheduled 10-year Td booster for adults. For adolescents and adults who have not had a complete series (at least 3 doses) of tetanus or diphtheria toxoid vaccines, Tdap should be given followed by 2 doses of Td at least 4 weeks apart. Tdap should be used in place of Td for wound management for all individuals who have not previously had a dose.

Postpartum women who have never received Tdap should receive a dose before discharge from the hospital. The recommended interval since the last dose of Td is 2 years, but shorter intervals may be used if there is no history of moderate-to-severe adverse reactions to previous doses of tetanus and diphtheria toxoid–containing vaccines. The dose of Tdap "resets the clock" for the next decennial dose of tetanus and diphtheria toxoid vaccines. Pregnant women who are not immune to tetanus or who require a diphtheria booster should receive either Td or Tdap. Pregnant women who are likely to be tetanus immune should either receive Tdap or have vaccination deferred until after delivery, when they should receive Tdap. Tetanus immunity is likely in the following situations:

- Women ≤30 years of age who received a complete childhood series of tetanus toxoid–containing vaccine and at least 1 booster as an adolescent or adult (the primary series in childhood consists of 4 or 5 doses, and in adolescents and adults, it consists of 3 doses)
- Women ≥31 years of age who received a complete childhood series and at least 2 boosters, or who received a primary series as an adolescent or adult
- Tetanus antibody level ≥0.10 IU/mL

The following should be taken into account when deciding whether or not a pregnant woman should receive Tdap during pregnancy:

- Tdap should be strongly considered if there is an increased risk of pertussis (the AAP favors giving Tdap to pregnant adolescents for this reason).
- There are no data on safety, immunogenicity, pregnancy outcomes, and protection of the infant against pertussis.
- There is the theoretic possibility that transplacental antibodies could interfere with infant immunization.
- If given, the second or third trimester is preferred.

The use of tetanus toxoid–containing vaccines and tetanus immune globulin for wound management is summarized in **Table 9.3**.

Haemophilus influenzae Type b

■ The Pathogen

H influenzae type b is an aerobic gram-negative bacterium that appears as pleomorphic coccobacilli on Gram's stain. The organism produces a polysaccharide capsule that contributes to virulence by inhibiting complement-mediated lysis and phagocytosis by neutrophils. Colonization of the nasopharynx is facilitated by factors that mediate adherence to respiratory epithelium and interfere with ciliary clearance, as well as immune evasion mechanisms such as IgA1 protease. Disease results from bacteremia and spread to distant sites like the meninges.

Clinical Features

The most common forms of invasive *H influenzae* type b disease are *meningitis*, *bacteremia*, *epiglottitis*, *pneumonia*, *arthritis*, and *periorbital* and *buccal cellulitis*. Meningitis is the most common clinical manifestation, accounting for 50% to 65% of cases in the prevaccine era. Hallmark presenting features include fever, altered mental status, and stiff neck. The mortality rate is 2% to 5%, even with appropriate antimicrobial therapy, and neurologic sequelae occur in 15% to 30% of survivors. Osteomyelitis and pericarditis are less common. Otitis media and acute bronchitis due to *H influenzae* are generally caused by nontypable (nonencapsulated) strains.

Epidemiology and Transmission

Humans are the only natural hosts and transmission occurs by direct person-to-person contact or via respiratory droplets. The organism does not survive on fomites. Asymptomatic nasopharyngeal colonization was seen in 2% to 5% of children in the prevaccine era, but widespread use of *H influenzae* conjugate vaccine (Hib) has resulted in much lower colonization rates. Invasive disease now is extremely rare. *H influenzae* type b disease was more frequent in boys, African-Americans, Alaska Eskimos, Apache and Navajo Indians, child care center attendees, children living in overcrowded conditions, and children who were not breast-fed. Unimmunized children, particularly those <4 years of age who were in prolonged close (eg, household) contact with an infected child, were at high risk. Other factors predisposing to invasive infection included sickle cell disease, asplenia, HIV infection, certain immunodeficiency syndromes, and malignant neoplasms.

Many laboratories are now relatively inexperienced in identifying *H influenzae* type b, and many isolates that are labeled as such turn out to be other serotypes or nontypable strains when subjected to molecular genetic analysis.

Background on Immunization Program

Prior to the introduction of routine childhood immunization, *H influenzae* type b was a major cause of invasive bacterial infection in the United States, with an estimated 12,000 cases of meningitis and 8000 other invasive syndromes annually. A striking one out of every 200 children in the first 5 years of life developed invasive *H influenzae* type b infection, with peak incidence in 6- to 12-month-olds. In high-risk populations, disease rates were even higher.

Since 1988, when Hib was first introduced in the United States, the incidence of invasive disease in infants and young children has declined by >99%. This remarkable reduction in disease burden was partly due to the ability of conjugate vaccines to reduce nasopharyngeal carriage, leading to reduced rates of exposure and infection even in those not immunized (this is an example of herd immunity; see Chapter 1, *Introduction to Vaccinology*). Today,

TABLE 9.3 — Tetanus Prophylaxis in Wound Management

Primary Series of Tetanus-Toxoid Vaccine[c]	Age (Years)	Time Since Last Dose of Vaccine	Clean, Minor Wounds		Tetanus-Prone Wounds[a]	
			Vaccine	TIG[b]	Vaccine	TIG[b]
Complete[c]	≤6	<5 years	No	No	No	No
		>5 years	DTaP[d,e]	No	DTaP[e]	No
	7 to 10	<5 years	No	No	No	No
		>5 years	Td[f]	No	Td[f]	No
	≥11	<5 years	No	No	No	No
		>5 years	Tdap[g]	No	Tdap[h]	No
Unimmunized, unknown, incomplete, or HIV-infected[i]	≤6	Not relevant	DTaP[d,e]	No	DTaP[e]	Yes
	7 to 10		Td[f]	No	Td[f]	Yes
	≥11		Tdap[g]	No	Tdap[h]	Yes

a Includes puncture, avulsion, crush, necrotic, and burn wounds; frostbite; and wounds contaminated with dirt, feces, soil, saliva. Wounds should be cleaned, necrotic tissue debrided, and foreign material removed.

b The dose of TIG is 250 units given intramuscularly. Immune globulin intravenous can be used if TIG is not available. Equine tetanus antitoxin is not available in the United States. Vaccine and TIG should be given at separate sites.

c The primary series is considered complete if the patient has received ≥3 doses of an adsorbed (not fluid) tetanus toxoid. HIV-infected individuals should be considered *unimmunized* even if they have received the vaccine series.

d A booster dose of DTaP is routinely indicated for all children at 4 to 6 years of age, so a dose should be given for children ≤6 years of age who have not received a routine booster, even for clean, minor wounds (vaccination here is for catch-up, not wound management).

e Use DT if pertussis immunization is contraindicated.

f Td is preferred but tetanus toxoid can be used; only adsorbed products are indicated.

g One dose of Tdap is routinely indicated for all adolescents and adults, so a dose should be given (if not previously received) even for clean, minor wounds (vaccination here is for catch-up, not wound management). Use Td if pertussis immunization is contraindicated.

h If Tdap is not available or has been given previously, Td (or tetanus toxoid, if Td is not available) should be used. No Tdap is licensed for use in patients >64 years of age. Use Td if pertussis immunization is contraindicated.

i For infants <6 months of age who have not received the 3-dose primary series, decisions about the use of TIG should be based on the mother's vaccination history.

invasive *H influenzae* type b disease is seen primarily in underimmunized children and infants too young to have completed the primary series.

■ **Available Vaccines**

Characteristics of the Hib vaccines licensed in the United States are given in **Table 9.4**.

■ **Efficacy and/or Immunogenicity**

Efficacy of PRP-OMPC (PedvaxHIB) was first demonstrated in Navajo infants who had very high rates of invasive infection. After a primary 2-dose regimen given at 2 and 4 months of age, 91% of infants had anti-PRP antibody levels >0.15 mcg/mL and 60% had levels >1 mcg/mL, and efficacy at 15 to 18 months of age was 93% (see *Chapter 1* for discussion of serologic correlates of protection). In infants drawn from the general US population who received the 2-dose primary series, 97% achieved anti-PRP antibody levels >0.15 mcg/mL and 80%, >1 mcg/mL; the levels after a booster at 12 to 15 months were 99% and 95%, respectively. PedvaxHIB is the only vaccine that induces significant antibody levels after a single injection in infants <6 months of age.

Licensure of PRP-T (ActHIB) was based on immunogenicity that was comparable to that of the other licensed products. Overall, about 90% of infants achieve anti-PRP antibody levels of ≥1 mcg/mL after the primary series of 3 doses, and 98% achieve this level after a booster dose.

Children ≥15 months of age respond well to a single dose of either vaccine.

■ **Safety**

Local reactions such as redness, swelling and pain occur in 5% to 30% of recipients, but typically are mild and last <24 hours. Systemic reactions, such as fever and irritability, are infrequent. Serious adverse events such as anaphylaxis are rare.

- *Contraindications*
  - Allergic reaction to previous dose of vaccine or any vaccine component (risk of recurrent allergic reaction)
  - Age <6 weeks (risk of induction of immune tolerance)
- *Precautions*
  - Moderate or severe acute illness (difficulty distinguishing illness from vaccine reaction)

■ **Recommendations for General Use**

All infants should be vaccinated against *H influenzae*. The primary series for ActHIB consists of doses at 2, 4, and 6 months of age; the primary series for PedvaxHIB consists of doses at 2 and 4 months of age. For both vaccines, booster doses are given at 12 to 15 months of age. Previously unimmunized children 15 to 59 months should receive a single dose of either vaccine.

Hepatitis A

■ The Pathogen

Hepatitis A virus (HAV) is a small, nonenveloped, single-stranded RNA virus in the Picornaviridae family. There is only one known serotype. Initial infection occurs in the pharynx and lower GI tract, with hematogenous spread to the liver, where the virus replicates in hepatocytes and Kupffer cells (resident macrophages). It is believed that most of the injury to the liver is immune mediated rather than the direct result of viral replication. Virus is excreted in the bile and ultimately shed in the stool. Unlike HBV, HAV does not establish chronic infection and does not cause chronic liver disease.

■ Clinical Features

Ninety percent of children <5 years of age with HAV infection are asymptomatic, whereas 90% of adults experience symptoms such as jaundice. The incubation period ranges from 15 to 50 days. Onset is usually abrupt, with low-grade fever, myalgia, poor appetite, nausea, vomiting, malaise, and fatigue, followed by dark-colored urine, scleral icterus, pale stools, jaundice, and weight loss. Diarrhea is more common in children. Hepatomegaly, right upper quadrant tenderness, and occasionally splenomegaly or rash may be present. Symptoms generally subside within 3 to 4 weeks, although 10% to 15% of patients experience prolonged or relapsing disease for up to 6 months. Fulminant hepatitis is rare. Extrahepatic manifestations include arthralgias, pruritus, cutaneous vasculitis, cryoglobulinemia, hemophagocytic syndrome, and Guillain-Barré syndrome.

■ Epidemiology and Transmission

Humans are the only natural hosts and transmission occurs by the fecal-oral route. Peak infectivity occurs during the 2-week period before the onset of jaundice, and infants and children can shed the virus for several months. Since infants and young children often have clinically silent infection and exposure to their feces may be unavoidable, they are often the source of infection for adults in households or day care centers. Contaminated water and undercooked food (especially shellfish) are also common sources of transmission—often a food handler somewhere down the line is infected. Transient viremia in a blood donor occasionally leads to transmission through transfusion of blood products.

Hepatitis A is most prevalent in Southeast Asia, Africa, and Latin America. In countries with high endemnicity, the infection is usually acquired in childhood, whereas in developed countries many adults have not yet been exposed. Childhood disease often correlates with overcrowding, poor sanitation, limited access to clean water, and inadequate sewage systems. Prior to the institution of a universal immunization program in the United States, the incidence of *disease* was highest among children 5 to 14 years of

TABLE 9.4 — Hib Vaccines[a]

Trade name	ActHIB[b,c]	PedvaxHIB[b,d]
Abbreviation	PRP-T	PRP-OMPC
Manufacturer/distributor	Sanofi Pasteur	Merck
Type of vaccine	Inactivated, engineered subunit	Inactivated, engineered subunit
Composition	Polyribosylribitol phosphate (10 mcg) conjugated to tetanus toxoid (24 mcg)	Polyribosylribitol phosphate (7.5 mcg) conjugated to *Neisseria meningitidis* serogroup B (strain B11) outer-membrane protein (125 mcg)
Adjuvant	None	Aluminum hydroxide (0.225 mg aluminum)
Preservative	None	None
Excipients and contaminants	Sucrose (8.5%)	Sodium chloride (0.9%)
Latex	Vial stopper contains dry natural rubber	None
Labeled indications	Immunization against invasive *Haemophilus influenzae* type b disease	Immunization against invasive *H influenzae* type b disease
Labeled ages	2 to 18 months	2 to 71 months
Dose	0.5 mL	0.5 mL
Route of administration	Intramuscular	Intramuscular
Usual schedule	2, 4, 6, 12 to 15 months of age	2, 4, 12 to 15 months of age[e]
How supplied (number in package)	1-dose vial (5), lyophilized, with diluent	1-dose vial (10)

Storage	Vaccine: refrigerate, do not freeze	Refrigerate
	Diluent: refrigerate, do not freeze	Do not freeze
	Reconstituted vaccine: use within 24 hours	
Reference package insert	December 2005	January 2001

[a] ProHIBit (PRP-D; Connaught) and HibTITER (HbOC; Wyeth) are no longer available.

[b] ActHIB and PedvaxHIB are considered interchangeable. However, if either the 2-month or 4-month dose is given as ActHIB, a dose of either product must be given at 6 months. If the first 2 doses are PedvaxHIB, the 6-month dose is omitted.

[c] ActHIB is also available in combination with DTaP (TriHIBit; Sanofi Pasteur); in this case, ActHIB is reconstituted with liquid DTaP (Tripedia) that is packaged with the product. TriHIBit is indicated only for the fourth dose of DTaP. ActHIB is also available in combination with DTaP and IPV (Pentacel; Sanofi Pasteur); in this case, ActHIB is reconstituted with liquid DTaP-IPV that is packaged with the product. Pentacel is indicated at 2, 4, 6, and 15 to 18 months of age.

[d] PedvaxHIB is also available in combination with HepB (Comvax; Merck). Comvax is indicated at 2, 4, and 12 to 15 months of age.

[e] The primary series for PedvaxHIB consists of only 2 doses.

9

age, but the incidence of *infection* was highest in those <4 years of age. Infection was more common among American Indians, Alaska natives, and Hispanics. Disease rates were substantially higher in the western United States; between 1987 and 1997, half of all cases occurred in 11 states west of the Mississippi. The majority of patients in the United States in 2006 (65.2%) had no known risk factor for hepatitis A. The most important *known* risk factor was international travel (14.7% of cases); other risk factors were sexual or household contact with a case (10.2%), male homosexual activity (9.3%), food- or waterborne outbreaks (7.5%), employment or attendance at a day care center (4.2%), contact with a day care employee or attendee (4.3%), injection drug use (2.1%), and other known contact with a case (12.7%).

■ Background on Immunization Program

In the prevaccine era, there were 22,000 to 36,000 annual reported cases of hepatitis A and an estimated 271,000 annual HAV infections in the United States. Up to 22% of patients were hospitalized, and the average work lost for these patients was 33 days. Annual direct and indirect costs were as high as $488 million (1997 dollars).

In 1996, HepA was recommended for high-risk groups and children living in communities with the highest rates of infection. In 1999, universal vaccination of all children ≥2 years of age was recommended in states, counties, and communities whose average annual reported incidence of hepatitis A was ≥20 cases per 100,000 population (at least twice the national average between 1987 and 1997). At the time, those states were Arizona, Alaska, Oregon, New Mexico, Utah, Washington, Oklahoma, South Dakota, Idaho, Nevada, and California. Routine immunization was also considered for children living in areas where the average annual reported incidence was ≥10 but <20 cases per 100,000 population; those states were Missouri, Texas, Colorado, Arkansas, Montana, and Wyoming. For areas with high rates of disease, routine vaccination of children beginning at 2 years of age, catch-up vaccination of preschool children, and vaccination of older children (10 to 15 years of age) was recommended.

After these recommendations were instituted, hepatitis A declined dramatically in the United States, a demonstration of the remarkable ability of childhood immunization to prevent disease in an entire population (see *Chapter 1* and **Figure 1**.6 for discussion of herd immunity related to vaccination against hepatitis A). By 2006, there were only 3579 symptomatic cases reported, for an incidence of 1.2 per 100,000, the lowest ever recorded (the estimated number of infections was 32,000). As might have been expected, the disease burden decreased and the highest incidence of disease moved from the West to other regions of the country. In 2006, new age indications for both available vaccines (down to 12 months) made it easier to consider incorporation of HepA into the routine childhood schedule, and the final step in the incremental national strategy to control hepatitis A was taken—the recommendation to immunize all young children. This was seen as creating the foundation for eventual elimination of indigenous transmission.

■ Available Vaccines

Characteristics of the hepatitis A vaccines licensed in the United States are given in **Table 9.5**.

■ Efficacy and/or Immunogenicity

Nearly 100% of individuals who receive 2 doses of either vaccine achieve protective levels of antibody to HAV. Seroconversion rates within 1 month of the first dose exceed 95%. Based on kinetic models of antibody decay, protective antibody may persist for up to 20 years in children and ≥25 years in adults.

The efficacy of Havrix was evaluated in a study of 40,119 school children in Thailand aged 1 to 16 years. Two doses of vaccine (360 ELISA units each) or placebo were administered 1 month apart. Two children in the vaccine group and 32 in the control group developed hepatitis A, indicating an efficacy of approximately 94%. In children 2 to 19 years of age (N=314), 1 dose (720 ELISA units) resulted in seroconversion rates of 96.8% to 100%, and 2 doses given 6 months apart resulted in seroconversion rates of 100%. In studies involving over 400 adults, 1 dose (1440 ELISA units) resulted in seroconversion rates of >96%; 100% of adults (N=269) were seropositive 1 month after a booster dose. In children immunized with 2 doses 6 months apart beginning at 11 to 13 months of age (N=218), the vaccine response rate was 99%. Persistence of antibody was evaluated in a study of 1016 subjects who had received a 3-dose schedule as adults; 10 years out, 98.3% still had protective levels of antibody.

The efficacy of Vaqta was evaluated in a study of 1037 healthy seronegative children 2 to 16 years of age in Monroe County, New York, a small community with a historically high infection rate. A single dose of vaccine (25 units) or placebo was administered. Beyond the immediate postvaccination period, there were no cases of hepatitis A in the vaccine group and 21 confirmed cases in the placebo group, for an efficacy of 100%. After this study, a subset of vaccinees received a booster dose of vaccine. No cases of hepatitis A occurred among these individuals in the 9 years they were monitored. In Butte County, CA, a mass immunization campaign in children 2 to 12 years of age between 1995 and 2000 resulted in a 93.5% decline in cases in the entire county population (see **Figure 1.6**).

In studies of children 12 to 23 months of age, seroconversion rates were 96% of 471 and 100% of 343, respectively, for 1 or 2 doses of Vaqta (25 units). In studies of children 2 to 18 years of age, seroconversion rates were 97% in 1230 and 100% in 1057, respectively, for 1 or 2 doses (25 units). In studies of adults, seroconversion rates were 95% in 1411 and 99.9% in 1244, respectively, for 1 or 2 doses (50 units).

TABLE 9.5 — HepA Vaccines

Trade name	Havrix[a,b]	Vaqta[b]
Abbreviation	HepA	HepA
Manufacturer/distributor	GlaxoSmithKline	Merck
Type of vaccine	Inactivated, whole agent	Inactivated, whole agent
Composition:[c]		
Virus	HM175 strain	CR326F strain
Propagation culture	Human diploid (MRC-5) cells	Human diploid (MRC-5) cells
Inactivation	Formalin	Formalin
Pediatric/adolescent formulation	720 ELISA units/0.5 mL	25 U/0.5 mL
Adult formulation	1440 ELISA units/mL	50 U/mL
Adjuvant	Aluminum hydroxide (0.25 mg/0.5 mL aluminum)	Aluminum hydroxide (0.225 mg/0.5 mL aluminum)
Preservative	None	None
Excipients and contaminants	Amino acid supplement (0.3%)	Formaldehyde ($\leq$0.8 mcg/mL)
	Phosphate-buffered saline	Nonviral protein (<0.1 mcg/mL)
	Polysorbate 20 (0.05 mg/mL)	DNA ($<4 \times 10^{-6}$ mcg/mL)
	Residual MRC-5 cellular proteins ($\leq$5 mcg/mL)	Bovine albumin ($\leq$0.0001 mcg/mL)
	Formalin ($\leq$0.1 mg/mL)	Sodium borate (70 mcg/mL)
	Neomycin ($\leq$40 ng/mL)	Sodium chloride (0.9%)

Latex	Tip cap and plunger of prefilled syringe contain dry natural rubber	Vial stopper and plunger of prefilled syringe contain dry natural rubber
Labeled indications	Immunization against disease caused by HAV	Immunization against disease caused by HAV
Labeled ages	≥12 months	≥12 months
Dose:[d]		
Pediatric (1 to 18 years)	0.5 mL	0.5 mL
Adult (≥19 years)	1.0 mL	1.0 mL
Route of administration	Intramuscular	Intramuscular
Usual schedule	0, 6 to 12 months	0, 6 to 18 months
How supplied (number in package):		
Pediatric/adolescent formulation	1-dose vial (10) Prefilled syringe (5)	1-dose vial (1, 10) Prefilled syringe (6)
Adult formulation	1-dose vial (10) Prefilled syringe (5)	1-dose vial (1, 10) Prefilled syringe (1, 6)
Storage	Refrigerate Do not freeze	Refrigerate Do not freeze
Reference package insert	December 2006	December 2007

[a] Havrix is also available in combination with HepB (Twinrix; GlaxoSmithKline).
[b] Havrix and Vaqta are considered interchangeable.
[c] The units used to measure antigen content for these vaccines are different and cannot be directly compared.
[d] The patient's age at the time of the dose determines which formulation is used.

■ Safety

Reactions are usually mild and subside within 24 hours. Mild injection-site reactions, including erythema, swelling, pain, or tenderness, occur in 20% to 50% of patients. Systemic reactions, including low-grade fever, malaise, and fatigue, are reported in <10% of vaccinees. No serious adverse events have been reported.

- *Contraindications*
  - Allergic reaction to previous dose of vaccine or any vaccine component (risk of recurrent allergic reaction)
- *Precautions*
  - Moderate or severe acute illness (difficulty distinguishing illness from vaccine reaction)
  - Pregnancy (theoretic risk to the fetus or attribution of birth defects to vaccination, although no deleterious effects from HepA administered during pregnancy have been demonstrated)

■ Recommendations for General Use

Pre-exposure Prophylaxis

All children should be vaccinated against hepatitis A during the second year of life. The first dose of HepA is usually given at 12 months of age and the second at 18 to 23 months of age. Vaccination for children 2 to 18 years of age should continue in areas that had catch-up programs in place based on the 1999 recommendations; catch-up vaccination for children 2 to 18 years of age in other communities is optional.

The following persons are at increased risk for hepatitis A and *should be routinely vaccinated*:

- Persons traveling to or working in countries with high or intermediate endemnicity
- Men who have sex with men (the risk is thought to relate to fecal-oral contact)
- Injection and noninjection illegal drugs users (transmission probably occurs through percutaneous and fecal-oral routes)
- Persons who work with HAV-infected primates or with HAV in a research laboratory
- Persons who have clotting-factor disorders (outbreaks presumably due to blood from donors who were viremic at the time of donation were reported in the early 1990s)
- Persons who have chronic liver disease, including those who are waiting for or have received liver transplants (these individuals are particularly susceptible to severe disease)

Vaccination *should be considered* for juveniles in correctional facilities. For most travelers to endemic areas, vaccination is now preferred to the use of immune globulin (see *Chapter 7*).

Routine vaccination is *not* considered necessary for the following:

- Health care workers
- Persons attending or working in child care centers
- Caretakers in institutions for the developmentally challenged
- Persons working in correctional facilities
- Persons working in waste management
- Food service workers, unless recommended by state or local authorities

Postexposure Prophylaxis

In the past, prophylaxis with immune globulin was recommended for susceptible individuals after exposure to hepatitis A. However, immune globulin is expensive, relatively painful, difficult to obtain, and only offers transient protection. A randomized, double-blind trial results published in 2007, as well as experience from other countries, suggest that postexposure vaccination also is effective. The recommendations below are for *unimmunized individuals* exposed to hepatitis A (individuals who received at least 1 dose of vaccine at least 1 month before exposure are considered immune). Prophylaxis should be initiated as soon as possible after exposure, but preferably within 2 weeks (efficacy beyond 2 weeks is questionable). Only monovalent HepA should be used for the following indications:

- *12 months to 40 years of age*: Vaccination is preferred.
- *>40 years of age*: Immune globulin (0.02 mL/kg intramuscularly) is preferred but vaccine can be given if immune globulin is not available. If the person has other reasons to be vaccinated with HepA, he or she should receive a dose of the vaccine simultaneously (at a separate site) and receive the second dose at the appropriate interval.
- *<12 months of age, immunocompromised individuals, those with chronic liver disease, and those in whom vaccination is contraindicated*: Immune globulin (0.02 mL/kg intramuscularly) should be given. Immunocompromised individuals and those with chronic liver disease should receive a dose of the vaccine simultaneously (at a separate site) and receive the second dose at the appropriate interval.

The following situations constitute a high risk of exposure to hepatitis A and warrant postexposure prophylaxis (if the individuals were not previously immunized):

- Household and sexual contacts of a case (consider also for individuals with ongoing close personal contact such as occurs with regular babysitting)
- Persons who have shared illicit drugs with a case
- Staff members and attendees at day care centers and day care homes if there has been one or more case in employees or attendees, or if two or more cases occur in the households of attendees. If the center does not have children who are in diapers, prophylaxis should be given only to classroom contacts of the index case. If three or more families are affected,

prophylaxis should be considered for members of households that have children in diapers who attend the center.

- Other food handlers at an establishment where there is an index case in a food handler. Prophylaxis of patrons should be considered if the index case could have contaminated food because of diarrhea and poor hygienic practices, and only if the patrons can be identified and treated within 2 weeks of exposure. Institutional cafeterias might represent a higher risk to patrons than other establishments. In a common-source outbreak, prophylaxis should not be given once cases begin to occur since by then, the 2-week window for effective prophylaxis will have been exceeded.
- Prophylaxis is indicated in the school or hospital setting only if transmission from an index case has been demonstrated.

Hepatitis B

■ The Pathogen

HBV is a nonenveloped, partially double-stranded DNA virus in the Hepadnaviridae family. The virus infects hepatocytes but is not directly cytopathic; instead, damage occurs through the action of cytotoxic T cells directed against virus-infected hepatocytes. Immune tolerance leads to persistent infection in some individuals; hallmark features include low-grade chronic hepatitis and HBsAg (a surface protein of the virion that is overproduced) in the serum, as well as an increased lifetime risk of hepatocellular carcinoma. One factor that contributes to carcinogenesis is chronic inflammation, with attendant regeneration, fibrosis, and the accumulation of cellular mutations. Another factor is the random integration of HBV DNA into the host chromosome, resulting in mutations that either inactivate tumor suppressor genes or activate oncogenes. Finally, much attention has focused on the viral X protein, which can upregulate the expression of host cell oncogenes.

■ Clinical Features

The incubation period ranges from 6 weeks to 6 months and averages 120 days. The clinical course of acute infection is indistinguishable from that of other types of viral hepatitis. While infants and children are usually asymptomatic, clinical signs and symptoms occur in about 50% of adults. The prodromal phase usually lasts 3 to 10 days and is characterized by the insidious onset of malaise, anorexia, nausea, vomiting, right upper-quadrant abdominal pain, fever, headache, myalgia, rash, arthralgia, arthritis, and dark urine. The icteric phase, which usually lasts from 1 to 3 weeks, is characterized by jaundice, elevated hepatic transaminases, light or gray-colored stools, liver tenderness, and hepatomegaly (splenomegaly is less common). During convalescence, malaise and fatigue may persist for weeks to months, while jaundice, anorexia, and other symptoms disappear.

Most acute hepatitis B infections in adults result in complete recovery, with disappearance of HBsAg from the blood and the production of HBsAb (antibody directed against HBsAg), which provides for lasting immunity. However, 90% of infants, 30% of young children, and <5% of adults with acute infection become persistently infected (so-called "chronic carriers"). Premature death from cirrhosis, liver failure, or hepatocellular carcinoma occurs in 25% of those who become persistently infected in childhood and in 15% of those who become persistently infected after childhood.

■ Epidemiology and Transmission

Humans are the only natural hosts and transmission occurs by contact with contaminated secretions, including semen, vaginal secretions, blood, and saliva; through percutaneous inoculation (eg, accidental needlesticks or sharing of needles with infected people); or by maternal-neonatal transmission (the risk is about 10% if the mother is a chronic carrier). Almost half of the world's population lives in areas where ≥8% of the population is persistently infected; in China, southeast Asia, most of Africa, most of the Pacific Islands, parts of the Middle East, and the Amazon basin, 8% to 15% of the population are chronic carriers, and most individuals are infected at birth or in early childhood. The lifetime risk of infection in these areas exceeds 60%. An estimated 2 billion people worldwide have been infected with HBV and 350 million are chronic hepatitis B carriers.

Between 2001 and 2005 in the United States, 39% of newly acquired adult cases were associated with heterosexual activity, 24% with male homosexual activity, and 16% with injection drug use. Occupational, household, travel, and health care–related exposures accounted for 5% of new cases, and no identified risk factor was found in 16%. From 1988 to 1994, the age-adjusted prevalence of HBV infection in the United States population was about 5%; approximately 1 million people, or 0.4%, were chronically infected.

■ Background on Immunization Program

While acute hepatitis B can cause significant morbidity and even death, a major rationale for immunization is to prevent chronic carriage. This is because chronic carriers are often asymptomatic, can infect others over long periods of time, and are at increased risk for developing cirrhosis and primary hepatocellular carcinoma. Each year in the United States there are up to 4000 deaths from hepatitis B–related cirrhosis and 1500 from liver cancer. Data from Alaska show that universal childhood immunization can decrease the prevalence of chronic carriage, and data from Taiwan demonstrate that universal HepB immunization can decrease the incidence of hepatocellular carcinoma. This makes HepB vaccine the first vaccine that prevents a human cancer.

Selective vaccination of high-risk populations in the 1980s failed to impact disease burden. The rationale for universal vaccination at birth, which was recommended in 1991, includes the following:

- The vaccine is immunogenic in infants.
- Potentially reduces the number of concurrent injections that must be given at the 2-month visit
- Increases the likelihood that the entire 3-dose series will be completed
- Protects infants born to carrier mothers whose HBsAg status is not known at delivery (because such a high proportion of infected infants develop chronic carriage, preventing perinatal infection can have a major impact on the incidence of cirrhosis and hepatocellular carcinoma later in life)
- Emphasizes the importance of immunization for new parents and lays the groundwork for the routine schedule in infancy

In 2006, there were 4713 reported cases of acute hepatitis B, for an overall incidence of 1.6 per 100,000 population. This was the lowest rate ever recorded and represents an 81% decline since 1990.

In situations where exposure has occurred, the long incubation period allows for postexposure prophylaxis through vaccination. However, even an accelerated vaccine series requires a minimum of 4 months to complete, and the series cannot be completed in neonates until 24 weeks of age. Therefore, passive immunization with hepatitis B immune globulin (HBIG) is a necessary adjunct to active vaccination for immediate protection after exposure.

■ Available Vaccines

Characteristics of the hepatitis B vaccines licensed in the United States are given in **Table 9.6**.

■ Efficacy and/or Immunogenicity

Engerix-B was found to be 95% effective in preventing perinatal infection when given without immunoglubulin to newborns ($N=58$; 0, 1, 2 month schedule) of mothers who were chronic carriers. Of neonates ($N=52$) given the vaccine at 0, 1, and 6 months of age, 97% achieved a seroprotective level of antibody (≥ 10 mIU/ mL). Seroprotection rates of 98% were seen in children 6 months to 10 years of age ($N=242$) and 97% in adolescents ($N=119$) after a 3-dose schedule. Studies in adolescents and adults demonstrate seroprotection rates of >95% after 3 doses, although responses are somewhat lower in those >40 years of age.

Recombivax HB was found to be 95% effective in preventing perinatal transmission among 130 high-risk infants who were given concomitant HBIG. With 3 doses of vaccine, protective levels of antibody were achieved in 100% of infants ($N=92$), 99% of children ($N=129$), and 99% of adolescents ($N=112$). Response rates in adults were 98% in those 20 to 29 years of age ($N=787$), 94% in those 30 to 39 years of age ($N = 249$), and 89% in those

≥40 years of age ($N=177$). Seroprotection rates in adolescents who received the 2-dose regimen ($N=255$) were 99%.

Although antibody titers after HepB vaccination wane with time, immune memory and protection remain intact for >20 years. A study from The Gambia, for example, showed that 50% of individuals followed for ≥15 years had antibody levels that fell below 10 mIU/mL. Despite this, efficacy was 83% against infection and 97% against chronic carriage.

■ Safety

The most common adverse reaction following HepB vaccination is pain at the site of injection, reported in 13% to 29% of adults and 3% to 9% of children. Mild systemic complaints, such as fatigue, headache, and irritability, have been reported in 11% to 17% of adults and up to 20% of children. Low-grade fever is seen in 1% of adults and in up to 6% of children. It should be noted that well over 1 billion doses of HepB have been given worldwide since the 1980s, and serious systemic adverse events and allergic reactions have rarely been reported.

- *Contraindications*
  - Allergic reaction to previous dose of vaccine or any vaccine component, including baker's yeast (risk of recurrent allergic reaction)
- *Precautions*
  - Moderate or severe acute illness (difficulty distinguishing illness from vaccine reaction)
  - Infant weight <2000 g, unless the mother is HBsAg-positive (risk of poor response to vaccination)

■ Recommendations for General Use

Universal Infant, Child, and Adolescent Immunization

All infants should be vaccinated against hepatitis B. The usual schedule for HepB is a dose at birth (before hospital discharge), 1 to 2 months of age, and 6 to 18 months of age (6 to 12 months of age for high-risk groups such as Alaska natives, Pacific Islanders, and immigrants from areas like Asia and Africa). Only monovalent vaccine may be used for the birth dose. Infants who receive subsequent doses as DTaP-HepB-IPV (Pediarix) or HepB-Hib (Comvax) may receive an extra dose at 4 months of age; this does not increase reactogenicity or impair the immune response. The birth dose should be implemented by *standing order* and should be deferred only by a physician's order, with a copy of the mother's *recent* negative HBsAg test result on the infant's chart. If the birth dose is deferred, the first dose of HepB should be administered before 2 months of age. The birth dose *should not be deferred* if the mother is HBsAg-positive (see below), had any behavioral risk factors for HBV infection during pregnancy, or if the infant is unlikely to return for follow-up. However, the birth dose *should be deferred* for preterm infants weighing <2000

TABLE 9.6 — HepB Vaccines

	Engerix-B[a,b]	Recombivax HB[b,c]
Trade name	Engerix-B[a,b]	Recombivax HB[b,c]
Abbreviation	HepB	HepB
Manufacturer/distributor	GlaxoSmithKline	Merck
Type of vaccine	Inactivated, engineered subunit	Inactivated, engineered subunit
Composition:	HBsAg expressed in yeast (Saccharomyces cerevisiae)	HBsAg (adw subtype) expressed in yeast (S cerevisiae)
Pediatric/adolescent formulation	10 mcg/0.5 mL	5 mcg/0.5 mL
Adult formulation	20 mcg/mL	10 mcg/mL
Dialysis formulation	—	40 mcg/mL
Adjuvant	Aluminum hydroxide (0.25 mg/0.5 mL aluminum)	Aluminum hydroxide (0.25 mg/0.5 mL aluminum)
Preservative	None	None
Excipients and contaminants	Yeast protein (≤5%) Sodium chloride (9 mg/mL) Disodium phosphate dihydrate (0.98 mg/mL) Sodium dihydrogen phosphate dihydrate (0.71 mg/mL)	Yeast protein (≤5%)
Latex	Tip cap and plunger of prefilled syringe contain dry natural rubber	Not reported

	Immunization against infection caused by all known subtypes of HBV	Immunization against infection caused by all known subtypes of HBV
Labeled indications		
Labeled ages	All ages	All ages
Dose:		
Pediatric/adolescent formulation (≤19 years)	0.5 mL[d]	0.5 mL
Adult formulation (≥20 years)	1 mL[d]	1 mL[g]
Hemodialysis formulation	2 simultaneous adult doses of 1 mL each[e,f]	1 mL[f]
Route of administration	Intramuscular[h]	Intramuscular[h]
Usual schedule:	0, 1, 6 months of age[i]	0, 1, 6 months of age[i]
Hemodialysis patients	0, 1, 2, and 6 months; periodic boosters[f,j]	0, 1, 6 months; periodic boosters[f,j]
Alternate dosing for 11 to 15 years of age	—	Adult formulation at 1, 4 to 6 months[g]
How supplied (number in package):		
Pediatric/adolescent formulation	1-dose vial (10)	1-dose vial (10)
	Prefilled syringe (5)	Prefilled syringe (6)
Adult formulation	1-dose vial (10)	1-dose vial (1, 10)
	Prefilled syringe (5)	Prefilled syringe (1, 6)
Hemodialysis formulation	—	1-dose vial (1)
Storage	Refrigerate	Refrigerate
	Do not freeze	Do not freeze
Reference package insert	December 2006	December 2007

Continued

9

TABLE 9.6 — *Continued*

[a] Engerix-B is also available in combination with DTaP and IPV (Pediarix; GlaxoSmithKline) and with HepA (Twinrix; GlaxoSmithKline).

[b] Engerix-B and Recombivax HB are considered interchangeable except for the 2-dose schedule in adolescents, for which only Recombivax HB is approved.

[c] Recombivax HB is also available in combination with Hib (Comvax; Merck).

[d] Adolescents 11 to 19 years of age may receive the adult formulation.

[e] There is no specific hemodialysis formulation. The 40-mcg/2 mL dose can be constituted by 2 separate injections of the adult (20-mcg/mL) formulation at the same site or by combining 2 adult doses in the same syringe.

[f] Hemodialysis patients need higher doses to respond.

[g] An adult dose (10 mcg/mL) may be constituted by 2 separate injections of the pediatric (5 mcg/0.5 mL) formulation at the same site or by combining 2 pediatric doses in the same syringe.

[h] May be administered subcutaneously in patients who are at risk of hemorrhage with intramuscular injections (eg, hemophiliacs). However, reactogenicity may be increased and immunogenicity decreased.

[i] Other dosing regimens are contained in the package insert.

[j] Booster doses are given when annual testing shows that HBsAb levels have fallen below 10 mIU/mL. Annual testing with periodic booster doses may be indicated for other immunocompromised persons, such as those with HIV infection, hematopoietic stem-cell transplant recipients, and those receiving chemotherapy.

g whose mother is HBsAg-negative. These infants should be vaccinated at 1 month of age or at hospital discharge, whichever comes first (babies are assumed to be medically stable and gaining weight consistently if discharged before 1 month of age).

All children and adolescents ≤18 years of age who were not vaccinated as infants should receive HepB. Routine postvaccination testing for HBsAb is not recommended.

Adult Vaccination

Vaccination is recommended for the following:
- Sex partners of persons who are HBsAg-positive
- Persons with more than one sex partner in the past 6 months
- Persons seeking evaluation or treatment for a sexually transmitted disease
- Men who have sex with men
- Injection drug users
- Household contacts of HBsAg-positive persons
- Residents and staff of facilities for developmentally disabled persons
- Health care and public safety workers at risk for infection through exposure to blood or blood-contaminated body fluids, including hospital, institutional, and laboratory employees, students, contractors, physicians, emergency medical technicians, paramedics, and volunteers
- Patients with end-stage renal disease, including those on hemodialysis and peritoneal dialysis (vaccination of patients with renal failure is encouraged before they require hemodialysis)
- Patients with chronic liver disease
- Persons with HIV infection
- Travelers to regions where the prevalence of chronic infection is ≥2%
- Inmates undergoing medical evaluation at a correctional facility
- Anyone who wants protection from hepatitis B

Standing orders for HepB administration should be implemented in settings where high-risk individuals are seen, including sexually transmitted disease and HIV clinics, drug abuse treatment centers, correctional facilities, facilities that care for men who have sex with men, kidney disease programs, and facilities for the developmentally disabled. Prevaccination testing might reduce costs by avoiding vaccination of persons who are already immune, and is recommended for the following groups: persons born in areas where the prevalence of chronic infection is ≥8%; household, sex, and needle-sharing contacts of HBsAg-positive persons; HIV-infected persons; other populations in whom the prevalence of chronic infection exceeds 20%. The preferred test is for antibody to hepatitis B core antigen, since this identifies all people with previous infection. Testing for HBsAb can be used, but must be done along with testing for HBsAg, since chronic carriers may have negative tests for HBsAb.

Testing for HBsAb 1 to 2 months after vaccination is recommended for the following groups: health care and public safety workers at high risk for exposure to blood or body fluids; chronic hemodialysis patients; HIV-infected and other immunocompromised persons; and sex partners of HBsAg-positive persons. Levels ≥10 mIU/mL are considered protective. Patients with antibody levels <10 mIU/mL should receive a second 3-dose series of HepB, followed by repeat testing. If the result is still <10 mIU/mL, the person should be tested for HBsAg, since chronic carriage is a reason for nonresponse to vaccination. If they are negative for HBsAg, they are considered primary nonresponders; these individuals may respond to intradermal vaccination, although neither HepB product is labeled for this route of administration. Periodic (eg, annual) testing for HBsAb after vaccination is only recommended for dialysis patients and other immunocompromised persons, including those with HIV infection, hematopoietic stem-cell transplant recipients, and persons receiving chemotherapy.

Postexposure Prophylaxis for Infants of HBsAg-Positive and HBsAg-Unknown Mothers

All pregnant women should be tested for HBsAg early on in each pregnancy. Women who were not screened prenatally, those who are at high risk for infection, and those with clinical hepatitis should be tested at the time of delivery. A physical copy of the test results should be provided to the birthing hospital and the newborn's health care provider.

Infants born to mothers who are HBsAg-positive should receive HepB and HBIG (0.5 mL intramuscularly) at separate sites within 12 hours of birth. The vaccine series should be completed with dose 2 at 1 to 2 months of age and dose 3 at 6 months of age. For preterm infants weighing <2000 g, both vaccine and HBIG should be given as well, but the vaccine dose should not count toward the complete series, since responses are not reliable; the first valid dose is given at 1 month of age, the second at 2 to 3 months, and the third at 6 months. Both term and preterm infants of HBsAg-positive mothers should be tested for HBsAg and HBsAb at 9 to 18 months of age (not earlier than 4 weeks after the last dose). Those with protective levels of antibody and a negative HBsAg test need no further medical management. Those without protective levels of antibody who are HBsAg-negative should receive a second 3-dose vaccine series and should be tested again 1 to 2 months after completion. Those who are HBsAg-positive should receive appropriate medical management.

Infants born to mothers whose HBsAg status is unknown or not documented at the time of delivery should be vaccinated within 12 hours of birth, and the mother should be tested. If she is HBsAg-positive, the baby should receive HBIG before 7 days of age and should complete the HepB series at 6 months of age. If

302

she is HBsAg-negative, the HepB series should be completed by 6 to 18 months of age. If the mother is not tested, the baby should complete the HepB series by 6 months of age, but HBIG should not be given—unless the baby is preterm and weighs <2000 g. In this situation, if the mother's status will not be known within 12 hours of birth, both vaccine and HBIG should be given and the infant should be followed as if born to an HBsAg-positive mother.

Postexposure Prophylaxis in Other Settings

Recommendations for the management of potential occupational and nonoccupational exposures to HBV are given in **Tables 9.7** and **9.8**, respectively.

HBIG is a hyperimmune globulin preparation made from the plasma of donors who have high titers of HBsAb. The donors are screened for antibodies to HIV and hepatitis C virus, as well as for hepatitis C virus RNA. In addition, the manufacturing process inactivates known bloodborne viruses. HBIG is administered intramuscularly at the same time as HepB but at a different site (the deltoid or gluteal regions are preferred). Available products in the United States include Nabi-HB (North American Biologicals) and HepaGam B (Cangene). The only contraindication is a history of anaphylaxis to a previous dose of human immune globulin. Certain safety issues are common to all immune globulin products, including the possibility of allergic reaction to residual IgA in the product in IgA-deficient individuals and the possibility of transmission of bloodborne pathogens that are not killed in the manufacturing process.

Human Papillomavirus

■ The Pathogen

Human papillomavirus (HPV) is a small, nonenveloped, double-stranded DNA virus in the family Papillomaviridae that is tropic for epithelial surfaces. The virion capsid is composed of major and minor late proteins, L1 and L2. The oncogenic HPV types—most notably 16 and 18, but including as well types 33, 45, 31, 58, 52, and others—are a *necessary* but not *sufficient* cause of cervical cancer. In other words, the virus *must* be present for cervical cancer to develop, but the majority of women who acquire the virus do not develop cancer. Approximately 90% of new infections clear within 2 years, and it is only the remaining 10% of persistent infections that can lead to cancer. It is important to note that certain biologic factors put young women at particularly high risk for infection, persistence, and ultimately neoplasia. The most important of these is the presence of the *cervical transformation zone*, an area of immature metaplasia between the prepubertal squamocolumnar junction (where the squamous cells of the vagina meet the columnar epithelial cells of the endocervix, originally found peripheral to the cervical

TABLE 9.7 — Management of Potential Occupational Exposures to HBV[a]

Vaccination Status of Exposed Person	Response to Vaccination[b]	HBsAg Status of Source Individual		
		Positive	Negative	Unknown[c]
Not vaccinated or incompletely vaccinated (<3 doses)	—	Give HBIG[d] and initiate or complete HepB series[e]	Initiate or complete HepB series[e]	Initiate or complete HepB series[e]
Vaccinated	Responder[f]	No treatment	No treatment	No treatment
	Nonresponder[f]	Patients who *have not* received a second complete 3-dose HepB series: 1 dose of HBIG[d] and initiate second 3-dose HepB series[e] Patients who *have* received a second complete 3-dose HepB series: 2 doses of HBIG[d] separated by 1 month	No treatment	If high-risk, assume HBsAg-positive and treat accordingly
	Antibody level unknown—test exposed person for HBsAb:			
	Adequate response[f]	No treatment	No treatment	No treatment
	Inadequate response[f]	Give HBIG[d] and a booster dose of HepB[e,g]	No treatment	Give booster dose of HepB[e,h]

a Percutaneous exposures include needle sticks, lacerations, and bites. Permucosal exposures include splashes of blood, any fluid containing visible blood, other potentially infectious fluid (including semen; vaginal secretions; CSF; synovial, pleural, peritoneal, pericardial, or amniotic fluids; tracheal secretions; and saliva), or tissue onto any mucosal surface, including the conjunctival, oral, and buccal mucosa.

b Testing for HBsAb 1 to 2 months after vaccination is recommended for health care and public safety workers at high risk for exposure to blood or body fluids.

c Efforts should be made to test the source individual for HBsAg.

d The dose is 0.06 mL/kg given intramuscularly. HBIG should be given as soon as possible after exposure, preferrably within 24 hours. Intervals exceeding 7 days are unlikely to be of benefit after percutaneous exposure.

e The first dose should be given as soon as possible, preferably within 24 hours.

f An adequate response is ≥10 mIU/mL of HBsAb 1 to 2 months postvaccination.

g Test for HBsAb in 4 to 6 months. If the level is inadequate, give 2 more doses to complete a second 3-dose series.

h Test for HBsAb in 1 to 2 months. If the level is inadequate, give 2 more doses to complete a second 3-dose series.

Centers for Disease Control and Prevention. *MMWR.* 2001;50(RR-11):1-52.

TABLE 9.8 — Management of Potential Nonoccupational Exposures to HBV[a]

Status of Exposed Individual	Source HBsAg Status[b]	Management
Not vaccinated or incompletely vaccinated (<3 doses)	Positive	Initiate or complete HepB series[c] Give HBIG[d]
	Unknown[e]	Initiate or complete HepB series[c]
Vaccinated[f]	Positive	Give a booster dose of HepB[c]
	Unknown[e]	No treatment

[a] Percutaneous exposures include needle sticks (needle sharing), lacerations, and bites. Permucosal exposures include splashes of blood, any fluid containing visible blood, other potentially infectious fluid (including semen; vaginal secretions; CSF; synovial, pleural, peritoneal, pericardial, or amniotic fluids; tracheal secretions; and saliva), or tissue onto any mucosal surface, including the conjunctival, oral and buccal mucosa.

[b] Exposures to individuals who are known to be HBsAg-negative do not require prophylaxis.

[c] The first dose should be given as soon as possible, preferably within 24 hours.

[d] The dose is 0.06 mL/kg given intramuscularly. HBIG should be given as soon as possible after exposure, preferably within 24 hours. Intervals exceeding 7 days after percutaneous exposure and 14 days after sexual exposure are unlikely to be of benefit.

[e] Efforts should be made to test the source individual for HBsAg. Needles and syringes discarded in public places, presumably by injection drug users, pose a risk of transmission since HBV can survive on environmental surfaces for up to 7 days. However, the risk depends on the prevalence of hepatitis B in the drug-abusing population and the amount of blood in the needle. There is no consensus opinion regarding the use of HBIG in these situations.

[f] Written documentation of a complete 3-dose series of HepB should be provided.

Centers for Disease Control and Prevention. *MMWR*. 2006;55(RR-16):1-25.

opening) and the postpubertal junction, found inside the cervical opening.

HPV initially reaches dividing cells in the basal layer of the cervical epithelium, commonly at the transformation zone, through minute fissures and abrasions. DNA replication and early cell differentiation occur together, but expression of the viral proteins E6 and E7 prevents further cell differentiation and causes delayed cell-cycle arrest. These proteins also help the infected cell evade host-immune responses. The result is a vertical expansion of the dividing cell population. Integration of viral DNA into the host genome results in overexpression of E6 and E7, leading to further unchecked cell proliferation and the accumulation of germ-line mutations, which ultimately lead to invasive cancer.

Some HPV types—most notably 6 and 11—cause genital warts rather than cancer, although they may cause low-grade cervical dysplasia that eventually regresses.

■ Clinical Features

HPV is one of the few human viruses unequivocally linked to cancer (others include HBV and EBV). *Squamous cell carcinoma of the cervix* comprises 75% of cervical cancers in the United States; the remainder are *adenocarcinomas*. HPV 16 and 18 cause approximately 70% of squamous cell carcinomas and 80% of adenocarcinomas. Most HPV infections are asymptomatic and self-limited. In a minority of women, persistent infection leads to progressive dysplasia, referred to as *cervical intraepithelial neoplasia* grades 1 (CIN 1) through 3 (CIN 3). Approximately 60% of CIN 1 cases spontaneously regress and <1% lead to cancer. On the other hand, only 30% to 40% of CIN 2/3 lesions regress, and >12% develop into cancer. The Pap test is used to detect dysplasia early so treatment can be initiated. The duration of time from the first intraepithelial lesion to invasive cancer is 15 to 20 years.

HPV also causes *vaginal and vulvar intraepithelial neoplasia* (VaIN and VIN) that can progress to cancer; up to 50% of vulvar and vaginal cancers are caused by HPV. Up to 90% of *anal cancers*, 50% of *penile cancers*, and 20% of *oropharyngeal cancers* are also caused by HPV. For most of these tumors, types 16 and 18 predominate.

Approximately 90% of *anogenital warts* are caused by types 6 and 11. These are typically small, soft flesh-colored growths that are raised to varying degrees; some develop into large, cauliflower-like clusters called *condyloma acuminata*. In women, warts can be seen anywhere from the cervix to the vagina, urethra, inguinal region or upper thighs. In males, the most common site is the shaft of the penis. Most individuals are asymptomatic, but some experience itching, burning, pain, bleeding, and tenderness. *Recurrent respiratory papillomatosis*, defined by wart-like lesions that develop on the larynx, nasopharynx, oropharynx, trachea and/or esophagus, is also caused by types 6 and 11. The infection is seen most commonly in infants and children <5 years of age and is acquired from the mother during vaginal delivery. Infants may present with hoarseness, weak cry, stridor, feeding difficulties, and failure to thrive. Airway obstruction can result from enlarged lesions, and multiple surgical laser procedures are often necessary. Malignancy can develop, albeit rarely.

■ Epidemiology and Transmission

Whereas papillomaviruses are widely distributed in nature, HPV is only transmitted among humans. Direct *skin-to-skin* or *skin-to-mucosa* contact is required; generally, this means sexual activity where there is direct contact between the genitalia, anus, and/or mouth. Direct transfer of virus from the hands can occur. Not surprisingly, the risk of HPV infection correlates directly with sexual activity. Studies demonstrate that over half of young women acquire an HPV infection within 4 years of their first sexual intercourse, and it is estimated that in developed countries, >80% of sexually active women will have acquired HPV infection by 50 years of age. Estimates of the prevalence in men vary widely, but some are as high as 70%.

Worldwide there are 500,000 new cases of cervical cancer and 250,000 cervical cancer deaths each year—virtually all of these caused by HPV. In the United States, an estimated 6.2 million new HPV infections occur every year among teenagers and young adults. The annual disease burden includes approximately 5000 deaths, 17,000 cancers, 300,000 high-grade cervical dysplasias, 1,250,000 low-grade cervical dysplasias, and 1,400,000 cases of genital warts. The estimated direct medical costs are at least $4 billion (2004 dollars).

■ Background on Immunization Program

The quadrivalent HPV vaccine (HPV4) licensed in 2006 for females 9 to 26 years of age (Gardasil; Merck) provides protection against types 6, 11, 16, and 18. Prevention of cervical cancer due to types 16 and 18 is the most important anticipated outcome of a universal immunization program utilizing this vaccine in females. Prevention of anogenital warts due to types 6 and 11 would also be important, given the medical and psychologic costs of diagnosis and treatment. The potential benefits of vaccination could go beyond these to include reductions in the direct and indirect costs associated with cervical cancer screening, follow-up of abnormal Pap tests, as well as fewer cases of recurrent respiratory papillomatosis and reductions in the incidence of anal, penile, and oral cancers. Vaccination of males could potentially further reduce transmission and disease burden.

Studies show that 4% of girls in the United States are sexually active before 13 years of age; 25% are sexually active by 15, 40% by 16, and 70% by 18. Most sexually active teenage girls have had more than one partner. Since the benefits of vaccination can best be realized before sexual debut, adding HPV vaccine to the routine adolescent health care visit at 11 to 12 years of age makes sense. For those girls who will abstain from sex and ultimately enter a monogamous relationship, vaccination still makes sense because exposure through involuntary sexual contact is a possibility and the sexual history of the eventual partner may not be known.

Studies suggest that protection lasts at least 5 years without waning, and antibody levels achieved by young adolescents are actually higher that those achieved by older women. Vaccination does not lead to clearance of persistent HPV infection nor prevent neoplasia in women who are already infected with a particular serotype of HPV. However, sexually active women or those known to be infected with HPV can still benefit from vaccination due to protection against serotypes with which they are not infected.

Vaccination of an entire cohort of girls at 12 years of age would reduce the lifetime risk of cervical cancer by 20% to 66%. Depending on the assumptions made, the cost per quality-adjusted life year saved would be slightly more than $20,000; models that incorporate herd immunity effects yield estimates as low as $3000 per quality-adjusted life year saved.

■ Available Vaccines

Characteristics of the HPV vaccine licensed in the United States are given in **Table 9.9**.

■ Efficacy and/or Immunogenicity

Prelicensure efficacy studies of HPV4 involved >20,000 women between 16 and 26 years of age. These studies necessarily used CIN 2/3 and adenocarcinoma in situ as outcomes, since invasive cervical cancer was not a feasible or ethical end point. Two large phase 3 studies were conducted: FUTURE (Females United to Unilaterally Reduce Endo/Ectocervical Disease) I, which enrolled 5442 women, and FUTURE II, which enrolled 12,157. Licensure was based on pooled efficacy data from these trials as well as from two smaller phase 2 studies. Ninety-four percent of the women were sexually active at enrollment, 73% were HPV-naïve, and the median follow-up period ranged from 2 to 4 years.

The primary efficacy analyses (so-called *per protocol* analyses) included women who received all 3 doses of vaccine, had no major protocol deviations, and remained HPV-negative through 1 month after dose 3. Efficacy against types 16- or 18-related CIN 2/3 or adenocarcinoma in situ (AIS) was 100% no cases occurred among 8487 vaccinees and 53 occurred among 8460 placebees. Efficacy against any grade of CIN or AIS caused by any of the 4 types was 95%, and efficacy against genital warts was 99%. Among women who were already infected with one of the HPV types in the vaccine, efficacy against the remaining types was excellent. Efficacy against condyloma and VIN or VaIN of any degree was also estimated at 100%.

In practice, not all women will complete the full series of shots, and some women will already be infected with one or more HPV type at the time they start vaccination. *Intention-to-treat* analyses

TABLE 9.9 — HPV Vaccine[a]

Trade name	Gardasil
Abbreviation	HPV4
Manufacturer/ distributor	Merck
Type of vaccine	Inactivated, engineered subunit
Composition	Virus-like particles composed of self-assembled L1 major capsid protein molecules from serotypes 6, 11, 16, and 18 expressed in yeast (*Saccharomyces cerevisiae*) HPV 6 L1 (20 mcg) HPV 11 L1 (40 mcg) HPV 16 L1 (40 mcg) HPV 18 L1 (20 mcg)
Adjuvant	Aluminum hydroxide (0.225 mg aluminum)
Preservative	None
Excipients and contaminants	Sodium chloride (9.56 mg) L-histidine (0.78 mg) Polysorbate 80 (50 mcg) Sodium borate (35 mcg)
Latex	None
Labeled indications	Prevention of the following diseases caused by HPV types 6, 11, 16, and 18: • Cervical cancer • Genital warts • Cervical adenocarcinoma in situ • Cervical intraepithelial neoplasia grades 1, 2, and 3 • Vulvar intraepithelial neoplasia grades 2 and 3 • Vaginal intraepithelial neoplasia grades 2 and 3
Labeled ages	Females 9 to 26 years
Dose	0.5 mL
Route of administration	Intramuscular
Usual schedule	0, 2, 6 months
How supplied (number in package)	1-dose vial (1, 10) Prefilled syringe (6)
Storage	Refrigerate Do not freeze Protect from light
Reference package insert	December 2007

[a] Licensure of a 2-valent vaccine (Cervarix [HPV types 16 and 18]; GlaxoSmithKline) is pending as of October 2008.

were therefore performed to estimate the impact that a vaccine program would have in practice. Among women who received at least 1 vaccine dose, regardless of baseline HPV status, efficacy against 16- or 18-related CIN 2/3 or AIS was 39% and against any grade of CIN or AIS caused by any of the four types was 46%. The vast majority of cases in these analyses occurred in women who were HPV-infected at the time of first vaccination; these thus represent *prevalent*, not *incident*, disease.

Ongoing studies suggest that HPV4 may provide some protection against persistent infection and high-grade lesions caused by oncogenic types that are not contained in the vaccine (eg, 31 and 45). The vaccine is also immunogenic in boys. In addition, it appears to be immunogenic in older women.

Nearly 100% of vaccinated individuals develop antibodies to all four types after the 3-dose series, and antibody titers are higher than those seen after natural infection. Licensure for use in girls 9 to 15 years of age was based on immunogenicity bridging studies that demonstrated noninferiority of antibody responses compared with those in women 16 to 26 years of age. In fact, the antibody titers in young adolescents a year and a half postvaccination were 2- to 3-fold higher than those in the older women.

■ Safety

Prelicensure safety data were collected from approximately 12,000 HPV4 recipients, about 5100 of whom kept detailed diaries for 2 weeks after each dose. Pain at the injection site occurred in 84%, compared with 75% of controls who received an aluminum-containing placebo and 49% who received a saline placebo. Swelling and erythema were reported in about 25% of vaccinees. Fewer than 3% of local reactions were believed to be severe. Approximately 5% of female vaccinees reported a temperature of $\geq 100°F$ ($\geq 38°C$) after any dose, and temperatures $\geq 102°F$ ($\geq 38.9°C$) occurred in <1%. The rates of fever, other systemic adverse events (eg, nausea, nasopharyngitis, dizziness, diarrhea, vomiting, myalgia), serious adverse events, and new medical conditions arising within 4 years were similar in vaccinees and placebees.

In prelicensure trials, there were 10 deaths among vaccinees and 7 among placebees—none of these were considered to be vaccine related. Seven deaths were caused by motor vehicle accidents, three by intentional drug overdose or suicide, two by thromboembolic disease, two by sepsis, and one each by cancer, arrhythmia, and asphyxia.

The number of syncopal events reported to VAERS has increased since licensure of HPV4, although the reporting rate remains well below one in 1 million (see Chapter 4, *Vaccine Practice*). Between licensure and April 2008, after the distribution of >13 million doses, 7802 VAERS reports had been received describing events after vaccination with HPV4. Less than 7% of these reports described serious events, which is less than half of the average for VAERS reports after administration of other vaccines. Despite the well-publicized case of a 14-year-old girl who developed a peripheral motor neuropathy 4 months after dose 3 of HPV4, no other cases of lower motor-neuron disease were found in the VAERS database. There were 15 reports of death, 10 of which contained sufficient data for analysis; none of these were linked to the vaccine. There were 31 reports of Guillain-Barré syndrome, 10 of which were confirmed; the reporting rate was not above the expected background rate.

- *Contraindications*
  - Allergic reaction to previous dose of vaccine or any vaccine component, including baker's yeast (risk of recurrent allergic reaction)
- *Precautions*
  - Moderate or severe acute illness (difficulty distinguishing illness from vaccine reaction)
  - Pregnancy (theoretic risk to the fetus or attribution of birth defects to vaccination, although no deleterious effects from HPV4 administered during pregnancy have been demonstrated)

■ Recommendations for General Use

All adolescent girls and young women should be vaccinated against HPV. The usual schedule is 3 doses of HPV4 (given at 0, 2, and 6 months) at 11 to 12 years of age. The series may be started as early as 9 years of age. All females 13 to 26 years of age also should be vaccinated, whether or not they are sexually active. Screening for HPV infection before vaccination is not needed, and the vaccine should be given regardless of history of HPV infection, cervical, vaginal, or vulvar dysplasia, Pap test results, and history or presence of genital warts. As of October 2008, the vaccine was not labeled or recommended for administration to females <9 or >26 years of age or males of any age.

Vaccination against HPV should not change protocols for cervical cancer screening in the near future, which include initial testing 3 years after the onset of vaginal intercourse (but no later than 21 years of age) and continued annual testing for women <30 and testing every 2 to 3 years for women ≥30 who have had three negative tests.

A bivalent (types 16 and 18) HPV vaccine (Cervarix; GlaxoSmithKline) that utilizes a novel adjuvant was filed with the FDA in April 2007; action was still pending as of October 2008.

Influenza

■ The Pathogen

Influenza viruses are enveloped viruses with a segmented, single-stranded RNA genome. Antigenic types A and B are the most important causes of human disease. Influenza A viruses are characterized by two major surface proteins that are involved in infectivity and generation of protective immune responses: hemagglutinin (HA or H), which mediates attachment, and neuraminidase (NA or N), which mediates release from cells. Proteolytic cleavage of the HA molecule is required for infectivity. HA and NA types are designated by numbers—since 1977, the predominant circulating influenza A viruses have been A (H1N1) and A (H3N2). The HA and NA molecules undergo minor changes from year to year that result in slight variation in antigenicity, something termed *antigenic drift*. This accounts for the fact that an individual's experience with influenza in the prior year does not prevent infection with the current year's strain, although severity of illness might be mitigated (depending on how much drift has occurred). Occasionally, a major change in antigenicity occurs, resulting in pandemic strains that express novel HA or NA molecules to which few people have immunity—this is termed *antigenic shift*.

Antigenic shift can occur when an animal host (most likely a pig) is simultaneously infected with an animal strain of influenza A (most likely an avian strain) and a human strain (pigs can be infected with animal as well as human strains and they are in a position to be exposed to both). Through *ressortment*, the human strain may accidentally package the RNA segment encoding the avian HA or NA molecule, creating a human virus with the avian HA or NA type. If this reassortant is capable of spreading from person to person, a pandemic may ensue. Pandemic strains could also theoretically emerge if an animal influenza virus learns how to infect humans and spread from person to person.

Influenza virus infects columnar epithelial cells of the respiratory tract, causing necrosis, edema, and inflammation. Systemic symptoms are likely caused by circulating interleukin-6 and interferon-alpha induced by the infection. Influenza A virus infects all age groups and causes the most severe disease. Influenza B is milder and occurs more often in children. Influenza C is rarely seen and does not cause epidemic disease.

■ Clinical Features

The incubation period is 1 to 4 days. Classic symptoms include abrupt onset of fever, myalgia, headache, sore throat, photophobia, tearing, rhinitis, and nonproductive cough. Older children may experience nausea and vomiting, and infants may present with a sepsis-like syndrome. Fever is usually 101° to 102°F (38.3° to 38.9°C) and may be accompanied by prostration. Uncomplicated illness lasts from 3 to 7 days, and while recovery is usually rapid, some patients may have lingering cough and fatigue for several weeks.

Secondary bacterial infection (eg, pneumonia, sinusitis, and otitis media) is the most common complication of influenza. The risk of complications and hospitalization with influenza are highest among persons ≥65 years of age, the very young, and in persons with certain underlying medical conditions. The virus itself may cause pneumonia, encephalitis, myocarditis, myositis, and exacerbation of underlying chronic medical conditions such as cardiopulmonary disease.

■ Epidemiology and Transmission

Influenza virus is transmitted person to person through large-particle respiratory droplets that are expelled during coughing or sneezing. Maximum communicability occurs from 1 day before the onset of illness to 5 days thereafter. Disease activity peaks between December and March in temperate climates. During 1976 to 2006, peak influenza activity in the United States occurred most frequently in January (19% of seasons) and February (45% of seasons). However, peak activity occurred in March, April, or May in 19% of seasons. During average interpandemic years, anywhere from 5% to 15% of the population may become infected, and up to half of these infections will result in medical attention. Illness rates are highest among school-aged children, sometimes as high as 30%. Among adults, influenza illness results in an average of 2 lost work days per episode.

School-aged children are at low risk for complications, but they play a key role in spreading the virus throughout the community. This was demonstrated in a classic study in Houston showing that school absenteeism during the influenza season preceded workplace absenteeism by several weeks. Moreover, routine vaccination of school children in Japan between the 1960s and early 1980s resulted in dramatic reductions in excess (influenza-related) mortality among the elderly and other high-risk groups.

Annual hospitalization rates for laboratory-confirmed influenza are around 20 per 100,000 for children 2 to 5 years of age, but as high as 240 to 720 per 100,000 for infants <6 months of age. The rate of hospitalization for infants is similar to the rate for children with high-risk conditions and is comparable to that for adults ≥65 years of age. The annual outpatient burden of influenza may be as high as 100 clinic visits and 30 emergency department visits per 1000 children.

During the 1980s and 1990s in the United States, influenza resulted in an average of 226,000 hospitalizations and 34,000 deaths. In fact, the number of deaths increased over that period of time, due in large part to the aging of the population (90% of deaths occur in persons ≥65 years of age). Although the number of deaths in children is small (153 in the 2003 to 2004 season), it is notable that nearly two thirds occur in children without underlying medical conditions.

Influenza peaks between April and September in temperate regions of the Southern Hemisphere and occurs throughout the year in tropical areas. Traveling with large tourist groups (eg, on cruise ships) that include persons from these areas increases the risk of infection during the summer.

■ Background on Immunization Program

The first influenza vaccines became commercially available in 1945. Between then and 2008, the focus was on protecting individuals from complications, hospitalization, and death related to influenza. High-risk groups were identified and recommended for annual immunization, and increasing emphasis was placed on immunizing close contacts of those individuals. Immunization of all adults ≥65 years of age was recommended until 2000, when the recommendation was broadened to include all adults ≥50 years of age. In 2002, immunization of all children 6 to 23 months of age was encouraged; in 2004, this was strengthened to a full recommendation. In 2006, all children 24 to 59 months of age were added to the routine vaccination list.

In 2008, an unprecedented step was taken in the fight against influenza—going beyond protecting individuals to protecting entire communities through herd immunity. The recommendation was made to extend routine childhood immunization to include all children 6 months to 18 years of age. As noted earlier, there is good reason to believe that preventing influenza in school-aged children will change the epidemiology of influenza transmission in the community.

Studies suggest that influenza immunization reduces health care–provider visits and lost workdays by nearly 50%. A 2004 analysis suggested that the cost of influenza immunization among persons 18 to 64 years of age was $4500 per illness averted in a typical season; the cost decreased to $60 when the attack rate and vaccine effectiveness were high. Another study was done that looked at the direct and indirect costs of both vaccination and disease, assuming that vaccination occurred in a low-cost setting, such as the workplace. This analysis demonstrated that routine vaccination of healthy working adults would result in an average cost saving of $13.66 per person vaccinated (1998 dollars). Studies looking at vaccination of persons ≥65 years of age demonstrate net savings or very low cost (<$1000 [2000 dollars]) per quality-adjusted life year saved. The costs per quality-adjusted life year saved in healthy children 6 to 23 months of age are estimated to be around $12,000 (2003 dollars), and for adolescents around $119,000. The additional benefits that would accrue from the herd-immunity effects of immunizing all school-aged children are difficult to assess.

■ Available Vaccines

Characteristics of the influenza vaccines licensed in the United States are given in **Table 9.10**.

■ Efficacy and/or Immunogenicity

Practically speaking, vaccine-induced immunity to influenza is good for only 1 year because antibody wanes. In addition, the circulating strains vary from year to year, and the vaccine strains chosen for a given year may not be a good antigenic match with the prevailing strains. For example, during the 2007 to 2008

TABLE 9.10 — Influenza Vaccines[a]

Trade name	Afluria	Fluarix	Flulaval	FluMist	Fluvirin	Fluzone
Abbreviation	TIV	TIV	TIV	LAIV	TIV	TIV
Manufacturer/distributor	CSL Biotherapies	GlaxoSmithKline	GlaxoSmithKline	MedImmune	Novartis	Sanofi Pasteur
Type of vaccine	Inactivated, purified subunits (split virus)	Inactivated, purified subunits (split virus)	Inactivated, purified subunits (split virus)	Live attenuated, engineered	Inactivated, purified subunits (split virus)	Inactivated, purified subunits (split virus)
Composition[b]	Influenza A (H1N1) Influenza A (H3N2) Influenza B Propagated in embryonated eggs Inactivated with beta-propiolactone Hemagglutinin (15 mcg of each strain)	Influenza A (H1N1) Influenza A (H3N2) Influenza B Propagated in embryonated eggs Inactivated with formaldehyde Hemagglutinin (15 mcg of each strain)	Influenza A (H1N1) Influenza A (H3N2) Influenza B Propagated in embryonated eggs Inactivated with ultraviolet light and formaldehyde Hemagglutinin (15 mcg of each strain)	Cold-adapted, temperature-sensitive, attenuated reassortants expressing influenza A (H1N1), influenza A (H3N2), and influenza B antigens[c] Propagated in specific pathogen-free eggs $10^{6.5\text{-}7.5}$ fluorescent focus units of each reassortant strain	Influenza A (H1N1) Influenza A (H3N2) Influenza B Propagated in embryonated eggs Inactivated with beta-propiolactone Hemagglutinin (15 mcg of each strain)	Influenza A (H1N1) Influenza A (H3N2) Influenza B Inactivated with formaldehyde
Adjuvant	None	None	None	None	None	None

Preservative	Thimerosal (24.5 mcg mercury) or none	None	Thimerosal (25 mcg mercury)	None	Thimerosal (24.5 mcg mercury) or none	Thimerosal (25 mcg mercury) or none
Excipients and contaminants	Sodium chloride (4.1 mg) Monobasic sodium phosphate (80 mcg) Dibasic sodium phosphate (300 mcg) Monobasic potassium phosphate (20 mcg) Potassium chloride (20 mcg) Calcium chloride (1.5 mg) Sodium taurodeoxycholate (≤10 ppm) Ovalbumin (≤0.1 mcg) Neomycin sulfate (≤0.2 pg)	Octoxynol-10 (≤0.085 mg) Alpha-tocopherol hydrogen succinate (≤0.1 mg) Polysorbate 80 (≤0.415 mg) Thimerosal (trace) Hydrocortisone (≤0.0016 mcg) Gentamicin sulfate (≤0.15 mcg) Ovalbumin (≤20 mcg) Formaldehyde (≤1 mcg) Sodium deoxycholate (≤50 mcg)	Ovalbumin (≤1 mcg) Formaldehyde (≤25 mcg) Sodium deoxycholate (≤50 mcg)	Monosodium glutamate (0.188 mg) Hydrolyzed porcine gelatin (2 mg) Arginine (2.42 mg) Sucrose (13.68 mg) Dibasic potassium phosphate (2.26 mg) Monosodium phosphate (0.96 mg) Gentamicin sulfate (<0.015 mcg/mL)	Phosphate buffered saline (0.01 M) Preservative-free formulation: thimerosal (≤0.98 mcg mercury)	Sodium phosphate buffered isotonic sodium chloride Gelatin (0.05%)

Continued

TABLE 9.10 — *Continued*

Trade name	Afluria	Fluarix	Flulaval	FluMist	Fluvirin	Fluzone
Excipients and contaminants *(continued)*	Polymyxin B ($\leq$0.03 pg) Beta-propiolactone (<25 ng)					
Latex	None	Tip cap and plunger of prefilled syringe contain dry natural rubber	None	None	None	None
Labeled indications	Immunization against influenza	Immunization against influenza	Immunization against influenza	Immunization against influenza	Immunization against influenza	Immunization against influenza
Labeled ages	$\geq$18 years	$\geq$18 years	$\geq$18 years	2 to 49 years	$\geq$4 years	Thimerosal-containing formulation: $\geq$6 months Preservative-free, pediatric formulation: 6 to 35 months Preservative-free formulation: $\geq$36 months

Dose	0.5 mL	0.5 mL	0.5 mL	0.2 mL (0.1 mL per nostril)	0.5 mL	Preservative-free, pediatric formulation: 0.25 mL Other formulations: 0.5 mL
Route of administration	Intramuscular	Intramuscular	Intramuscular	Intranasal[d]	Intramuscular	Intramuscular
Usual schedule	1 dose annually	1 dose annually	1 dose annually	1 dose annually[e]	1 dose annually[e]	1 dose annually[e]
How supplied (number in package)	Thimerosal-containing formulation: 10-dose vial (1) Preservative-free formulation: prefilled syringe (10)	Prefilled syringe (5)	10-dose vial (1)	Prefilled sprayer (10)	Thimerosal-containing formulation: 10-dose vial (1) Preservative-free formulation: prefilled syringe (1)	Thimerosal-containing formulation: 10-dose vial (1) Preservative-free, pediatric formulation: prefilled syringe (10) Preservative-free formulation: prefilled syringe (10)
Storage	Refrigerate Do not freeze Protect from light	Refrigerate Do not freeze Protect from light	Refrigerate Do not freeze Protect from light	Refrigerate Do not freeze	Refrigerate Do not freeze	Refrigerate Do not freeze

Continued

TABLE 9.10 — *Continued*

Trade name	Afluria	Fluarix	Flulaval	FluMist	Fluvirin	Fluzone
Storage *(continued)*	Multidose vial should be discarded 28 days after first use		Multidose vial should be discarded 28 days after use			
Reference package insert	September 2007	August 2007	August 2007	September 2007	April 2007	June 2007

[a] Influenza vaccines are interchangeable in the sense that one product (any inactivated vaccine or LAIV) can be used 1 year and another product the next year. Although no data are available regarding 2 consecutive doses of different products in the same year, it is assumed that this is acceptable. Other inactivated or live vaccines may be given at any time in relation to inactivated influenza vaccine; other inactivated vaccines may be given at any time in relation to LAIV and other live vaccines should not be given within 4 weeks of each other.

[b] The strains used vary from year to year depending on the strains that are anticipated to circulate during the influenza season.

[c] LAIV is produced from a master donor virus that is *cold adapted* (replication is efficient at 25°C), *temperature sensitive* (replication is restricted at 37°C to 39°C), and *attenuated*. Each season, the type A and type B master donor viruses are co-cultured with the relevant wild-type influenza A and B strains, respectively. Reassortants are selected that retain the attenuated phenotype (and relevant gene segments) of the master donor virus but express (and contain the gene segments for) the wild-type HA and NA. The reassortant viruses are capable of replicating in the nasopharynx, where they induce immunity but produce little disease; they are incapable of replicating lower in the respiratory tract.

[d] If the patient sneezes after administration, the dose should not be repeated. Influenza antiviral medications should be avoided in the 48 hours before and 2 weeks after vaccination. No data exist regarding concomitant use of intranasal medications. Severely immunocompromised individuals should not administer LAIV.

[e] Children <9 years of age who are receiving influenza vaccine for the first time, or who were vaccinated for the first time in the previous season and only received 1 dose, need 2 doses separated by 4 weeks.

influenza season, the circulating A (H3N2) and B viruses (A/Brisbane/10/2007-like and B/Florida/04/2006-like, respectively) were substantially different from the strains in the vaccine (A/Wisconsin/67/2005-like and B/Malaysia/2506/2004-like, respectively). Effectiveness against medically-attended influenza A infection was 58% but no effectiveness against influenza B was seen.

TIV

Most vaccinees develop serum hemagglutination inhibition and neutralizing antibodies, considered immunologic correlates of protection. Children 6 months to 8 years of age require 2 doses in the same season to ensure protective responses. In a study among children conducted between 1985 and 1990, annual vaccination with TIV reduced laboratory-confirmed influenza A by 77% to 91%. A 1-year placebo-controlled study yielded efficacy estimates of 56% among healthy children 3 to 9 years of age and 100% among adolescents, and a retrospective study of 30,000 young children showed approximately 50% effectiveness against medically-attended, clinically diagnosed pneumonia or influenza. TIV may also reduce episodes of otitis media in children by as much as 30%.

Randomized controlled trials demonstrate efficacy against laboratory-confirmed influenza illness of 70% to 90% among healthy adults <65 years of age. Whereas estimates of efficacy drop to 50% to 77% when the vaccine and circulating strains are not well matched, protection against hospitalization appears to be preserved. Efficacy against illness is lower among adults >65 years of age, but protection against influenza-related death may be as high as 80%.

Immunogenicity may be lower among immunocompromised individuals and those with chronic medical conditions.

LAIV

Immunologic correlates of protection after administration of LAIV have not been established but probably include antibodies in nasal secretions. LAIV was evaluated in a placebo-controlled study between 1996 and 1998 involving 1602 healthy children 15 to 71 months of age. Efficacy against culture-confirmed influenza was 89% for those who received 1 dose and 94% for those who received 2 doses. In the second year, despite a poor match with the circulating A (H3N2) strain, efficacy was 86%. Efficacy against pneumonia, other lower respiratory tract disease, and influenza-associated otitis media was also demonstrated. In a multinational blinded trial conducted during the 2004 to 2005 influenza season, 3916 children <5 years of age were randomized to receive LAIV and 3936 received TIV. Culture-confirmed influenza illness caused by any strain was reduced by 55% in recipients of LAIV compared with recipients of TIV; for matched strains, the reduction was 45% and for mismatched strains it was 58%, suggesting that LAIV provides broader cross-protection.

Other studies also suggest that LAIV is more effective than TIV in children. Additional prelicensure, placebo-controlled trials involving >4000 children demonstrated efficacy of 73% to 93% for culture-confirmed influenza due to any strain.

A multicenter placebo-controlled trial among 4561 healthy, working adults was conducted during 1997 to 1998, a season when the A (H3N2) strain in the vaccine was not well matched with the circulating strain. Febrile illnesses were not reduced among vaccinees, but severe febrile illnesses (19% reduction) and febrile upper respiratory tract illnesses (24% reduction) were. There were also reductions in days of illness (23% for febrile illnesses, 27% for severe febrile illnesses), days of work lost (18% for severe febrile illnesses, 28% for febrile respiratory tract illnesses), days with health care–provider visits (25% for severe febrile illnesses, 41% for febrile upper respiratory tract illnesses). Use of prescription antibiotics and over-the-counter medications was also reduced. Studies suggest that LAIV and TIV have similar efficacy in adults.

In experiments using LAIV as a challenge, subjects previously immunized with LAIV shed less virus than those previously immunized with inactivated vaccine. These results suggest that LAIV may reduce carriage of natural influenza virus and help to control spread of infection in the community.

■ Safety

TIV

Inactivated influenza vaccine cannot cause influenza. Less than one third of vaccinees have been reported to develop local redness or induration for 1 to 2 days at the site of injection. Fever, chills, headache, and malaise, although infrequent, most often affect children who have had no previous exposure to the antigens contained in the vaccine. These reactions generally begin 6 to 12 hours after vaccination and persist for only 1 to 2 days. Immediate reactions, presumably allergic, may consist of hives, angioedema, allergic asthma, or systemic anaphylaxis. These are rare and probably result from hypersensitivity to a vaccine component, most likely residual egg protein. If influenza vaccines have any association with Guillain-Barré syndrome, it is on the order of one case per million vaccinees, well below the background rate in the population (see *Chapter 8*).

In a retrospective study of 45,000 children 6 to 23 months of age, vaccination was not associated with any medically attended outcome, but several diagnoses, such as acute upper respiratory tract illness, otitis media, and asthma, were significantly *reduced*. Some studies in adults show similar rates of systemic symptoms, such as fever, malaise, myalgia, and headache, between vaccinees and placebees. There is no evidence that TIV has any deleterious impact on HIV infection or immunocompetence.

During the 2000 to 2001 season in Canada, a discrete oculo-respiratory syndrome was reported with TIV. Symptoms were mild and self-limited, began within 24 hours of injection, and included hoarseness, sore throat, difficulty swallowing, cough, sore and/or itchy eyes, bilateral conjunctival erythema, facial edema, and nasal congestion. Microaggregates of unsplit virus were implicated as the cause.

LAIV

Children report rhinorrhea or congestion (20% to 75%), headache (2% to 46%), fever (up to 26%), vomiting (3% to 13%), abdominal pain (2%), and myalgias (up to 21%). Symptoms are more often associated with the first dose and are self-limited. In a study of 8352 children 6 to 59 months of age who were randomized to receive either TIV or LAIV, rhinorrhea among first-time vaccinees was reported in 57% of LAIV recipients and in 46.3% of TIV recipients. Temperature >100°F (37.8°C) was reported in 5.4% of LAIV and in 2% of TIV recipients. Among children <24 months of age, 3.2% of LAIV recipients and 2.0% of TIV recipients had medically significant wheezing after 1 dose.

Adult vaccinees report rhinorrhea (44%, vs 27% in placebees), headache (40% vs 38%), sore throat (28% vs 17%), tiredness (26% vs 22%), muscle aches (17% vs 15%), cough (14% vs 11%), and chills (9% vs 6%).

Serious adverse events are rare. Shedding of vaccine virus is common among children; in one study, at least one vaccine strain was recovered from 80% of young children from 1 to 21 days postvaccination. However, horizontal transmission appears to be rare—the estimated probability of a young child acquiring a vaccine virus from a vaccinated child in the day care setting is 0.6% to 2.4%. Up to 50% of adults may have viral antigen in nasal secretions for the first 7 days after vaccination. Person-to-person transmission among adults has not been assessed.

- *Contraindications for TIV*
  - Allergic reaction to previous dose of vaccine or any vaccine component, including eggs (risk of recurrent allergic reaction). Being able to eat eggs (even in baked goods) without adverse effects is a reasonable indication of a very low risk of anaphylaxis. Mild or local manifestations of allergy to eggs or feathers are not a contraindication. Skin testing can be done and desensitization may be possible.
- *Precautions for TIV*
  - Moderate or severe acute illness (difficulty distinguishing illness from vaccine reaction)
  - Guillain-Barré syndrome within 6 weeks of a prior dose of influenza vaccine (risk of recurrent Guillain-Barré syndrome)
- *Contraindications for LAIV*
  - Allergic reaction to previous dose of vaccine or any vaccine component, including eggs (risk of recurrent allergic reac-

tion). Being able to eat eggs (even in baked goods) without adverse effects is a reasonable indication of a very low risk of anaphylaxis. Mild or local manifestations of allergy to eggs or feathers are not a contraindication.

- Underlying medical conditions that place patients at high risk for complications and serve as an indication for influenza vaccination, including asthma or equivalent, chronic cardiopulmonary disease, diabetes, renal dysfunction, hemoglobinopathies, immunodeficiency, or immunosuppression (risk of exacerbating underlying condition or causing influenza-like disease)
- Children or adolescents receiving aspirin or other salicylates (risk of Reye syndrome)
- History of Guillain-Barré syndrome (risk of recurrent Guillain-Barré syndrome)
- Pregnancy (theoretic risk of live virus vaccine to the fetus or attribution of birth defects to vaccination)
- Household or health care contacts of severely immunosuppressed individuals, eg hematopoietic stem-cell transplant recipients who are confined to protective environments with regulated airflow, filtration, etc (risk of transmission of live virus vaccine to immunosuppressed person). Individuals who receive LAIV should avoid contact with severely immunosuppressed patients for 7 days (contact with patients who have lesser degrees of immunosuppression is acceptable).

• *Precautions for LAIV*
  - Moderate or severe acute illness (difficulty distinguishing illness from vaccine reaction)
  - Severe nasal congestion (interference with delivery of vaccine)

■ Recommendations for General Use

Influenza vaccine is given annually, usually beginning in October in the United States. It is never too late in the season to vaccinate, even if influenza season has already begun. In general, vaccination efforts should continue well into March.

Technically speaking, the only people who should *not* be immunized against influenza each year (excluding infants <6 months of age for whom there is no licensed vaccine) are those who *want* to get the flu or who *want to take the risk* of infecting others. This sounds sarcastic, but influenza vaccine is officially recommended for any person who wishes to reduce the likelihood of becoming ill with influenza or transmitting influenza to others should they become infected. TIV may be used for anyone; LAIV should only be used for healthy persons 2 to 49 years of age.

Beyond this, all persons ≥50 years of age, regardless of underlying conditions, should receive TIV each year. In addition, all children and adolescents 6 months to 18 years of age should be immunized against influenza each year; LAIV is an option for those 2 to 18 years of age who do not have contraindications.

While asthma is a contraindication for LAIV, there are children in the 2- to 4-year age group who have had episodes of wheezing but who have not (yet) been diagnosed with asthma. The following screening question for parents has been suggested: "In the past 12 months, has a health care provider ever told you that your child had wheezing or asthma?" If the answer is yes, or if there is a wheezing episode documented in the medical record in the past 12 months, the child should receive TIV instead of LAIV.

Persons in the following high-risk groups should be given TIV every year:

- Women who will be pregnant during influenza season (there is no preference for products that do not contain thimerosal; see *Chapter 8*)
- Patients with chronic conditions involving the following systems:
  - Pulmonary (eg, emphysema, chronic bronchitis, and asthma)
  - Cardiovascular (eg, congestive heart failure)
  - Metabolic diseases (eg, diabetes mellitus)
  - Renal (eg, nephrotic syndrome, hemodialysis)
  - Hepatic (eg, cirrhosis)
  - Hematologic (eg, sickle cell disease, other hemaglobinopathies)
  - Immunologic (eg, immunosuppressive medications, congenital immunodeficiency, HIV infection)
  - Neurologic (eg, cognitive dysfunction, spinal cord injury, seizure disorder, neuromuscular disorder that compromises respiratory function or handling of secretions)
- Persons 6 months to 18 years of age on long-term aspirin therapy (to reduce the risk of Reye syndrome)

Persons in the following groups who are at increased risk for infection or who might spread influenza to high-risk individuals should be immunized every year (either TIV or LAIV may be used, depending on the age and presence or absence of contraindications):

- Household contacts of and persons who provide care for children <5 years of age, adults ≥50 years of age, and individuals with any of the high-risk conditions listed earlier. LAIV should not be used for those who have contact with severely immunosuppressed patients (eg, hematopoietic stem-cell transplant recipients who are confined to protective environments with regulated airflow, filtration, etc)
- Health care personnel (this includes physicians, nurses, residents, students, medical emergency response workers, and other workers in hospitals and clinics)
- Residents and employees of assisted-living residences, chronic or long-term care facilities, correctional facilities, nursing homes, and similar residential institutions
- College students

Consideration should be given to vaccinating healthy foreign travelers at least 2 weeks before departure, especially if the individual falls into a high-risk group and was not vaccinated the preceding fall or winter. Those who are vaccinated in the summer should be revaccinated with the current vaccine the following fall.

Measles, Mumps, Rubella

■ The Pathogens

Measles

Measles (rubeola) virus is an enveloped, single-stranded RNA virus in the Paramyxoviridae family. There is only one antigenic type. Two proteins—the hemagglutinin, which mediates attachment, and the fusion protein, which facilitates cell-to-cell spread of the virus—are important in generating neutralizing antibodies. The virus infects the respiratory epithelium of the nasopharynx, then spreads to regional lymph nodes, where replication leads to a primary viremia. Continued replication in the reticuloendothelial system leads to a secondary viremia about a week after infection; this leads to replication in the respiratory tract, skin, and viscera. Pathologic changes include lymphoid hyperplasia, mononuclear cell infiltration of the respiratory tract, and multinucleated giant cells.

Mumps

Mumps virus is an enveloped, single-stranded RNA virus in the Paramyxoviridae family. The virus contains a hemagglutinin and fusion protein, and there is only one antigenic type. Initial infection occurs in the respiratory epithelium of the nasopharynx, then spreads to regional lymph nodes, where replication leads to viremia and spread to glandular epithelia, including the salivary glands, testes, ovaries, and pancreas. Pathologic changes include interstitial edema and lymphocytic infiltration. Infarcts in the testes can lead to atrophy of the germinal epithelium. The virus also spreads to the CNS, where it infects the choroidal epithelium and ependymal lining of the ventricles, resulting in aseptic meningitis, and, in some cases, encephalitis.

Rubella

Rubella virus is an enveloped, single-stranded RNA virus in the Togavirus family. The virus has two major surface glycoproteins—E1 and E2. E1 is a hemagglutinin that engenders neutralizing antibodies. Infection occurs in the respiratory epithelium of the nasopharynx, then spreads to regional lymph nodes, where replication leads to viremia. The virus then spreads throughout the body, including the respiratory tract, skin, lymph nodes, and body fluids. While postnatal infection is relatively benign, infection of the fetus, which occurs transplacentally, leads to a persistent infection and progressive, generalized vasculitis, affecting organ development.

◼ Clinical Features

Measles

Measles is characterized by a several-day prodrome of malaise, fever, anorexia, coryza, cough, and conjunctivitis. Temperature usually increases for 5 or 6 days and can be as high as 104°F (40°C). In uncomplicated cases, the temperature drops 2 to 3 days after the onset of exanthem. At some point between the second and fourth days after onset of symptoms, but before rash appears, characteristic Koplik's spots appear on the buccal mucosa. The rash generally appears around the ears and hairline 3 to 5 days into the illness and spreads downward and outward to cover the face, trunk, and extremities over the next 3 to 4 days. It is initially erythematous and maculopapular and tends to become confluent as it spreads, especially on the face and neck. The rash usually lasts about 5 days and resolves in the order of appearance.

Measles is most frequently complicated by diarrhea, middle ear infection, or bronchopneumonia. Encephalitis occurs in approximately one out of every 1000 cases, and survivors often have permanent brain damage. Death, usually from pneumonia or acute encephalitis, occurs in one to two out of every 1000 cases; the risk is greater for infants, young children, and adults than it is for older children and adolescents. Subacute sclerosing panencephalitis is a rare, fatal degenerative disease of the CNS that appears years after measles infection (5 to 10 per million cases) and is associated with persistent infection with a mutant form of the virus.

In developing countries, measles is often more severe, with case-fatality rates as high as 25%. Measles can be severe and prolonged in immunocompromised persons, particularly those who have leukemia, lymphoma, or HIV infection. In these patients, the typical rash may be absent and the patient may shed virus for several weeks.

Mumps

Mumps usually presents as bilateral, or less commonly unilateral, parotitis, which may be preceded by fever, headache, malaise, myalgia, and anorexia. Only 30% to 40% of mumps infections produce typical acute parotitis; 15% to 20% are asymptomatic and up to 50% are associated with respiratory or nonspecific symptoms. Parotitis occurs more commonly among children aged 2 to 9 years, and inapparent infection may be more common among adults. Serious complications can occur without evidence of parotitis.

Mumps is usually self-limited but complications do occur. Orchitis is the most common complication in postpubertal males, occurring in up to 50% of cases; half of patients are left with some degree of testicular atrophy, but sterility is rare. Aseptic meningitis is common, occurring asymptomatically in 50% to 60% of patients and associated with headache and stiff neck in up to 15%. Adults are at greater risk for this complication than children, and boys are more often affected than girls. Encephalitis is rare, occurring in <2 per 100,000 cases. Mumps was a leading cause of acquired sensorineural deafness in the prevaccine era, with an estimated incidence of one per 20,000 cases.

Rubella

Rubella is characterized by nonspecific signs and symptoms including transient, erythematous and sometimes pruritic rash, postauricular or suboccipital lymphadenopathy, arthralgia, and low-grade fever. Twenty-five percent to 50% of infections are subclinical. The disease is generally considered benign and self-limited.

The most severe effects of rubella occur in the fetuses of pregnant women who contract the infection during the first trimester of pregnancy. Infants born with congenital rubella syndrome may have deafness, cataracts, microophthalmia, cardiac defects, and CNS abnormalities.

■ Epidemiology and Transmission

Measles

Humans are the only natural hosts. In temperate climates, measles occurs primarily in late winter and spring. Transmission is primarily person to person via large respiratory droplets. Airborne transmission has been documented in closed areas (such as office examination rooms) for up to 2 hours after the presence of an infected person. Measles is highly contagious, with secondary household attack rates exceeding 90%. It is estimated that before the introduction of the first vaccine in 1963, there were 3 to 4 million cases of measles each year in the United States. That number had fallen to about 1500 by 1983.

However, between 1989 and 1991, there were almost 56,000 reported cases and 123 deaths. This resurgence was primarily due to pockets of low vaccine coverage in the population. Another contributing factor was the fact that infants <1 year of age were more susceptible than in previous eras—their mothers had vaccine-induced immunity rather than natural immunity, and their transplacental antibody inheritance was lower. Finally, primary vaccine failure may have contributed—2% to 5% of children fail to respond to a single dose of MMR.

Renewed efforts to vaccinate young children and the institution of a second vaccination at school entry effectively reversed the resurgence such that by 2000, measles was considered to be no longer endemic in the United States. This is not to say that importation-related outbreaks do not continue to occur. For example, from January through April of 2008, 64 measles cases were reported; 54 were associated with importation from other countries. Most of the cases occurred during outbreaks in New York, Arizona, and California, and 22% of the patients were hospitalized. All but one case occurred in unvaccinated individuals or persons with unknown vaccination status. This experience underscores the importance of maintaining immunization rates despite the absence of endemic disease.

Mumps

Humans are the only natural hosts. Mumps incidence peaks in winter and spring, but disease has been reported throughout the year. Transmission occurs through airborne droplet nuclei or direct contact with saliva. Contagiousness is similar to that of influenza and rubella but less than that for measles and chickenpox. The infectious period is considered to be from 3 days before to 4 days after the onset of active disease.

In 1964 there were 212,000 cases in the United States; by 1983, after the vaccine had been licensed for 16 years, the number had fallen to 3000. There was a resurgence of disease among teenagers in the late 1980s that peaked a few years before the measles resurgence. A major contributing factor was the fact that this cohort of teenagers had missed the universal infant vaccination recommendation. The resurgence was reversed by institution of the second MMR vaccine at school entry, and the number of cases reached a low point of 258 in 2004. However, 2006 saw a multistate outbreak of 6584 cases, mostly in college students and other young adults, many of whom had 2 doses of the vaccine. Contributing factors may have been failure of 2 doses to produce immunity in some individuals and waning immunity from childhood vaccination.

Rubella

Humans are the only natural hosts. In temperate climates, rubella occurs in late winter and early spring. There is no carrier state per se, but infants with congenital rubella syndrome may shed large quantities of virus for up to a year. Rubella is only moderately contagious and spreads from person to person via airborne droplet nuclei shed from the respiratory tract. Transmission by subclinical cases, which constitute 20% to 50% of all infections, can occur. The disease is most contagious when the rash is erupting, but virus may be shed from 7 days before to 7 days after rash onset. Between 1964 and 1965, there were >12 million cases of rubella in the United States and 20,000 babies were born with congenital rubella syndrome. After vaccination was initiated in 1969, the number of cases declined dramatically, such that by 2004, rubella was considered to be no longer endemic in the United States. Disease, however, is still seen, especially in immigrants from Latin America.

■ Background on Immunization Program

The rationale for measles and mumps immunization is to prevent complications and death due to those diseases in children and adults. The rationale for rubella immunization is to prevent infection in pregnant women, thereby preventing congenital rubella syndrome. The first live-attenuated measles vaccine was licensed in 1963; mumps vaccine was licensed in 1967, and rubella vaccine in 1969. The first MMR vaccine was licensed in 1971; in 1979, a rubella vaccine grown in human diploid fibroblasts (RA 27/3) was licensed and replaced the duck embryo–passaged strain that was in MMR. Since 1980, MMR has been the preferred vaccine against these three diseases. A single dose was recommended for all children during the second year of life until 1989, when the measles resurgence discussed above prompted recommendations for a second dose. In 2005, a combination vaccine containing MMR and varicella vaccine was licensed.

Use of MMR in the United States has been remarkably successful, leading to the elimination of endemic transmission of measles and rubella and drastically reducing the annual number of reported cases of mumps. However, since 1998 these successes have been threatened by the false belief that MMR vaccine causes autism (see *Chapter 8*).

■ Available Vaccines

Characteristics of the MMR vaccine licensed in the United States are given in **Table 9.11**.

■ Efficacy and/or Immunogenicity

Measles

Antibodies develop in approximately 95% of children vaccinated at 12 months of age and 98% of children vaccinated at 15 months of age. Studies show that >99% of persons who receive 2 doses of vaccine (separated by at least 1 month) at ≥1 year of age develop serologic evidence of measles immunity. Although vaccine-induced antibody titers are lower than those following natural disease, immunity is probably lifelong in most people. Individuals who lose antibody over time have demonstrable anamnestic responses to revaccination, indicating that they are most likely still protected. A small percentage of vaccinated individuals may lose protection after several years.

Mumps

More than 97% of vaccinees develop protective antibody titers, albeit lower than those following natural infection. In postlicensure studies conducted between 1973 and 1989, efficacy of a single dose was 75% to 91%, and efficacy of 2 doses during the 2006 outbreak in the United States was estimated at 76% to 88%. A study published in 2008 showed that 94% of university students and staff had antibody to mumps virus after having received 2 doses of vaccine. The level of antibody was lower among those vaccinated ≥15 years earlier as compared with those vaccinated in the preceding 5 years, but seronegative subjects mounted anamnestic responses after repeat vaccination.

Rubella

At least 95% of vaccinees ≥12 months of age develop protective antibody titers. Vaccine-induced rubella antibodies have persisted in >90% of vaccinees at least 15 years after receipt of the RA 27/3 vaccine. Lifelong protection against clinical reinfection, asymptomatic viremia, or both usually results from a single dose of vaccine early in childhood. In some cases, vaccinees exposed to natural rubella develop an asymptomatic increase in antibody titer (reinfection with wild-type rubella virus has been observed in individuals with previous natural rubella). Infection of vaccinees is rarely associated with viremia or pharyngeal shedding, and person-to-person transmission has not been reported. Among vaccinated women, the risk of congenital rubella syndrome from rubella infection during pregnancy is extremely low.

■ Safety

Five to 15% of vaccinees develop fever ≥103°F (39.4°C) and about 5% develop a mild morbilliform rash, usually within 7 to 10 days. Transient lymphadenopathy sometimes occurs following MMR, and parotitis has been reported rarely. Arthralgia, which is reported in up to 25% of susceptible adult women given MMR, is attributed to the rubella component; persistent or recurrent joint symptoms have been reported but are rare. It should be mentioned that the incidence of joint problems after immunization is lower than that after natural infection at the same age.

One case of immune thrombocytopenic purpura, defined as a platelet count ≤50,000 per microliter with clinical bleeding, occurs for every 40,000 doses; this is much less than the incidence after natural measles or rubella. Febrile seizures, seen in the second week after vaccination, are estimated to occur in 25 to 34 per 100,000 vaccinees and are not associated with subsequent seizures or neurodevelopmental disabilities. Most allergic reactions are minor and consist of a wheal and flare or urticaria at the injection site, and anaphylactic reactions are extremely rare. The vaccine does not contain significant amounts of egg protein and can safely be given to patients with allergies to eggs, chickens, and feathers without prior skin testing and without incremental dosing.

The viruses in MMR are not transmitted from person to person after vaccination and therefore the vaccine can be given to contacts of immunosuppressed and pregnant individuals.

- *Contraindications*
  - Allergic reaction to previous dose of vaccine or any vaccine component, including gelatin and neomycin (risk of recurrent allergic reaction)
  - Severe immunodeficiency or immunosuppression (risk of disease caused by live virus; see *Chapter 7*)
  - Pregnancy (theoretic risk of live virus vaccine to the fetus or attribution of birth defects to vaccination)

TABLE 9.11 — MMR Vaccine[a]

Trade name	M-M-R II
Abbreviation	MMR
Manufacturer/distributor	Merck
Type of vaccine	Live attenuated, classic
Composition	Measles virus, Moraten strain (derived from the Edmonston B strain), propagated in chick embryo cells, at least 1000 $TCID_{50}$ Mumps virus, Jeryl Lynn strain (actually consists of two distinct strains), propagated in chick embryo cells, at least 12,500 $TCID_{50}$ Rubella virus, RA 27/3 strain, propagated in human diploid lung fibroblast (WI-38) cells, at least 1000 $TCID_{50}$
Adjuvant	None
Preservative	None
Excipients and contaminants	Sorbitol (14.5 mg) Sodium phosphate Sucrose (1.9 mg) Sodium chloride Hydrolyzed gelatin (14.5 mg) Recombinant human albumin ($\leq$0.3 mg) Fetal bovine serum (<1 ppm) Neomycin (25 mcg) Buffer and media ingredients
Latex	None
Labeled indications	Immunization against measles, mumps, and rubella
Labeled ages	$\geq$12 months
Dose	0.5 mL
Route of administration	Subcutaneous
Usual schedule	12 to 15 months of age Revaccination before school entry
How supplied (number in package)	1-dose vial (10), lyophilized, with diluent
Storage:	
Vaccine	Refrigerate, protect from light
Diluent	Refrigerate or room temperature, do not freeze
Reconstituted vaccine	Refrigerate for up to 8 hours, protect from light
Reference package insert	December 2007

TABLE 9.11 — *Continued*

ª The components of MMR are licensed as separate vaccines: measles vaccine (Attenuvax; Merck); mumps vaccine (Mumpsvax; Merck); rubella vaccine (Meruvax II; Merck); measles and mumps vaccine (M-M-Vax; Merck; this vaccine is no longer available in the United States). MMR is also available in combination with varicella vaccine (ProQuad; Merck).

- *Precautions*
  - Moderate or severe acute illness (difficulty distinguishing illness from vaccine reaction)
  - History of thrombocytopenia or thrombocytopenic purpura (risk of recurrent thrombocytopenia)
  - Recent receipt of antibody-containing blood product (risk of impaired response to vaccine; see *Chapter 5*)
  - Untreated, active tuberculosis (risk of exacerbation of tuberculosis). Measles vaccine virus replication can suppress the response to a tuberculin skin test. If not given before or on the same day as a tuberculin skin test, MMR should be delayed 4 weeks after the tuberculin skin test is done.

■ Recommendations for General Use

All individuals who do not have evidence of immunity to measles, mumps, and rubella should be vaccinated (the criteria for immunity are given in **Table 9.12**). MMR is the preferred vaccine, and there are very few reasons (if any) to give the monovalent vaccines separately (even if one or two of the components are not needed). For children, the first dose is usually given at 12 to 15 months of age and the second dose at 4 to 6 years of age. The second dose may be given any time ≥1 month following the first dose. High-risk adults (health care personnel, international travelers, and students at postsecondary educational institutions) who lack evidence of immunity should receive 2 doses of MMR separated by ≥1 month (those who have a history of 1 dose in the past should have a second dose). For health care personnel born before 1957, 1 dose of MMR should be considered. Women who might become pregnant and who lack evidence of immunity should receive 1 dose of MMR (pregnancy should be deferred at least 4 weeks after vaccination). Rubella vaccine may be given after anti-Rho(D) immune globulin administration, but testing for seroconversion should be performed 6 to 8 weeks later.

During measles outbreaks, when the likelihood of exposure is high, measles vaccine can be given to infants as young as 6 months of age. Doses given before the first birthday, however, *do not count* in the series, and these children should receive 2 subsequent doses according to the usual schedule. Although measles vaccination is not a requirement for entry into any country, measles and mumps are still endemic in many parts of the world. Persons who lack evidence of immunity and are planning travel to these areas should receive 2 doses of MMR (separated by ≥4

TABLE 9.12 — Immunity to Measles, Mumps, and Rubella[a]

Criteria	Persons to Whom the Criteria Apply		
	Measles	Mumps	Rubella
Birth before 1957	Everyone except health care personnel	Everyone except health care personnel	Everyone except health care personnel and women who might become pregnant
Personal history of disease	Persons with a history of *physician-diagnosed* disease	Persons with a history of *physician-diagnosed* disease	Not considered reliable evidence of immunity in anyone
Written history of at least 1 dose of vaccine	Children 1 year of age to school-aged	Children 1 year of age to school-aged	Anyone ≥1 year of age
Written history of 2 doses of vaccine	School-aged children (grades K-12) High-risk adults (health care personnel, international travelers, students at postsecondary educational institutions)	School-aged children (grades K-12) High-risk adults (health care personnel, international travelers, students at postsecondary educational institutions)	Not required
Serology	Positive measles-specific IgG antibody test	Positive mumps-specific IgG antibody test	Positive rubella-specific IgG antibody test

[a] Any one criterion is considered sufficient.

Centers for Disease Control and Prevention. *MMWR.*1998;47(RR-8):1-57; Centers for Disease Control and Prevention. *MMWR.* 2006;55:629-630.

weeks) before leaving. Infants 6 to 12 months of age who will be traveling anywhere outside the United States should receive 1 dose, but should be revaccinated according to the routine schedule when they reach 12 months of age (vaccination of infants <6 months of age is not necessary because most will be protected by maternal antibodies).

Measles vaccine given within 72 hours of exposure to measles may prevent infection, but this is not true for mumps and rubella vaccines. Immunocompromised individuals who are exposed to measles should receive intramuscular immune globulin, 0.5 mL/kg (maximum 15 mL), within 6 days of exposure. The AAP recommends immune globulin prophylaxis for *all* HIV-infected children and adolescents exposed to measles, regardless of vaccination status, degree of symptoms, and level of immune suppression (the dose for asymptomatic HIV-infected individuals is 0.25 mL/kg, maximum 15 mL); the ACIP specifies prophylaxis only for *symptomatic* HIV infection. Susceptible household contacts of measles cases, especially those <1 year of age, should receive immune globulin as well (0.25 mL/kg, maximum 15 mL). Immune globulin is not recommended for postexposure prophylaxis against rubella or mumps.

Neisseria meningitidis

■ The Pathogen

N meningitidis is a gram-negative bacterium that typically takes the appearance of intracellular diplococci on Gram's stain. The organism produces a polysaccharide capsule that is the basis for classification into serogroups, the most important of which in causing disease are A, B, C, Y, and W-135. The capsule contributes to virulence by inhibiting complement-mediated lysis and phagocytosis by neutrophils. Pathogenicity is enhanced by the production of endotoxin. *N meningitidis* often colonizes the nasopharynx—disease results from bacteremia and bacteremic spread to distant sites such as the meninges.

■ Clinical Features

Meningococcemia (bloodstream infection with *N meningitidis*) is characterized by the sudden onset of fever, lethargy, myalgia, rash, and vomiting, followed by altered mental status, high fever or hypothermia, tachypnea, and hypotension. Initially, the rash may be macular or maculopapular, but there is rapid transition to petechiae and/or purpura. *Purpura fulminans* is characterized by rapid progression to disseminated intravascular coagulation, hypotension, shock, and possibly death within hours despite antimicrobial therapy and supportive measures. Death is common, and survivors may lose extensive areas of skin or extremities due to ischemia. Interestingly, some individuals experience transient meningococcal bacteremia that resolves spontaneously without treatment.

Meningitis presents with fever, vomiting, headache and photophobia. It is distinguished from other forms of pyogenic meningitis by the association with petechial or purpuric rash in two thirds of patients. Neurologic sequelae include deafness, cranial nerve palsies, hydrocephalus, and developmental delay. Meningococcus also causes pneumonia, myocarditis, pericarditis, arthritis, conjunctivitis, endophthalmitis, urethritis, and pharyngitis. Immune mediated arthritis, cutaneous vasculitis, and pericarditis can occur late in the course of infection, after antibiotic therapy is instituted. *Chronic meningococcemia* occurs rarely and is characterized by recurrent episodes of fever, chills, rash, arthralgias, and headache over a 6- to 8-week period.

■ Epidemiology and Transmission

Humans are the only natural hosts and transmission occurs by direct person-to-person contact or via respiratory droplets. Whereas asymptomatic carriage of *N meningitidis* in the general population is common, <5% of individuals carry pathogenic strains. In contrast, nasopharyngeal colonization with invasive strains approaches 50% in closed settings where a case has occurred. The secondary attack rate in households is 3% to 4%, and the risk to household members is 500 to 800 times the risk in the general population (this is why chemoprophylaxis is used for close contacts).

The highest incidence of invasive disease occurs in infants <1 year of age, once maternal antibodies have waned. A second peak occurs in adolescence and young adulthood, when intimate contact with other people increases. Disease occurs predominantly in late winter and early spring, and outbreaks may parallel increases in influenza activity. Risk factors include active and passive smoking, respiratory illness, steroid use, new residence, new school, lower socioeconomic status, and household crowding. Individuals with congenital or acquired immunodeficiency, especially complement deficiency (classically terminal component deficiency), asplenia, antibody deficiency, and HIV infection are also at increased risk. During outbreaks, alcohol use and patronizing bars and nightclubs are implicated as risk factors.

Epidemics caused by serogroup A most commonly occur in the meningitis belt of sub-Saharan Africa, central Asia, the Indian subcontinent, and Saudi Arabia. Such epidemics are rare in developed countries. In the United States, the vast majority of cases are sporadic, but localized outbreaks have increased. In the late 1980s, most US cases were due to serogroups B and C, and only 2% were due to serogroup Y. By the late 1990s, serogroups B, C, and Y each accounted for about one third of cases. The majority of cases in those <1 year of age are due to serogroup B, for which no vaccine is currently available in the United States.

■ Background on Immunization Program

Prior to the initiation of a universal adolescent immunization program in the United States, up to 2800 cases of invasive disease occurred each year. The overall case-fatality rate was as high as 14%, and up to 20% of survivors had some form of permanent disability. Half of patients had meningitis, making meningococcus the most common cause of bacterial meningitis in persons 2 to 18 years of age.

Since licensure in 1981, MPSV4 was used in individuals with medical conditions that placed them at high risk for meningococcal disease, as well as in persons traveling to endemic areas, and laboratory workers and for outbreak control. The vaccine was never recommended for universal use for a number of reasons, including the limited duration of protection, absence of herd-immunity effects, and the low incidence of disease in the general population. In the late 1990s, studies showed that college freshmen living in dormitories were at increased risk for meningococcal disease, of the order of 2- to 5-fold higher than the general population. Upward of 80% of these cases were caused by serotypes A, C, Y, or W-135. In 2000, it was recommended that all college students be informed about the risk of meningococcal disease, and that MPSV4 be made available to those who requested it. It was estimated that vaccination of all college freshmen living in dormitories would prevent 16 to 30 cases and one to three deaths, at a cost of $617,000 to $1.85 million per case prevented and $6.8 to $20.4 million per death prevented.

The licensure of MCV4 in 2005 prompted reassessment of the meningococcal prevention strategy in the United States. As a conjugate vaccine, MCV4 was expected to result in more effective and longer-lived antibody responses, as well as the potential to reduce nasopharyngeal colonization and result in herd immunity. Moreover, the reality of herd effects was borne out in the experience with serogroup C conjugate vaccines in the United Kingdom. There, a universal immunization program for children 12 months to 17 years of age that began in 1999 resulted in dramatic declines in disease among both vaccinated and unvaccinated individuals, as well as decreases in nasopharyngeal carriage. It was estimated that a universal MCV4 program in the United States for children 11 years of age plus a catch-up campaign for adolescents would (assuming herd effects) prevent >5000 cases over a 10-year period, at a cost of $532,000 per case prevented and $5.9 million per death prevented.

These estimates make routine MCV4 vaccination more costly per health outcome than the programs for prevention of disease due to *H influenzae* type b and *S pneumoniae*. Nevertheless, recommendations for universal immunization of adolescents at 11 to 12 years of age, with limited catch-up of adolescents at 15 years of age, were released in 2005; the idea was to provide protection against the exposures that would occur in high school (more aggressive catch-up was not recommended because of anticipated supply issues). It was felt that immunization at 11 to 12 years of age would anchor the recommended routine preadolescent health care visit and would lay a foundation for the adolescent vaccination platform, which has since been rounded out with Tdap and the HPV vaccine. MCV4 also was recommended as a replacement for MPSV4 in high-risk individuals within the labeled age group, from 11 to 55 years of age, and the recommendation for college freshmen living in dormitories was strengthened from "educate" to "vaccinate."

In June 2007, when supply was sufficient, catch-up of all adolescents 11 to 17 years of age with MCV4 was recommended. In October 2007, with the extension of the label down to 2 years of age, the recommendation was made to substitute MCV4 for MPSV4 in high-risk children. In February 2008, the decision was made *not* to recommend universal immunization of children 2 to 10 years of age, for the following reasons: 1) it was not clear that immunization at younger ages would provide protection when it would be needed most, ie, at high school entry; 2) the burden of disease in that age group was lower than in infants and adolescents, and a smaller proportion of cases were due to vaccine serogroups; and 3) vaccinating children at 2 years of age would be much less cost-effective than vaccinating children at 11 years of age.

■ **Available Vaccines**

Characteristics of meningococcal vaccines licensed in the United States are given in **Table 9.13**. Biologic differences between conjugate and polysaccharide vaccines are discussed in *Chapter 1* and are summarized in **Table 1.3**.

■ **Efficacy and/or Immunogenicity**

Serogroup A polysaccharide vaccines induce an antibody response in infants as young as 3 months of age, but responses are not comparable to those in adults and efficacy declines within 3 years. Serogroup C polysaccharide is poorly immunogenic in children <18 months of age. In children <5 years of age, antibodies to serogroups A and C wane by 3 years after receipt of a single dose. In healthy adults, antibody concentrations after polysaccharide vaccine decrease with time but may be detectable for as long as 10 years after vaccination.

Serogroup C polysaccharide vaccine was tested in 20,000 US Army troops between 1969 and 1970. Efficacy was 90%, even in the face of ongoing epidemics. During an epidemic of serogroup C disease in Sao Paulo, Brazil, in 1974, efficacy among 67,000 infants and young children was 67% in those aged 24 to 36 months of age. During an epidemic of serogroup A disease in Finland in 1975 and 1976, nearly 50,000 young children were given a serogroup A vaccine in a controlled trial, with a demonstrated efficacy of 100%. Efficacy of 100% against serogroup A was also observed in a New Zealand study in 1985 and 1986, where 2 doses were given to children 3 to 23 months of age and 1 dose was given to those >2 years of age. In children 3 to 23 months of age who failed to return for their second dose, efficacy was only 52% and fell to 16% after 1 year. In the infants, however, antibody declined by 50% after 2 years and by 90% after 3 years.

Administration of serogroup C vaccine to all US troops since 1972 resulted in the elimination of serogroup C disease in this population. During a mass immunization campaign among individuals 6 months to 20 years of age in Quebec in 1992 and 1993, 1.6 million doses of vaccine were distributed; 24% of these contained serogroups A, C, Y and W-135 and 76% contained serogroups A and C only. Protection against serogroup C was 65% in the first 2 years but 0% in the next 3 years. Efficacy was strongly related to age, ranging from 83% for ages 15 to 20 years to 41% for ages 2 to 9 years. In Rwanda, a serogroup A epidemic was halted with the use of a serogroup A and C vaccine, although the carrier rate remained unchanged.

Some studies suggest that multiple doses of serogroup A and C polysaccharides (but not conjugated polysaccharides) can cause immunologic hyporesponsiveness, which means that the response to subsequent doses is reduced. The clinical significance of this phenomenon has not been addressed.

Licensure of MCV4 was based on immunologic noninferiority to MPSV4 rather than demonstrated efficacy. In a randomized trial of adolescents who received either MCV4 ($N=423$) or MPSV4 ($N=423$), the percentage of subjects in each group achieving a ≥4-fold rise in bactericidal antibody titer was approximately ≥90% for serogroups A, C, and W-135; responses to serogroup Y were lower but similar for both vaccines (81.8% and 80.1%, respectively). The percentage of subjects achieving a serum bactericidal titer of ≥128—the presumed protective level in assays using *rabbit* complement (see *Chapter 1* for a discussion of correlates of protection)—was >98% for all serogroups for each vaccine. In a similar study of adults, those who received MCV4 ($N=1280$) less often had ≥4-fold rises in antibody as compared with those who received MPSV4 ($N=1098$); however, the percentage achieving titers ≥128 were similar and the criteria for noninferiority were met. Again, 4-fold responses for serogroup Y were lower than for other serogroups (73.5% and 79.4%, respectively).

In a study involving children 2 to 3 years of age, antibody responses to each serogroup were higher among MCV4 recipients ($N=48$ to 52) than MPSV4 recipients ($N=50$ to 53). The percentage of MCV4 subjects achieving a serum bactericidal titer of ≥8—the presumed protective level in assays using *human* complement—was 73% for serogroup A, 63% for C, 88% for Y, and 63% for W-135. Similarly, responses were higher among

TABLE 9.13 — Meningococcal Vaccines

Trade name	Menactra	Menomune—A/C/Y/W-135
Abbreviation	MCV4	MPSV4
Manufacturer/distributor	Sanofi Pasteur	Sanofi Pasteur
Type of vaccine	Inactivated, engineered subunits	Inactivated, purified subunits
Composition	Group-specific polysaccharides (4 mcg each) from *Neisseria meningitidis* serogroups A, C, Y, and W-135, conjugated to diphtheria toxoid (48 mcg)	Group-specific polysaccharides (50 mcg each) from *N meningitidis* serogroups A, C, Y, and W-135
Adjuvant	None	None
Preservative	None	Thimerosal (1:10,000) or none
Excipients and contaminants	None reported	Lactose (2.5 to 5 mg)
Latex	Vial stopper contains dry natural rubber	Vial stopper contains dry natural rubber
Labeled indications	Immunization against invasive meningococcal disease	Immunization against invasive meningococcal disease
Labeled ages	2 to 55 years	≥2 years
Dose	0.5 mL	0.5 mL
Route of administration	Intramuscular	Subcutaneous
Usual schedule	1 dose	1 dose
		Revaccination in 2 to 5 years

How supplied (number in package)	1-dose vial (5) Prefilled syringe (1, 5)	Preservative-free formulation: 1-dose vial (1, 5), lyophilized, with diluent Thimerosal-containing formulation: 10-dose vial (1), lyophilized, with diluent
Storage	Refrigerate Do not freeze	Vaccine: refrigerate Diluent: refrigerate or room temperature Reconstituted vaccine: 1-dose vial, use within 30 minutes; 10-dose vial, refrigerate for up to 35 days
Reference package insert	October 2007	December 2005

9

children 4 to 10 years of age who received MCV4 ($N=84$) as compared with those who received MPSV4 ($N=84$). The percentage of MCV4 subjects achieving a serum bactericidal titer (human complement assay) of ≥ 8 was 81% for serogroup A, 79% for C, 99% for Y, and 85% for W-135.

■ **Safety**

Reactions to both MPSV4 and MCV4 are generally mild and consist primarily of pain and erythema at the injection site, occurring in around half of recipients. Mild systemic reactions, such as headache and malaise, are seen in somewhat over half of patients, but fever is unusual.

See *Chapter 8* for a discussion of Guillain-Barré syndrome following receipt of MCV4.

- *Contraindications*
  - Allergic reaction to previous dose of vaccine or any vaccine component (risk of recurrent allergic reaction)
- *Precautions*
  - Moderate or severe acute illness (difficulty distinguishing illness from vaccine reaction)
  - Personal history of Guillain-Barré syndrome (risk of recurrent Guillain-Barré syndrome)

■ **Recommendations for General Use**

All adolescents should be vaccinated against *N meningitidis*. The usual schedule is 1 dose of MCV4 at 11 to 12 years of age, but adolescents ≤ 18 years of age who have not been vaccinated should receive a dose at the earliest opportunity.

In all situations where vaccination against *N meningitidis* is called for, MCV4 is preferred to MPSV4 if the individual is 2 to 55 years of age. In addition to age-based routine use, MCV4 *is recommended* for the following individuals or situations.

- College freshmen living in dormitories
- Microbiologists routinely exposed to *N meningitidis*
- Military recruits
- Travelers to or residents of countries in which *N meningitidis* is hyperendemic or epidemic
- Persons with terminal complement component deficiencies (properdin deficiency also increases the risk of meningococcal disease and might be considered in this category)
- Persons with anatomic or functional asplenia (in elective situations, such as planned splenectomy, vaccination should occur at least 2 weeks earlier, if possible)

Immunization also is used for outbreak control. In general, outbreaks are defined as ≥ 3 cases in 3 months, resulting in a primary attack rate of ≥ 10 cases per 100,000 population. For short-term protection of infants 3 to 23 months of age during outbreaks of serogroup A, 2 doses of MPSV4 may be given 3 months apart.

Immunization *should be considered* for persons with HIV infection, although the risk of meningococcal disease is not as great as the risk for invasive pneumococcal disease. In addition, anyone who wants to reduce their risk of meningococcal disease should be offered vaccination.

Individuals who previously received MPSV4 because they were at increased risk for meningococcal disease should receive a dose of MCV4 if they remain at increased risk. For children 2 to 10 years of age, the dose of MCV4 should be given as close as possible to 3 years after the dose of MPSV4. For example, a sickle cell patient who received MPSV4 at 2 years of age should receive a dose of MCV4 at 5 years of age. For adolescents and adults, a minimum of 5 years should elapse. For example, an adult who received MPSV4 5 years ago before relocating to sub-Saharan Africa should receive MCV4 if he continues to reside there. Revaccination after receipt of MCV4 is not recommended.

Meningococcal conjugate vaccines that can be used in infancy, as well as vaccines for serogroup B, are in the late stages of clinical development.

Polio

9

■ The Pathogen

Poliovirus is small, nonenveloped, single-stranded RNA virus in the Picornaviridae family. Initial replication occurs in the pharynx and lower GI tract as well as in associated lymph nodes. This leads to primary viremia that seeds peripheral sites, including the viscera and skeletal muscle. Most infections are contained at this point and are therefore subclinical. In a minority of individuals, replication at peripheral sites leads to secondary viremia associated with nonspecific symptoms, such as fever and malaise; in about one in 100 infections, the CNS is involved, either through hematogenous spread or axonal transport from muscle. Once in the CNS, poliovirus can cause a self-limited aseptic meningitis, but more importantly can replicate in and destroy anterior horn cells of the spinal cord, leading to lower motor-neuron paralysis.

■ Clinical Features

Approximately 95% of poliovirus infections are asymptomatic. Minor, nonspecific illness with low-grade fever and sore throat occurs in 4% to 8% of infected people; aseptic meningitis, sometimes with paresthesias, occurs in 1% to 2% of patients a few days after these symptoms resolve. The CSF may show mild pleocytosis with a lymphocytic predominance. Less than 1% of patients experience the rapid onset of asymmetric flaccid paralysis and areflexia; the proximal lower extremity muscles are most often involved, and some patients have cranial nerve involvement. Prior to the availability of modern assisted ventilation, most deaths occurred from respiratory failure. In the past, patients who survived the acute illness but failed to recover respiratory muscle function were condemned to live out the remainder of their lives in an iron lung; today, tracheostomy and positive-pressure ventilation are used. Somewhat more than half of patients who developed limb paralysis have permanent functional deficits. Adults who contracted paralytic polio during childhood may develop postpolio syndrome, characterized by muscle pain and exacerbation of weakness 30 to 40 years later.

■ Epidemiology and Transmission

Humans are the only natural hosts and transmission occurs by the fecal-oral route, although pharyngeal secretions may be involved. Communicability is greatest shortly before and after onset of clinical illness, but patients may be contagious in the absence of symptoms and fecal excretion may persist for weeks. Immunodeficient patients can excrete the virus for >6 months.

Infection is more common in infants and young children and occurs at an earlier age among children living in poor hygienic conditions. The risk of paralytic disease increases with age. In temperate climates, poliovirus infections are most common during the summer and autumn. In the tropics, the seasonal pattern is variable with a less-pronounced peak of activity.

The last reported indigenous case of polio in the United States occurred in 1979, and the only identified imported case of paralytic polio since 1986 occurred in a child transported here for medical care in 1993. Since 1979, all other cases of polio, an average of eight per year between 1980 and 1996, were caused by OPV-derived strains. While OPV has not been used in the United States since 2000, infections with OPV-derived strains still occur. In 2005, four unimmunized children in an Amish community in Minnesota were found to be infected with an OPV-derived strain of poliovirus. The index case was an infant with severe combined immunodeficiency disease, and the other three children were otherwise healthy siblings in a separate household. Genetic analysis suggested that the strain had been imported by someone vaccinated with OPV in another country. Vaccine-derived poliovirus that has reverted to virulence can emerge because of continuous replication in immunodeficient individuals or continuous circulation in unimmunized populations. The latter phenomenon was highlighted during an outbreak of paralytic polio in the Caribbean in 2000 to 2001, which was caused by a strain of OPV that had reverted to virulence in areas of very low vaccine coverage.

■ Background on Immunization Program

Because of widespread vaccination, worldwide eradication of polio is now on the horizon. In the United States, the annual number of wild-type cases fell from >18,000 to zero in about 2 decades. In 1988, the World Health Assembly resolved to eradicate polio through the Global Polio Eradication Initiative. As a result, the number of cases worldwide has been reduced from 350,000 in 1988 to 1310 in 2007. The number of countries that have never succeeded in interrupting wild poliovirus transmission has been reduced from 125 to just 4: Afghanistan, India, Nigeria, and Pakistan.

In 2006, Global Polio Eradication Initiative partners immunized 375 million children in 36 countries with 2.1 billion doses of vaccine, and the technical feasibility of polio eradication was affirmed. We may soon be living in a world free of circulating wild-type polioviruses. After global eradication, however, it will be difficult to decide when or if polio immunization should be discontinued. Live-attenuated vaccine strains could still be circulating. In addition, reservoirs of wild-type virus could still exist (eg, in laboratories that have frozen stool specimens from the polio era), and infectious virus that can be used in bioterrorism can be reconstructed from the genetic material of the virus.

These astonishing accomplishments have occurred primarily through the use of OPV. This was the vaccine of choice for children in the United States since the early 1960s because it induced optimal intestinal immunity, was relatively inexpensive, was painless, required little training to administer, and contributed to immunity at the population level through fecal-oral spread. For these same reasons, OPV continues to be used in the worldwide eradication effort. However, the continued use of OPV, with the attendant five to ten cases of vaccine-associated polio per year, was felt to be unjustified in the United States in the absence of wild-type disease. IPV is known to be highly effective, incapable of causing polio, and is used routinely in several countries that had controlled or eliminated polio. Accordingly, expanded use of IPV was recommended beginning in 1997, and as of January 2000, the recommendation was made to substitute IPV for OPV in the United States.

■ **Available Vaccines**

Characteristics of the polio vaccines licensed in the United States are given in **Table 9.14**.

■ **Efficacy and/or Immunogenicity**

Ninety-percent or more of vaccinees develop protective antibody to all three serotypes after 2 doses, and ≥99% are immune after 3 doses. Protection against paralytic disease correlates with the presence of serum antibody. IPV appears to induce less mucosal immunity than does OPV, so persons who receive IPV are more readily infected in the GI tract with wild poliovirus. Thus a person immunized with IPV could become infected in an endemic area and shed virus upon return to the United States. The infected person would be protected from paralytic polio, but the wild virus shed in the stool could be transmitted to a contact. The duration of immunity from IPV is not known with certainty but is probably many years after a complete series.

TABLE 9.14 — Polio Vaccine[a]

Trade name	IPOL[b]
Abbreviation	IPV
Manufacturer/ distributor	Sanofi Pasteur
Type of vaccine	Inactivated, whole agent
Composition	Type 1 (Mahoney), 40 D antigen units
	Type 2 (MEF-1), 8 D antigen units
	Type 3 (Saukett), 32 D antigen units
	Propagated in Vero (African Green Monkey kidney) cells
	Inactivated with formalin
Adjuvant	None
Preservative	2-phenoxyethanol (0.5%) and formaldehyde ($\leq$0.02%)
Excipients and contaminants	Neomycin (<5 ng)
	Streptomycin (<200 ng)
	Polymyxin B (<25 ng)
	Calf serum protein (<1 ppm)
Latex	None
Labeled indications	Immunization against poliomyelitis
Labeled ages	$\geq$6 weeks
Dose	0.5 mL
Route of administration	Intramuscular or subcutaneous
Usual schedule	2, 4, 6 to 18 months, 4 to 6 years of age
How supplied (number in package)	10-dose vial (1)
	Prefilled syringe (10)
Storage	Refrigerate
	Do not freeze
Reference package insert	December 2005

[a] An IPV that is very similar to IPOL is available in combination with DTaP and HepB (Pediarix; GlaxoSmithKline). This IPV is not licensed or distributed separately in the United States. Pediarix is indicated at 2, 4, and 6 months of age. The same IPV is available in combination with DTaP (Kinrix; GlaxoSmithKline). Kinrix is indicated for the booster doses of DTaP and IPV at 4 to 6 years of age. The IPV in Pediarix and Kinrix is considered interchangeable with IPOL.

[b] An IPV that is very similar to IPOL (Poliovax; Sanofi Pasteur) is also available in combination with DTaP and Hib (Pentacel; Sanofi Pasteur). Pentacel is indicated at 2, 4, 6, and 15 to 18 months of age.

■ Safety

Minor local reactions, such as pain and redness, may occur following IPV. No serious adverse events have been associated with use of the currently available vaccine.

- *Contraindications*
  - Allergic reaction to previous dose of vaccine or any vaccine component (risk of recurrent allergic reaction)
- *Precautions*
  - Moderate or severe acute illness (difficulty distinguishing illness from vaccine reaction)
  - Pregnancy (theoretic risk to the fetus or attribution of birth defects to vaccination, although no deleterious effects from IPV administered during pregnancy have been demonstrated)

■ Recommendations for General Use

All children should be vaccinated against polio. The primary series of IPV consists of 3 doses, usually given at 2, 4, and 6 to 18 months of age. A fourth dose is given around the time of school entry, between 4 and 6 years of age. If the fourth dose is given before 4 years of age, a fifth dose is not necessary, unless the state requires a dose on or after the child turns 4. Routine immunization of US adults ≥18 years of age is not recommended. However, a 3-dose series of IPV (0, 1 to 2, and 6 to 12 months) *is* recommended for *previously unvaccinated adults in the following circumstances* (an accelerated schedule consisting of doses at 0, 1, and 2 months can be used if necessary):

- Travel to countries where polio is epidemic or endemic
- Members of a community experiencing wild-type poliovirus disease
- Health care workers who will come into close contact with patients potentially excreting wild-type poliovirus
- Laboratory workers who will come in contact with specimens that may contain poliovirus

Adults who have received a primary series of at least 3 doses who are at increased risk of exposure to polio should receive a single supplemental dose of IPV (this does not need to be repeated for subsequent travel). Those who have had <3 doses (of either OPV or IPV) should complete the primary series of 3 doses using IPV, regardless of the interval since the last dose and the type of vaccine that was previously given.

Rotavirus

■ The Pathogen

Rotavirus is a nonenveloped virus with a wheel-like appearance in the Reoviridae family. The genome is divided into 11 double-stranded RNA segments, most of which encode only one viral protein. Infection of the GI tract causes diarrhea by several mechanisms: increased fluid secretion due to the effects of a virus-encoded enterotoxin (NSP4) and stimulation of the enteric nervous system, and increased osmotic load caused by destruction of villus epithelial cells, decreased absorption of salt and water, and decreased disaccharidase activity. Protection against disease is mediated by immune responses to the G, or coat, protein (also known as VP7) and the P, or spike, protein (also known as VP4). Any given rotavirus strain has a specific G type, designated by a serotype number (as in "G1") and a P type, designated by a serotype number (as in "P1a") and/or a genotype number in brackets (as in "P[8]"). Certain combinations of G and P types are found more commonly than others, eg, G1P[8] and G2P[4].

■ Clinical Features

The incubation period is 1 to 4 days. Illness begins abruptly with fever and vomiting, and diarrhea ensues shortly thereafter. There may be >20 daily episodes of vomiting and/or diarrhea during the peak of the illness. Severe vomiting may lead to dehydration even before the diarrhea begins, and associated symptoms include irritability and lethargy. The illness lasts for about a week and appears to be more severe than other forms of gastroenteritis in infants. For example, in one study of outpatients with acute gastroenteritis, children with rotavirus more often had fever (60% vs 43%) as well as both vomiting *and* diarrhea (75% vs 50%) when compared with those with other etiologies; more days of work were lost by the parents (median of 2 vs 0) and more days of day care were lost by the children (median of 3 vs 1).

Risk factors for hospitalization include low birth weight, child care attendance, and absence of breast-feeding. Common complications of severe rotavirus infection include isotonic dehydration, electrolyte disturbances, metabolic acidosis, and temporary milk intolerance. Rare complications include necrotizing enterocolitis and hemorrhagic gastroenteritis. Immunocompromised patients may develop particularly severe or fatal illness and may shed virus in the stool for months. When infected, adults are usually asymptomatic, but outbreaks in nursing homes have led to symptomatic disease and fatalities in the elderly.

■ Epidemiology and Transmission

Animal strains of rotavirus exist, but transmission of those strains to humans is rare. Transmission of human rotavirus occurs from person to person through the fecal-oral route, airborne droplets, and contaminated fomites. Infected children shed as much as 100 billion viral particles per milliliter of stool. Since the infectious dose is around 10,000 particles, it only takes one ten-millionth of a milliliter of stool to transmit the infection. This makes rotavirus one of the more contagious forms of gastroenteritis. Because rotavirus is not spread through contaminated food or water, improvements in sanitation and public hygiene do not affect the incidence of disease; this explains why the proportion of severe gastroenteritis caused by rotavirus is the same in developed countries as it is in developing countries.

Rotavirus causes approximately 70,000 hospitalizations and 700,000 outpatient visits each year in the United States. The numbers worldwide are staggering—2 million hospitalizations and approximately 25 million outpatient visits. Virtually all children experience at least one rotavirus infection by 5 years of age. First infections and those occurring in infants are the most severe, and it is worth noting that rotavirus causes about 10% of all first-time pediatric hospital admissions in the United States. Death, while unusual in the United States (approximately 60 per year) and other developed countries, is common in developing countries (nearly 500,000 per year) where the infrastructure to support hydration of infants during the acute illness is lacking. Reinfection is common, but disease is usually mild or asymptomatic, and repeated reinfections reduce the likelihood of subsequent infections. Outbreaks and nosocomial spread occur frequently in day care centers, pediatric hospital wards, and nurseries.

In the United States, annual epidemics begin in the late fall in the Southwest and spread to the North and East by the end of winter or early spring. In the tropics, rotavirus may occur at any time of the year. The predominant circulating strains vary from year to year, but the most prevalent serotype is G1P[8]. Other important serotypes are G2P[4], G3P[8], G4P[8], and G9P[8].

■ Background on Immunization Program

The first vaccine against rotavirus, rhesus rotavirus vaccine, tetravalent (RRV-TV), was licensed in 1998 under the trade name RotaShield (Wyeth). The vaccine was made from a rhesus rotavirus strain that was naturally attenuated for humans. Three reassortants were constructed, each of which expressed a different human G serotype (G1, G2, and G4); the native rhesus strain, which had a G3-like serotype, was also carried through into the final product. Thus RRV-TV consisted of four live viruses— three reassortants and the parental rhesus strain—representing G serotypes 1 through 4 (each strain also expressed the rhesus P[3]). The vaccine was administered orally at 2, 4, and 6 months of age, was 70% to 95% effective at preventing severe rotavirus gastroenteritis, and was recommended for all infants in the United States.

Within a year of licensure, RRV-TV was found to be associated with intussusception, a form of bowel obstruction in which a portion of the intestine telescopes into itself, resulting in swelling and vascular compromise (see discussion of the vaccine safety net in Chapter 2, *Vaccine Infrastructure in the United States*). The attributable risk was estimated at about one in 11,000 vaccinees, with most cases occurring in the first 2 weeks after dose 1, the time when viral replication peaks. RRV-TV was withdrawn in 1999; the mechanism whereby it caused intussusception is still not clear, but it was felt to be related to certain biologic characteristics of the native rhesus rotavirus strain.

The disease burden continues to justify a vaccination program, as does the cost of rotavirus disease—>$1 billion each year in the United States alone in direct medical and societal costs. It was estimated that a universal vaccination program instituted in a single US birth cohort—assuming only 70% coverage and looking at outcomes over 5 years—would reduce the number of domiciliary episodes of rotavirus gastroenteritis by 48%, office visits by 60%, emergency department visits by 64%, hospitalizations by 66%, and deaths by 44%. The cost per case averted would be $138, cost per serious case averted would be $3024, and cost per year of life saved would be $197,190.

Pentavalent rotavirus vaccine (PRV), a live, oral, bovine reassortant vaccine marketed under the trade name RotaTeq (Merck), was licensed in February 2006. Prelicensure clinical trials demonstrated safety, efficacy, and importantly, no association with intussusception, and the vaccine was recommended for all infants in the United States. By May 2008, coverage for 1 dose in infants 3 months of age was estimated to be 56% and coverage for 3 doses in children 13 months of age was estimated to be 34%. Laboratory surveillance demonstrated that the 2007-2008 rotavirus season was delayed by several months when compared with the previous 15 seasons, and the magnitude (in terms of the number and proportion of positive tests for rotavirus) was diminished by >50%. This indicates substantial impact of the vaccination program on the epidemiology of the disease, despite incomplete uptake.

Human rotavirus vaccine (HRV), a live, attenuated, oral vaccine made from a human strain of rotavirus and marketed under the trade name Rotarix (GlaxoSmithKline), was licensed in April 2008. Both PRV and HRV have been licensed and distributed in other countries.

■ Available Vaccines

Characteristics of the rotavirus vaccines licensed in the United States are given in **Table 9.15**.

■ Efficacy and/or Immunogenicity

Prelicensure studies of PRV involved >70,000 infants in many countries throughout the world; half of the subjects were enrolled in the United States, a third in Finland, and the rest in Latin America, Europe, and Taiwan. Detailed information about efficacy came from about 7000 of these infants. The pivotal trial, a placebo-controlled study called the Rotavirus Efficacy and Safety Trial (REST), consisted of a large-scale safety study ($N=69,625$), a detailed safety substudy ($N=9605$), and an efficacy substudy ($N=5673$); efficacy against rotavirus-related hospitalizations and emergency department visits was determined in the entire cohort. Efficacy against rotavirus gastroenteritis of any severity due to serotypes G1 through G4 during the first season after vaccination was 74%, and against severe disease was 98% (efficacy was still

98% against severe disease when the data were looked at without regard to serotype). Efficacy against disease of any severity was 71% though two seasons; in the second season alone, efficacy was 63% against disease of any severity and 88% against severe disease. Emergency department visits due to rotavirus serotypes G1 through G4 were reduced by 94% during the 2 years following dose 3, and hospitalizations were reduced by 96%; in a separate post hoc analysis, efficacy against hospitalizations and emergency department visits due to G9P[8] strains was 100%.

The prelicensure studies of HRV also involved >70,000 infants (efficacy was evaluated in about 24,000). Two pivotal trials were done—3994 infants were enrolled in a European trial and slightly over 63,225 in a trial in Latin America and Finland. Efficacy in the European study against rotavirus gastroenteritis of any severity through one season was 87% and through two seasons was 79%; the respective efficacies against severe disease were 96% and 90%. Hospitalizations were reduced by 100% through one season and 96% through two seasons. In the Latin America/ Finland study, efficacy against severe rotavirus gastroenteritis through one season was 85% and through two seasons was 81%; hospitalizations were reduced by 85% and 83%, respectively. Type-specific efficacy was evaluated in about 4000 infants. The vaccine was highly effective against G1P[8] strains. For non-G1 strains, efficacy through one season against any severity of disease ranged from 76% for G9P[8] to 90% for G3P[8] but was not significant for G2P[4] (very few cases occurred). Efficacy through two seasons against any severity of disease ranged from 58% for G2P[4] to 85% for G3P[8]. Efficacy through one season against severe disease ranged from 95% for G9P[8] to 100% for G3P[8] and G4P[8] but was not significant for G2P[4] (again, very few cases occurred). Efficacy through two seasons against severe disease ranged from 85% for G9P[8] to 95% for G4P[8].

■ Safety

In REST, 11 cases of intussusception occurred within 42 days of any dose of PRV—six among vaccinees and five among place-bees, a difference that was not statistically significant. No clustering of cases was seen after any dose. Following licensure, VAERS reports of intussusception occurring among vaccinees were not increased above the expected background rates, and postmarketing surveillance (15 million doses had been distributed in the United States by May 2008) showed no association between the vaccine and intussusception. Prelicensure trials showed a slight excess of vomiting (6.7% vs 5.4%) and diarrhea (10.4% vs 9.1%) after dose 1 among vaccinees as compared with placebees, and a slight excess of diarrhea (8.6% vs 6.4%) after dose 2. Vaccine virus is shed in the stool in about 9% of vaccinees after dose 1 but is rarely shed after subsequent doses. Horizontal transmission, while not formally evaluated, has not been reported.

TABLE 9.15 — Rotavirus Vaccines

Trade name	Rotarix	RotaTeq
Abbreviation	HRV	PRV
Manufacturer/distributor	GlaxoSmithKline	Merck
Type of vaccine	Live attenuated, classic	Live attenuated, engineered
Composition	Human rotavirus strain 89-12, serotype G1P1[8]	5 naturally attenuated bovine rotavirus reassortants expressing the following serotypes:
	Propagated in Vero (African Green Monkey kidney) cells	Human G1, bovine P7[5]
	10^6 median cell culture infective dose	Human G2, bovine P7[5]
		Human G3, bovine P7[5]
		Human G4, bovine P7[5]
		Bovine G6, human P1[8]
		Propagated in Vero (African Green Monkey kidney) cells
		2.0 to 2.8×10^6 infectious units of each virus
Adjuvant	None	None
Preservative	None	None
Excipients and contaminants	Lyophilized vaccine:	Sucrose
	Amino acids	Sodium citrate
	Dextran	Sodium phosphate monobasic monohydrate
	Dulbecco's Modified Eagle Medium	Sodium hydroxide
	Sorbitol	Polysorbate 80
	Sucrose	Cell culture media

	Diluent: Calcium carbonate Xanthan	Fetal bovine serum (trace)
Latex	Tip cap and plunger of oral applicator contain dry natural latex rubber	None
Labeled indications	Immunization against rotavirus gastroenteritis caused by serotypes G1, G3, G4, and G9	Immunization against rotavirus gastroenteritis caused by serotypes G1, G2, G3, and G4
Labeled ages	6 to 24 weeks	6 to 32 weeks
Dose	1 mL	2 mL
Route of administration	Oral[a]	Oral[a]
Usual schedule	2, 4 months of age[b]	2, 4, 6 months of age[b]
How supplied (number in package)	1-dose vial (10), lyophilized, with diluent in prefilled oral applicator	1-dose squeezable, plastic tube (1, 10)
Storage	Vaccine: refrigerate, protect from light; Diluent: room temperature, do not freeze; Reconstituted vaccine: refrigerate or room temperature for up to 24 hr, do not freeze	Refrigerate; Protect from light; Administer as soon as possible after removing from refrigerator
Reference package insert	April 2008	April 2008

[a] The dose should not be repeated if it is spit out or regurgitated.

[b] According to the package inserts, the first dose of HRV may be given between 6 and 20 weeks of age, and no dose should be given beyond 24 weeks. Likewise, the first dose of PRV should be given at 6 to 12 weeks of age, and no dose should be given beyond 32 weeks. Provisional recommendations released July 2008 call for the first dose of either vaccine to be given between 6 weeks and 14 weeks 6 days of age, and all doses should be given by 8 months 0 days. If any dose in the series is PRV, 3 total doses should be given.

In the Latin America/Finland study of HRV, 13 cases of intussusception occurred within 31 days of any dose of HRV—six among vaccinees and seven among placebees, a difference that was not statistically significant. There were no confirmed cases within the 14-day period following dose 1, which was the highest risk period for RRV-TV. Solicited adverse events occurred at similar rates among HRV recipients and placebo recipients. HRV was, however, associated with slightly increased unsolicited reports of irritability (11.4% vs 8.7%) and flatulence (2.2% vs 1.3%) when compared with placebo. Vaccine virus is shed in the stool in about one fourth of patients after dose 1. Horizontal transmission, while not formally evaluated, has not been reported.

- *Contraindications*
  - Allergic reaction to previous dose of vaccine or any vaccine component (risk of recurrent allergic reaction)
- *Precautions*
  - Moderate or severe acute illness (difficulty distinguishing illness from vaccine reaction)
  - Moderate or severe acute gastroenteritis (risk of impaired immune response)
  - Immunodeficiency or immunosuppression (risk of disease caused by live virus)
  - Receipt of antibody-containing blood product (risk of impaired immune response). Do not defer vaccination if this would cause dose 1 to be given beyond of the recommended age (see *Chapter 5*).
  - Pre-existing GI disease such as congenital malabsorption syndrome, chronic diarrhea and failure to thrive, previous abdominal surgery, Hirschsprung's disease, short-gut syndrome, persistent vomiting of unknown cause (risk of exacerbation of GI disease; causality not established). History of uncorrected congenital malformation of the GI tract that might predispose to intussusception (eg, Meckel's diverticulum) is listed in the package insert as a contraindication for HRV.
  - Previous history of intussusception (risk of recurrent intussusception; causality not established)

■ Recommendations for General Use

All infants should be vaccinated against rotavirus. The usual schedule for PRV is 2, 4, and 6 months of age and the usual schedule for HRV is 2 and 4 months of age. According to recommendations published in 2006 after the licensure of PRV, vaccination *is recommended* in the following circumstances (publication of harmonized recommendations for both rotavirus vaccines is pending as of October 2008):

- Infants who have already had an episode of rotavirus gastroenteritis
- Breast-feeding

- Premature infants who are clinically stable and are being or have been discharged from the nursery (there are no clear-cut recommendations regarding vaccination of infants who will be residing in the nursery, but it seems prudent to administer the first dose before the window for dose 1 closes at 14 weeks 6 days of age; standard precautions should be followed to minimize horizontal transmission, which is a theoretic possibility)
- Infants living in the home of immunocompromised or pregnant individuals (standard precautions should be followed to minimize horizontal transmission, which is a theoretic possibility)

The series should be completed with the same product, but vaccination should not be deferred if the same product is unknown or not available. If any dose in the series is PRV, a total of 3 doses should be given.

Streptococcus pneumoniae

■ The Pathogen

S pneumoniae is a facultatively anaerobic, catalase-negative gram-positive bacterium that looks like lancet-shaped diplococci on Gram's stain. The organism produces a polysaccharide capsule that is the basis for serotyping (there are >90 known serotypes, although most invasive disease is caused by <20 of these). The capsule contributes to virulence by inhibiting complement-mediated lysis and phagocytosis by neutrophils. Other virulence factors include pneumolysin and pneumococcal surface protein A. *S pneumoniae* often colonizes the nasopharynx—disease results from contiguous spread to respiratory tract structures such as the middle ear space, hematogenous seeding of distant sites such as the meninges, or from bacteremia without focal infection. Resistance to penicillin and other antibiotics has increased dramatically since the early 1990s.

■ Clinical Features

Prior to the conjugate-vaccine era, bacteremia without focal infection accounted for 70% of invasive disease in those <2 years of age; bacteremic pneumonia accounted for another 12% to 16%. With the disappearance of invasive *H influenzae* type b disease from the United States in the 1990s, *S pneumoniae* became the leading cause of bacterial meningitis among children <5 years of age. *S pneumoniae* was also a common cause of acute otitis media (AOM), accounting for 28% to 55% of cases. By age 12 months, 62% of children had at least one episode of AOM, making this one of the more common reasons for sick visits to pediatric offices. Complications of otitis media include mastoiditis and suppurative intracranial infection.

Pneumonia is the most common presentation of pneumococcal disease in adults. Classically, there is abrupt onset of fever and a single episode of rigor. Other symptoms include pleuritic chest pain, productive cough yielding mucopurulent, rusty sputum, dyspnea, tachypnea, hypoxia, tachycardia, malaise, and weakness. Nausea, vomiting, and headaches occur less frequently. Complications include empyema, pericarditis, and abscess. Pneumococcal meningitis also occurs in adults. Symptoms include headache, lethargy, vomiting, irritability, fever, nuchal rigidity, cranial nerve signs, seizures, and coma. The spinal fluid profile and neurologic complications are similar to those in other forms of bacterial meningitis. One quarter of patients with pneumococcal meningitis also have pneumonia.

Mortality is highest in patients with bacteremia or meningitis, in patients with underlying medical conditions, and in the very young and the very old. In some high-risk groups, mortality from bacteremia is as high as 40% despite antibiotic therapy.

■ Epidemiology and Transmission

Humans are the only natural hosts and transmission occurs by direct person-to-person contact or via respiratory droplets. Spread within the household is facilitated by crowding and occurs more often in the late winter and early spring, when respiratory viral disease is more prevalent. In general, higher rates of nasopharyngeal carriage lead to higher rates of disease.

It is estimated that 1 million children worldwide die from invasive pneumococcal disease each year. In 1999, the year before the introduction of PCV7 in the United States, the overall incidence of invasive pneumococcal disease was 24 per 100,000 population. The rate was as high as 205 per 100,000 in children 1 year of age and as low as four per 100,000 in children between 5 and 17; adults ≥65 years of age had a rate of 62 per 100,000. It was estimated that there were a total of 64,400 cases of invasive disease and 7300 deaths. The most common serious clinical syndrome was bacteremic pneumonia (54%), followed by bacteremia without a focus (38%), and meningitis (5%), and pneumococcus was estimated to cause over one third of community-acquired and one half of hospital-acquired pneumonia in adults. In addition, an estimated 5 million cases of AOM due to pneumococcus occurred each year in children <5 years of age. Children with functional or anatomic asplenia, particularly those with sickle cell disease, and children with HIV infection were at particularly high risk for invasive disease, with rates in some studies >50 times those in age-equivalent children without these conditions. Alaska Native, American Indian, and African American children were also at increased risk. The reason for this is not known, but the same racial and ethnic predilection was seen for invasive *H influenzae* type b disease. Day care attendance was associated with a 2- to 3-fold increase in the risk of invasive pneumococcal disease and AOM among children ≤59 months of age.

■ Background on Immunization Program

At the time of its introduction in 2000, PCV7 covered 80% of the serotypes causing invasive disease in young children in the United States. By 2005, universal infant immunization had resulted in a 77% reduction in invasive disease among children <5 years of age. The largest percentage decline was among children 1 year of age. During 2001-2005, 62,000 children <5 years of age were spared invasive pneumococcal disease—59% through direct effects of the vaccine and the remainder through indirect effects (herd immunity as the result of decreased nasopharyngeal carriage rates). Overall decreases in pneumonia (not traditionally considered an invasive infection) and otitis media were seen as well, and rates of infection due to drug-resistant strains declined dramatically. Studies have demonstrated significant decreases in nasopharyngeal carriage of vaccine serotypes among vaccinated children, but there has been an increase in colonization with nonvaccine serotypes. This has been accompanied by increases in invasive disease due to those serotypes (so called *replacement disease*), particularly serotype 19A.

Declines in invasive pneumococcal disease due to vaccine serotypes also have been seen among older individuals as a result of herd immunity (see *Chapter 1* and **Figure 1.7**). While PPSV23 provides some protection for adults ≥65 years of age, conjugate vaccines that are approved for use in that age group, as well as higher valency conjugates for all age groups, are needed and are in development.

■ Available Vaccines

Characteristics of pneumococcal vaccines licensed in the United States are given in **Table 9.16**. Biologic differences between conjugate and polysaccharide vaccines are discussed in *Chapter 1* and are summarized in **Table 1.3**.

■ Efficacy and/or Immunogenicity

After 4 doses of PCV7, virtually all healthy infants develop antibody to all seven serotypes. PCV7 also is immunogenic in infants and children with sickle cell disease and HIV infection. In a controlled clinical trial involving nearly 40,000 children, the vaccine reduced invasive disease caused by vaccine serotypes by 97%; there was also an 89% reduction in invasive disease caused by all serotypes, including those not in the vaccine. The vaccine also reduced X-ray–confirmed pneumonia by 73%. Children who received PCV7 had 7% fewer episodes of AOM and underwent 20% fewer tympanostomy tube placements than unvaccinated children. In a Finnish study, efficacy against AOM caused by vaccine-related serotypes was 57%, but there was an increase of 33% in otitis episodes caused by nonvaccine serotypes. Despite this, there was a net reduction of 34% in AOM caused by *S pneumoniae*. A case-control study done after licensure demonstrated that ≥1 dose of PCV7 was 96% effective in preventing

TABLE 9.16 — Pneumococcal Vaccines

Trade name	Pneumovax 23	Prevnar
Abbreviation	PPSV23	PCV7
Manufacturer/distributor	Merck	Wyeth
Type of vaccine	Inactivated, purified subunits	Inactivated, engineered subunits
Composition	Capsular polysaccharides (25 mcg each) from *Streptococcus pneumoniae* serotypes 1, 2, 3, 4, 5, 6B, 7F, 8, 9N, 9V, 10A, 11A, 12F, 14, 15B, 17F, 18C, 19A, 19F, 20, 22F, 23F, 33F	Capsular polysaccharides from *S pneumoniae* serotypes 4, 9V, 14, 18C, 19F, and 23F (2 mcg each), and serotype 6B (4 mcg), conjugated to CRM$_{197}$, a nontoxic mutant diphtheria toxin (20 mcg)
Adjuvant	None	Aluminum phosphate (0.125 mg aluminum)
Preservative	Phenol (0.25%)	None
Excipients and contaminants	None reported	None reported
Latex	None	Vial stopper, syringe-plunger stopper and syringe-tip cap contain dry natural rubber
Labeled indications	Immunization against pneumococcal disease	Immunization against invasive disease caused by *S pneumoniae*
Labeled ages	≥2 years	6 months to 9 years
Dose	0.5 mL	0.5 mL
Route of administration	Intramuscular or subcutaneous	Intramuscular
Usual schedule	1 dose Revaccination in 5 years	2, 4, 6, 12 to 15 months of age

How supplied (number in package)	1-dose vial (10) 5-dose vial (1, 10)	1-dose vial (5) Prefilled syringe (10)
Storage	Refrigerate	Refrigerate Do not freeze
Reference package insert	September 2007	December 2007

9

invasive pneumococcal disease in healthy children 3 to 59 months of age and 81% effective in those with coexisting disorders. Effectiveness also was demonstrated against serotype 6A, which is not in the vaccine but is closely related to 6B, which is in the vaccine.

Protective efficacy of pneumococcal polysaccharide vaccines was initially demonstrated in healthy gold miners in South Africa. Postlicensure case-control studies estimate the efficacy of PPSV23 in preventing serious pneumococcal disease in immunocompetent persons to be 56% to 81%, but at least one meta-analysis suggested no protection against nonbacteremic pneumonia. A surveillance study demonstrated 57% overall effectiveness against invasive disease caused by vaccine serotypes; effectiveness was 65% to 84% in persons with underlying high-risk conditions and 75% in immunocompetent adults ≥65 years of age.

Antibody levels decline 5 to 10 years after vaccination, and may decline faster in the elderly. At least one study suggested that protection may last as long as 9 years. PPSV23 does not reduce nasopharyngeal carriage and does not protect children from otitis media.

■ Safety

Local reactions to PCV7, which are more common after dose 4, occur in 10% to 20% of recipients. Fewer than 3% of local reactions are considered to be severe (eg, tenderness that interferes with limb movement). In clinical trials, fever >100.4°F (38°C) within 48 hours of any dose of the primary series was reported in 15% to 24% of children. However, in these studies, DTwP was administered simultaneously with each dose and may have been responsible for the fever. In a study in which DTaP was given at the same visit as the booster dose of PCV7, 11% of recipients developed a temperature >102.2°F (39°C).

For persons ≥65 years of age receiving PPSV23, overall injection-site adverse experiences occur in about 50% after primary vaccination and in 80% after revaccination; moderate-severe pain and/or significant induration occur in about 10% of primary vaccinees and in 30% of revaccinees. Systemic adverse experiences such as fatigue, myalgia, and headache, are reported after primary vaccination in approximately 22% and after revaccination in 33%.

- *Contraindications*
  - Allergic reaction to previous dose of vaccine or any vaccine component (risk of recurrent allergic reaction)
- *Precautions*
  - Moderate or severe acute illness (difficulty distinguishing illness from vaccine reaction)

■ Recommendations for General Use

All children should be vaccinated against *S pneumoniae*. The primary series of PCV7 consists of doses at 2, 4, and 6 months of age, and a booster dose is given at 12 to 15 months of age. One dose of PCV7 should be given to all healthy children 24 to 59 months of age who have an incomplete schedule, including those who have never received PCV7. Age-dependent standard and catch-up schedules for healthy and high-risk children are given in **Table 9.17**. Note that PPSV23 is used to boost immunity in children ≥2 years of age with high-risk conditions who received PCV7 in infancy.

All adults ≥65 years of age should be vaccinated against *S pneumoniae*. One dose of PPSV23 is usually given at 65 years of age, and routine revaccination is not recommended. Those who received a dose before 65 years of age should receive a second dose if ≥5 years have elapsed since the first dose.

Persons ≥2 years of age at high risk for invasive pneumococcal disease should receive PPSV23. This includes persons in the following categories:

• *Increased risk*
  – Chronic cardiovascular disease, such as congestive heart failure or cardiomyopathy
  – Chronic pulmonary disease, such as cystic fibrosis (but not asthma)
  – Diabetes
  – Alcoholism
  – Cirrhosis
  – CSF leak
  – Cochlear implant
  – Asymptomatic HIV infection
• *Highest risk*
  – Chronic renal failure
  – Nephrotic syndrome
  – Functional, congenital, or surgical asplenia (this includes patients with sickle cell disease)
  – Symptomatic HIV infection
  – Immunosuppressive conditions, including Hodgkin's disease, lymphoma, multiple myeloma, generalized malignancy, organ or bone marrow transplantation, long-term high-dose corticosteroid therapy, and chemotherapy

In elective situations such as planned splenectomy, placement of a cochlear implant, or initiation of chemotherapy or immunosuppressive medication, vaccination should occur at least 2 weeks before the procedure, if possible. One-time revaccination is recommended for patients in the highest risk categories. The usual interval between doses is 5 years, but 3 years is recommended for children who would be ≤10 years of age at the time of revaccination. PPSV23 should be considered for persons living in special environments or social settings with increased risk of pneumococcal disease or its complications (eg, Alaska Native, Navajo, Apache populations). Women who are at high risk for

TABLE 9.17 — Pneumococcal Vaccine Schedule for Children

Condition	Current Age	Total Doses Already Received	Recommendation
Healthy	2 to 6 months	0	3 doses of PCV7 (2 months apart[a]), then PCV7 at 12 to 15 months
		1 dose of PCV7	2 doses of PCV7 (2 months apart[a]), then PCV7 at 12 to 15 months
		2 doses of PCV7	1 dose of PCV7 (2 months after most recent dose[a]), then PCV7 at 12 to 15 months
	7 to 11 months	0	2 doses of PCV7 (2 months apart[a]), then PCV7 at 12 months
		1 or 2 doses of PCV7 before 7 months	1 dose of PCV7,[a] then PCV7 at 12 to 15 months (≥2 months after last dose)
	12 to 23 months	0	2 doses of PCV7 (≥2 months apart)
		1 dose of PCV7 before 12 months	2 doses of PCV7 (≥2 months apart)
		1 dose of PCV7 at ≥12 months	1 dose of PCV7 (≥2 months after most recent dose)
		2 or 3 doses of PCV7 before 12 months	1 dose of PCV7 (≥2 months after most recent dose)
	24 to 59 months	Unvaccinated or any incomplete schedule	1 dose of PCV7 (≥2 months after most recent dose)
High-risk[b]	0 to 23 months	See recommendations for healthy children	See recommendations for healthy children
	24 to 59 months	4 doses of PCV7	1 dose of PPSV23 at 24 months (≥2 months after last dose of PCV7), then second dose of PPSV23 3 to 5 years after the first dose of PPSV23

3 doses of PCV7	1 dose of PCV7, then 1 dose of PPSV23 (≥2 months after last dose of PCV7), then second dose of PPSV23 3 to 5 years after the first dose of PPSV23
0 to 2 doses of PCV7	2 doses of PCV7 (2 months apart), then PPSV23 (≥2 months after last dose of PCV7), then second dose of PPSV23 3 to 5 years after the first dose of PPSV23
1 dose of PPSV23	2 doses of PCV7 (2 months apart, beginning 6 to 3 weeks after PPSV23), then second dose of PPSV23 3 to 5 years after the first dose of PPSV23

^a The minimum interval between doses of PCV7 <12 months of age is 4 weeks.

^b Includes sickle cell disease, congenital or acquired asplenia, or splenic dysfunction; HIV infection; congenital immune deficiency; chronic cardiac, pulmonary (including asthma), or renal disease; cerebrospinal fluid leak; cochlear implants; diabetes; and immunosuppressive therapy.

American Academy of Pediatrics. Pneumococcal infections. In: Pickering LK, ed. *2006 Red Book: Report of the Committee on Infectious Diseases.* 27th ed. Elk Grove Village, IL: American Academy of Pediatrics; 2006:525-537; Centers for Disease Control and Prevention; Advisory Committee on Immunization Practices. *MMWR Morb Mortal Wkly Rep.* 2008;57:343-344.

9

pneumococcal disease should be vaccinated before pregnancy, but may be vaccinated during pregnancy if necessary.

PPSV23 is often used to assess the adequacy of polysaccharide antibody responses in individuals ≥2 years of age who are suspected of having immune deficiency. A serum specimen is drawn, the vaccine is administered, and a second serum specimen is obtained 3 to 4 weeks later. The specimens are then tested in parallel for serotype-specific antibodies.

Varicella

■ **The Pathogen**

Varicella zoster virus (VZV) is a large, enveloped virus in the Herpesviridae family, subfamily Alphaherpesvirinae. It has a short reproductive cycle characterized by cellular destruction and release of free virus, as well as the ability to establish *latent infection*. After inoculation at mucosal surfaces, replication occurs in the regional lymph nodes, resulting in a primary viremia that seeds the liver and other reticuloendothelial organs. A secondary viremia then ensues, which infects epithelial cells of the skin, causing the vesicular lesions of *chickenpox*, as well as seeding of the respiratory mucosa, which facilitates contagion through respiratory droplets. Latent infection is invariably established in the dorsal root ganglia, where the linear, double-stranded DNA genome takes on a closed circular configuration. With reactivation, the genome linearizes and viral proteins are made and assembled into virions, which are then transported along sensory nerves to the skin, where replication causes *herpes zoster*, also known as *shingles*.

Cellular immunity is critical to limiting primary infection and preventing reactivation. Periodic re-exposure to exogenous natural varicella and/or subclinical reactivation of endogenous VZV may lead to boosts in immunity.

■ **Clinical Features**

The incubation period ranges from 10 to 21 days. In children, rash is often the first sign of disease, but adults may have a 1- to 2-day prodrome of fever and malaise. The rash is pruritic, usually beginning on the scalp or hairline, then moving to the trunk and the extremities. Lesions are 1 to 4 mm in diameter and appear in successive crops over several days; at any given time these crops are in different stages of development. Lesions characteristically evolve from macules to papules and then to superficial, delicate vesicles containing clear fluid on an erythematous base, so-called "dew drops on rose petals." They rapidly become pustules that crust and fall off, leaving shallow ulcers. Lesions can occur on mucous membranes and on the cornea. The average patient with primary varicella has malaise and fever for 2 to 3 days and develops 200 to 500 lesions, some of which may form a scar.

Varicella in vaccinated individuals, termed *breakthrough* or *vaccine-modified varicella*, is generally characterized by a shorter duration of illness and the absence of systemic symptoms and complications. There are usually <50 lesions, and these are often maculopapular rather than vesicular and difficult to recognize as chickenpox. However, up to 30% of children with breakthrough disease may have an illness that is similar to mild primary varicella.

In the prevaccine era, 5% to 10% of otherwise healthy children experienced complications. One half of these were secondary bacterial infections usually caused by *Staphylococcus aureus* or group A beta-hemolytic streptococcus (GABHS). Varicella increased the risk of severe GABHS infection among previously healthy children by 40- to 60-fold, and it was estimated that preventing varicella could prevent at least 15% of cases of severe pediatric GABHS infection. Otitis media occurred in up to 5% of cases. Serious secondary infections, such as pneumonia, bacteremia, osteomyelitis, septic arthritis, endocarditis, necrotizing fasciitis, and toxic shock syndrome, occurred much less frequently. Other complications included cerebellar ataxia, encephalitis, and Reye syndrome, which was associated with aspirin use during the illness.

Adults have more severe disease and higher complication rates. Slightly >1% of all adults with varicella are admitted to the hospital, and the case-fatality rate is 25 times higher than in children. In the prevaccine era, only 5% of cases, but 35% of annual deaths, occurred in adults; the majority of these had no identifiable risk factor for severe disease.

Immunocompromised individuals may develop *progressive varicella*, characterized by high fever, extensive vesicular eruption, and high complication rates. Mild hepatitis occurs in 20% to 50% of cases, but is usually asymptomatic. Similarly, 5% to 16% of patients develop thrombocytopenia, but bleeding is rare. *Hemorrhagic varicella* is characterized by thrombocytopenia and extensive purpuric lesions. Although rare, *congenital varicella syndrome*, characterized by birth defects and neurologic devastation, occurs in 1% of pregnancies complicated by varicella in the first or second trimester. Maternal varicella in the peripartum period can lead to overwhelming infection in the newborn because of a high inoculum and the absence of transplacental maternal antibody; the fatality rate is as high as 30%.

When immunity wanes (eg, as it does with aging), reactivation of latent VZV can result in herpes zoster, which is characterized by a unilateral, vesicular eruption and pain in a dermatomal distribution (usually on the trunk or the face). *Postherpetic neuralgia*, characterized by persistent pain in the affected area, is a distressing complication with no adequate therapy. Herpes zoster is common in patients undergoing immunosuppressive therapy and in infants with intrauterine exposure to varicella or infection in infancy. In immunocompromised patients, herpes zoster may disseminate, causing generalized skin lesions, and CNS, pulmonary, and hepatic complications.

■ Epidemiology and Transmission

Humans are the only natural hosts. Transmission occurs via respiratory droplets or by direct contact with or aerosolization of virus from vesicular skin lesions. Natural chickenpox is highly contagious, with attack rates among susceptible household contacts approaching 90%; contagiousness begins 1 to 2 days before onset of rash and lasts until the last lesion has crusted. Shingles is less contagious because there is less virus in the lesions and the respiratory tract is not involved. Vaccine-modified varicella also is less contagious than primary chickenpox, unless the number of lesions is >50, in which case contagiousness approaches that of primary disease.

Varicella is less common in tropical than in temperate areas. In the United States, the incidence is highest between March and May and lowest between September and November. Before universal immunization, essentially every child got chickenpox, most often by 4 years of age. Every year there were 4 million cases, 11,000 hospitalizations, and 100 deaths. Although the case-fatality rate in children was very low, the absolute number of childhood deaths was high (an average of 43 per year in the early 1990s) because there were so many cases. Ninety percent of children who died had no identifiable risk factors for severe varicella.

■ Background on Immunization Program

Varicella vaccine was licensed in the United States in 1995. Initial recommendations called for universal immunization of children 12 to 18 months of age and catch-up for children 19 months to 12 years of age who had not had chickenpox. Vaccination of susceptible persons ≥13 years of age (2 doses) was recommended if they were anticipated to have close contact with persons at high risk for serious complications; catch-up for other adolescents was considered desirable, but did not carry a strong recommendation. It was suggested that vaccination also be considered for certain susceptible individuals at high risk for exposure. Consideration was given as well to vaccination of susceptible nonpregnant women of childbearing age, who would be at risk for complications if they became pregnant and developed varicella. In 1999, stronger recommendations for these individuals were issued, essentially changing the language from "should be considered" to "recommended." Vaccination of all susceptible adolescents and adults living in households with children was recommended, as was postexposure vaccination. Use of varicella vaccine for outbreak control was suggested, as was vaccination of asymptomatic or mildly symptomatic HIV-infected children without evidence of immunosuppression.

Between 1997 and 2005, vaccine uptake among 2-year-olds increased to nearly 90%. Surveillance indicated approximately

90% declines in disease incidence, and the most affected age shifted from 3 to 6 years to 9 to 11 years. From 1994-2002, surveillance studies showed that hospitalization rates had declined 100% among infants, 91% among children <10 years of age, 92% among those 10 to 19 years of age, and 78% among adults 20 to 49 years of age. By 2003, the number of varicella-related deaths had declined to <20 per year, most of those occurring in persons with immunodeficiencies. This highlights an important fact about varicella—some people cannot be protected directly because they cannot be immunized with a live-attenuated vaccine. The only way to protect them as a population is to reduce transmission of the virus in the community, although passive immunization can be used for individuals after known exposure.

Despite the successes outlined above, outbreaks of varicella continued to occur, especially among elementary school students—even though the majority of them had been vaccinated. Granted, these were outbreaks of vaccine-modified varicella, which is less serious than primary disease. Nevertheless, it became clear that a 1-dose strategy would not eliminate transmission in the United States—either because a certain number of children fail to seroconvert after 1 dose or because immunity wanes with time. A randomized trial with 10 years of observation showed that 2 doses (separated by 3 months) reduced the breakthrough rate 3.3-fold as compared with 1 dose. Therefore, in 2007 a routine 2-dose strategy was adopted.

At the beginning of the program in 1995, it was estimated that every dollar spent on varicella vaccination resulted in a savings of $5.40, when both direct medical and indirect societal costs were considered. For the 2006 birth cohort (4.1 million children) followed over 40 years, it was estimated that without a vaccination program there would be $333 million in direct costs from varicella and $1.5 billion in societal costs. A 1-dose vaccination program would prevent 3.6 million cases and result in a net savings of $1.1 billion. A 2-dose program would prevent 375,000 additional cases at an incremental cost of $104 million; the cost per quality-adjusted life year saved would be $109,000.

■ Available Vaccines

Characteristics of the varicella vaccine licensed in the United States are given in **Table 9.18**.

■ Efficacy and/or Immunogenicity

Prelicensure studies showed seroconversion rates of 97% among children 1 to 12 years of age and 79% among adolescents after 1 dose. Adolescents and adults who received 2 doses separated by 4 to 8 weeks had seroconversion rates of 99%. In a study of children 12 months to 12 years of age conducted between 1988 and 2002, 86% of children who received 1 dose developed antibody levels ≥5 glycoprotein ELISA units/mL (this level is presumed to correlate with protection); nearly 100% achieved

TABLE 9.18 — Varicella Vaccine[a]

Trade name	Varivax
Abbreviation	—
Manufacturer/distributor	Merck
Type of vaccine	Live attenuated, classic
Composition	Oka/Merck strain
	Propagated in human diploid (MRC-5) cells
	At least 1350 plaque-forming units
Adjuvant	None
Preservative	None
Excipients and contaminants	Sucrose (25 mg)
	Hydrolyzed gelatin (12.5 mg)
	Sodium chloride (3.2 mg)
	Monosodium L-glutamate (0.5 mg)
	Sodium phosphate dibasic (0.45 mg)
	Potassium phosphate monobasic (0.08 mg)
	Potassium chloride (0.08 mg)
	Residual components of MRC-5 cells, including DNA and protein
	Sodium phosphate monobasic (trace)
	EDTA (trace)
	Neomycin (trace)
	Fetal bovine serum (trace)
Latex	None
Labeled indications	Immunization against varicella
Labeled ages	≥12 months
Dose	0.5 mL
Route of administration	Subcutaneous
Usual schedule	12 months to 12 years: 1 dose, with revaccination ≥3 months later
	≥13 years: 1 dose, with revaccination 4 to 8 weeks later
How supplied (number in package)	1-dose vial (1, 10), lyophilized, with diluent
Storage:	
Vaccine	Freeze, can be refrigerated for up to 72 hours before reconstitution, protect from light
Diluent	Refrigerate or room temperature
Reconstituted vaccine	Use within 30 minutes
Reference package insert	February 2007

[a] Varicella vaccine is also available in combination with MMR (ProQuad; Merck).

this level after a second dose, whether that was given 3 months or several years after the first dose. Antibodies have been detected as long as 9 years postvaccination in US studies and 20 years in Japanese studies; some studies show rising antibody levels over time, suggesting intermittent boosting by exposure to wild-type virus or perhaps reactivation of latent vaccine virus. Antibody persistence in the absence of natural boosting cannot be studied until endemic transmission is eliminated. Long-lived T-cell proliferative responses have been demonstrated in vaccinees.

In prelicensure trials, efficacy of a single dose against any disease was 70% to 90% and against severe disease was 95%. Most postlicensure studies show effectiveness of a single dose in the range of 70% to 90%, although some estimates have been lower, in the range of 44% to 56%. A case-control study set in pediatric offices from 1997-2003 demonstrated 1-dose effectiveness of 85%, and a study of household exposures demonstrated 79% effectiveness at preventing secondary disease. Severe varicella, characterized by >500 lesions, hospitalization, and complications, is extremely rare in vaccinees. A randomized trial in children showed 94% efficacy over 10 years of 1 dose ($N=1104$) compared with 98% efficacy of 2 doses given 3 months apart ($N=1017$). In adults and adolescents who have seroconverted, efficacy against disease is approximately 70% after household exposure.

Postexposure vaccination is ≥90% effective in preventing varicella if administered within 3 days of exposure; effectiveness drops to 70% by day 5, although effectiveness against severe disease remains 100%.

■ Safety

Injection-site reactions are reported in about 20% of vaccinees, and 15% may have low-grade fever. About 3% of children and 1% of adults get a few vesicles at the injection site, and up to 5% may experience a generalized varicella-like rash (median of 5 lesions, mostly maculopapular). The vaccine virus establishes latency, and herpes zoster due to the vaccine virus can occur. However, the overall incidence of herpes zoster appears to be lower in vaccinated children than in naturally infected children. Transmission of the vaccine virus from healthy vaccinees to susceptible individuals is extremely rare and is only known to occur when the vaccinee develops a rash after vaccination. In the few instances when transmission has occurred, mild disease has resulted and there is no evidence of reversion to virulence.

Ten years after licensure and the distribution of 55.7 million doses worldwide, 16,683 reports of adverse events (5054 of which were breakthrough disease) had been received, for a reporting rate of 3.4 per 10,000 doses distributed. Vesicular rashes occurring in the first 2 weeks after vaccination were mostly due to wild-type VZV, indicating that vaccinees had been exposed to or were incubating the natural infection when they were vaccinated. Among 95 reports of herpes zoster for which specimens were available,

57 were due to the vaccine strain and 38 were wild-type VZV. There were no primary neurologic events associated with vaccination. Household transmission was reported in three instances, and in each case the vaccinee had developed a vesicular rash. Disseminated infection was seen in seven patients, all but six of whom were immunocompromised.

- *Contraindications*
  - Allergic reaction to previous dose of vaccine or any vaccine component (risk of recurrent allergic reaction)
  - Severe immunodeficiency or immunosuppression (risk of disease caused by live virus; see *Chapter 7*)
  - Pregnancy (theoretic risk of live-virus vaccine to the fetus or attribution of birth defects to vaccination)
  - Untreated, active tuberculosis (risk of exacerbation of tuberculosis)
- *Precautions*
  - Moderate or severe acute illness (difficulty distinguishing illness from vaccine reaction)
  - Recent receipt of antibody-containing blood product (risk of impaired response to vaccine; see *Chapter 5*)
  - Salicylate therapy in children and adolescents (theoretic risk of Reye syndrome; the manufacturer recommends withholding salicylates at least 6 weeks after administration of vaccine, but other nonsteroidal anti-inflammatory agents can be used)

■ Recommendations for General Use

All people without evidence of immunity to varicella should be vaccinated. The criteria for evidence of immunity are listed in **Table 9.19**.

For children, the first dose is usually given at 12 to 15 months of age and the second dose at 4 to 6 years of age. The second dose may be given any time ≥3 months following the first dose. For persons ≥13 years of age, 2 doses are given 4 to 8 weeks apart. Anyone who received 1 dose in the past should receive a second dose. Evidence of immunity should be assessed in all individuals, and those without evidence of immunity should be vaccinated. Special attention should be paid to assessment of school-aged children, students in college and other postsecondary educational institutions, health care providers, household contacts of immunosuppressed persons, teachers, day care employees, residents and staff in institutional settings, inmates and staff of correctional facilities, military personnel, nonpregnant women of childbearing age, persons living in homes with children, and international travelers.

While there are no official recommendations, infants who had chickenpox before 6 months of age, and possibly before 9 months, should probably be vaccinated once they reach 12 months (there is no harm in giving the vaccine to someone who has already had chickenpox). This is because the immunity imparted by natural

TABLE 9.19 — Evidence of Immunity to Varicella[a]

- Documented age-appropriate vaccination:[b]
  - Preschool-aged children: 1 dose
  - School-aged children, adolescents, and adults: 2 doses
- Laboratory evidence of immunity[c]
- Laboratory confirmation of disease
- Birth in the United States before 1980 (exception: health care workers, pregnant women, and immunocompromised individuals)
- Typical varicella: diagnosis or verification of history by any health care professional (eg, school or occupational clinic nurse, nurse practitioner, physician assistant, physician)[d]
- Atypical or mild varicella: diagnosis or verification of history by a physician or physician's designee, utilizing the following information:
  - Epidemiologic link to a typical or laboratory-confirmed case
  - Laboratory confirmation performed at the time of acute disease
- Herpes zoster: diagnosis or verification of history by any health care professional

[a] Any one of these criteria constitute evidence of immunity.
[b] Appropriately vaccinated individuals who become immunosuppressed later in life are considered immune, except for hematopoietic stem-cell transplant recipients.
[c] Serologic testing of adults before vaccination may be cost-effective since approximately 80% will be found to be seropositive. Receipt of blood products can cause false-positive serologic test results because of passive transfer of antibodies.
[d] In general, immunocompromised individuals with a verified history of varicella are considered immune. The exception is hematopoietic stem cell transplant recipients, who are considered susceptible, regardless of their own personal history of varicella or a history of varicella in the donor. Transplant recipients who develop herpes zoster are subsequently considered immune.

Centers for Disease Control and Prevention. *MMWR*. 2007;56(RR-4):1-40.

disease in infants who have transplacental maternal antibodies may be suboptimal. Pregnant women without evidence of immunity should be vaccinated beginning in the postpartum period. HIV-infected persons without evidence of immunosuppression should be vaccinated. Susceptible household and other close contacts of immunocompromised persons also should be vaccinated; if the vaccinee develops a rash, contact with an immunocompromised person at risk for severe complications of varicella should be avoided.

Vaccination of individuals without evidence of immunity is recommended for outbreak control. Vaccination can also be used as postexposure prophylaxis for healthy, susceptible individuals if given within 3 to 5 days of exposure.

Exposed persons who lack evidence of immunity (**Table 9.19**), have contraindications to vaccination, and are at high risk for complications of varicella should receive passive immunoprophylaxis with varicella zoster immune globulin (VariZIG). Exposure is constituted by living in the same household as an infectious person with either chickenpox or herpes zoster; direct, indoor, face-to-face contact with an infectious person for >5 minutes (some experts say 1 hour); or sharing the same hospital room. A special case of exposure that carries high risk is the neonate whose mother develops chickenpox in the peripartum period. The following individuals should receive passive immunoprophylaxis if susceptible and exposed:

- Immunocompromised patients, including those with primary and acquired immunodeficiencies, receiving immunosuppressive medications, and those with cancer. Patients who receive regular immune globulin infusions do not need prophylaxis unless the last dose was ≤3 weeks before exposure.
- Neonates whose mothers have signs and symptoms of varicella from 5 days before to 2 days after delivery.
- Preterm neonates who are exposed postnatally
  - ≥28 weeks gestation whose mothers lack evidence of immunity
  - <28 weeks gestation or birth weight ≤1000 g, regardless of maternal immunity
- Pregnant women (VariZIG is indicated to protect the mother from complications of varicella; whether it will protect the fetus is not known)

The only high-titer immune globulin product available in the United States is VariZIG, but this must be obtained under an investigational new-drug protocol (FFF Enterprises, phone number 800-843-7477). VariZIG is supplied in 125-unit vials, and the dose is 125 units/10 kg intramuscularly; the minimum dose is 125 units and the maximum dose is 625 units. Intravenous immune globulin can be used if VariZIG is not available.

After intramuscular administration of VariZIG, varicella antibodies persist for about 6 weeks. Onset of action is very prompt, but the duration of protection is unknown. When given within 96 hours of exposure, VariZIG significantly reduces the morbidity and mortality from varicella among immunocompromised individuals. Attack rates are about one fifth as high as those in untreated, exposed individuals, and the severity of disease is reduced. Receipt of VariZIG may prolong the incubation period of varicella up to 28 days. If the patient develops varicella, antiviral therapy should be instituted.

The most frequent local adverse reactions to VariZIG are pain, redness, or swelling at the injection site, occurring in about 1%

of patients. Systemic reactions are less frequent and include GI symptoms, malaise, headache, rash, and respiratory symptoms. Certain safety issues are common to all immune globulin products, including the possibility of allergic reaction to residual IgA in the product in IgA-deficient individuals and the possibility of transmission of bloodborne pathogens that are not killed in the manufacturing process.

Zoster

■ The Pathogen

The biology of varicella zoster virus (VZV) is described in the section entitled *Varicella*. *Herpes zoster*, or *shingles*, results from the reactivation of latent VZV from sensory dorsal root or cranial nerve ganglia (it has nothing to do with herpes simplex virus, despite its name). The virus initially reaches these ganglia by retrograde axonal transport from the skin during an episode of chickenpox. In latency, which may last for many decades, there is restricted gene transcription and limited protein expression, but intact virions are not produced. What triggers release from latency and active, lytic infection is not clear, but it is clear that reduced VZV-specific (T cell) responder cell frequency characterizes all conditions associated with reactivation. In other words, normally there is enough constitutive immune surveillance for antigens associated with lytic infection that when active replication begins, infected cells are destroyed or replication is otherwise shut down.

When immune surveillance wanes, lytic infection in neuronal cell bodies can progress, and virions are transported back along sensory nerves to the skin, where lesions much like those of chickenpox are produced. Unlike with chickenpox, however, the lesions are restricted to a single dermatome (more than one dermatome may be involved in immunocompromised individuals). Moreover, they are associated with significant pain, the result of cell destruction and inflammation in the sensory ganglion. Pain often persists after regression of the lesions, a condition termed *postherpetic neuralgia* (PHN). This is associated with degeneration of primary afferent neuronal cell bodies and axons, scarring in the dorsal root ganglion, and *central sensitization*, which refers to changes in the dorsal horn of the spinal cord that generalize and perpetuate pain impulses.

Zoster is a re-immunizing event—immunity to VZV is boosted, and for this reason most people only have one lifetime episode.

■ Clinical Features

A prodrome of headache, photophobia, and malaise without fever may occur. Pain (often described as burning, shooting, stabbing, or throbbing), itching, or tingling precede skin lesions by 1 to 5 days. Lesions form over 3 to 5 days, usually in the distribution of a single dermatome, beginning as clusters of erythematous macules that rapidly become papules with superimposed clear vesicles, and—much like chickenpox—evolve to pustules and shallow ulcers with crusts that fall off within 2 to 4 weeks, often leaving scars and permanent changes in pigmentation. Thoracic, cervical, and ophthalmic dermatomes are most often involved, and the lesions do not cross the midline. Systemic symptoms occur in <20% of patients, and occasionally there are a few lesions outside the dermatome. Motor nerve involvement with associated paresis may be seen in 5% to 15% of patients (the mechanism for this is not clear). Involvement of the geniculate ganglion can lead to facial nerve paralysis (sensory and motor nerves are joined in nerve VII); the combination of lesions on the ear, hard palate, or tongue and facial paralysis is termed *Ramsay Hunt syndrome* and is associated with vertigo, hearing loss, tinnitus, and loss of taste. Occasionally, pain occurs without skin lesions, which is called *zoster sine herpete*.

Zoster tends to be more severe with advancing age. Subclinical involvement of the CNS is common in immunocompetent individuals; there may be CSF pleocytosis in up to half of patients and VZV can be detected in CSF in a third. Immunocompromised patients may experience severe localized zoster or *disseminated zoster* due to hematogenous spread of the infection outside of the original dermatome. The spectrum of illness ranges from generalized rash to life-threatening pneumonia, hepatitis, encephalitis, and disseminated intravascular coagulopathy.

PHN lasting ≥1 month occurs in 20% to 30% of patients with zoster, and about 10% have pain lasting ≥3 months. Pain may last for months or years, may be constant, intermittent, or triggered by trivial stimuli, and is described as excruciating in half of patients. The quality of life may be dramatically affected, leading to social withdrawal, depression, and even suicide. Advanced age correlates with the severity of PHN; in fact, PHN is rare in children.

Other complications of zoster include secondary bacterial infection, eye involvement with keratitis or retinitis, myelitis, and granulomatous angiitis.

■ Epidemiology and Transmission

Zoster only occurs in people who have had been infected with VZV; this includes >99.5% of the US population ≥40 years of age. Zoster is contagious in the sense that VZV from the lesions can cause chickenpox in a susceptible individual; however, zoster cannot directly cause zoster in another person, nor can chickenpox, because latency must first be established. Of note, the risk of contagion from zoster is less than that from chickenpox because there is less virus that can aerosolize from the lesions and there is no transmission (from respiratory sections) before the lesions erupt.

Estimates of age-adjusted incidence rates in the United States vary from 3.2 to 4.2 per 1000 population, or about 1 million cases annually. The rate is much higher—about 10 per 1000—in individuals ≥60 years of age. About one third of people in the United States will experience an episode of zoster in their lifetime. The most important risk factors are increasing age and conditions or medications that impair cell-mediated immunity; other risk factors include psychologic stress, female gender, white race, mechanical trauma, and genetic susceptibility. Exposure to varicella (eg, living or working in environments with young children) appears to be protective, as does varicella vaccination (the rates of zoster are much lower in vaccinated individuals than in naturally infected individuals). Zoster may be up to 10 times less common in children than in adults; when it does occur, a history of maternal varicella during pregnancy or chickenpox in the first year of life is often present. These are situations that can lead to immune tolerance, ie, blunting of immune memory to VZV.

Questions have been raised about how the universal varicella vaccination program will affect the incidence of zoster. Several competing factors are involved. First, as more and more people are vaccinated, fewer and fewer will become latently infected with wild-type VZV. Because wild-type VZV reactivates more readily than the attenuated vaccine strain (which, however, *does* establish latency), this might result in fewer people developing zoster as they age. However, less circulating virus in the community means fewer opportunities for boosted immunity in those who are already infected with wild-type VZV. Therefore, episodes of zoster could increase in one generation (those who are already infected with wild-type VZV and will not have the immunologic benefit of exposure to natural virus) while they decrease in another (those who received the varicella vaccine and never become latently infected with wild-type VZV). Studies done since 1995, when varicella vaccine was first licensed in the United States, have shown conflicting results regarding changes in the incidence of zoster.

■ Background on Immunization Program

The rationale for a zoster vaccine program is simple: Vaccination could mimic the effect of exposure to natural varicella in people who are latently infected, boosting cellular immune responses and thereby preventing reactivation. Zostavax (Merck), which was licensed in May 2006, consists of the same live-attenuated strain of VZV that is used in the varicella vaccine (Varivax), only in sufficiently high titer to overcome existing antibody and replicate in previously infected individuals.

It is estimated that each case of zoster results in up to three outpatient visits and from one to five medication prescriptions. Up to 4% of episodes result in hospitalization, with a mean duration of 5 days and average cost of $3221 to $7206 (2006 dollars). Annualized health care costs for PHN are as high as $5000. Assuming a vaccine cost of $150, a 1-dose vaccination program for healthy individuals ≥60 years of age would cost from $27,000 to $112,000 per quality-adjusted life year gained. This places the zoster vaccine in the intermediate-to-high end of cost-benefit when compared with other vaccination programs.

■ Available Vaccines

Characteristics of the zoster vaccine licensed in the United States are given in **Table 9.20**.

TABLE 9.20 — Zoster Vaccine

Trade name	Zostavax
Abbreviation	—
Manufacturer/distributor	Merck
Type of vaccine	Live attenuated, classic
Composition	Oka/Merck strain[a]
	Propagated in human diploid (MRC-5) cells
	19,400 plaque-forming units
Adjuvant	None
Preservative	None
Excipients and contaminants	Sucrose (31.16 mg)
	Hydrolyzed porcine gelatin (15.58 mg)
	Sodium chloride (3.99 mg)
	Monosodium L-glutamate (0.62 mg)
	Sodium phosphate dibasic (0.57 mg)
	Potassium phosphate monobasic (0.08 mg)
	Potassium chloride (0.10 mg)
	Residual components of MRC-5 cells, including DNA and protein
	Neomycin (trace)
	Bovine calf serum (trace)
Latex	None
Labeled indications	Prevention of herpes zoster
Labeled ages	≥60 years
Dose	0.65 mL
Route of administration	Subcutaneous
Usual schedule	1 dose
How supplied (number in package)	1-dose vial (1, 10), lyophylized, with diluent
Storage:	
Vaccine	Freeze, protect from light
Diluent	Refrigerate or room temperature
Reconstituted vaccine	Use within 30 minutes, do not freeze
Reference package insert	November 2007

[a] This is the same strain used in the varicella vaccine (Varivax; Merck).

■ Efficacy and/or Immunogenicity

Zoster vaccine was evaluated in a double-blind, randomized, placebo-controlled trial (the Shingles Prevention Study) involving 38,546 healthy adults ≥60 years of age who either had a personal history of varicella or who had resided in the United States for ≥30 years (and were therefore very likely to have been infected with VZV). The majority of suspected cases were confirmed by PCR. The mean duration of follow-up was 3.1 years, and patients with confirmed zoster were followed for at least 6 months. Remarkably, 95% of those enrolled completed the study.

There were 315 cases of zoster among 19,254 vaccinees and 642 among 19,247 placebees, for a risk reduction of 51%. Overall, vaccination reduced the risk of PHN in vaccinees by 67% when defined as ≥30 days of pain and by 73% when defined as ≥182 days of pain. Among subjects who developed zoster, the risk of PHN was reduced by 39%. Other complications, such as allodynia (a painful response to a normally nonpainful stimulus), bacterial superinfection, disseminated zoster, impaired vision, peripheral motor-nerve palsies, ptosis, scarring, and sensory loss occurred with similar frequency among vaccine and placebo cases of zoster but were less common among vaccinees than placebees. These results indicate that the main benefit of zoster vaccine is in preventing zoster rather than in modifying the severity and or complications should zoster occur. Efficacy at preventing zoster was highest among those 60 to 69 years of age, but the greatest effect in reducing the severity of illness was among persons 70 to 79 years of age. Efficacy declined during the first year following vaccination but stabilized thereafter at around 50%.

Anamnestic antibody and T-cell responses were seen in vaccinated subjects and persisted for 3 to 6 years. Immune responses were inversely related to the risk of zoster.

■ Safety

Erythema and pain at the injection site occur in about 35% of vaccinees; swelling occurs in 26%, and pruritus in 7%. Most of these reactions are mild and resolve within 4 days. A varicella-like rash occurs at the injection site within 3 to 4 days in 0.1% of vaccinees, and fever occurs in <1%. In the Shingles Prevention Study, serious adverse events such as death (which might be expected given the advanced age of the subjects) occurred with equal frequency among vaccine and placebo recipients.

On rare occasion, the vaccine strain of VZV has been detected in lesions that occurred after vaccination. Horizontal transmission, while not formally evaluated, has not been reported. Standard precautions should be adequate to protect susceptible individuals who are in contact with vaccinees who develop lesions.

- *Contraindications*
  - Allergic reaction to previous dose of vaccine or any vaccine component (risk of recurrent allergic reaction)

– Immunodeficiency or immunosuppression (risk of disease caused by live virus). The following may receive the zoster vaccine: patients with leukemia in remission who have not had chemotherapy or radiation for ≥3 months; patients receiving systemic steroids for <14 days or <20 mg/day; patients receiving low doses of methotrexate (≤0.4 mg/kg/week), azathioprine (≤3 mg/kg/day), or 6-mercaptopurine (≤1.5 mg/kg/day); HIV-infected persons with CD4 count ≥200/mL and CD4 percentage ≥15% of total lymphocytes; and persons with humoral immune deficiencies. Providers may consider immunizing hematopoietic stem cell transplant recipients who are immunocompetent and who are ≥24 months post-transplant.

– Pregnancy (theoretic risk of live virus vaccine to the fetus or attribution of birth defects to vaccination)

• *Precautions*

– Moderate or severe acute illness (difficulty distinguishing illness from vaccine reaction)

– Untreated, active tuberculosis (risk of exacerbation of tuberculosis)

■ Recommendations for General Use

All persons ≥60 years of age should be vaccinated against zoster. The usual schedule is 1 dose of zoster vaccine at 60 years of age, but catch-up vaccination is recommended (there is no upper age limit). Vaccination is recommended regardless of the personal history with respect to varicella. Patients who have had zoster should be vaccinated; while there is no minimum interval between an episode of zoster and vaccination, it would seem prudent to wait at least a year to vaccinate since immunity presumably will have been boosted by the episode. Patients with chronic medical conditions may be vaccinated, as long as those conditions are not associated with immunosuppression. The vaccine is not indicated to treat acute zoster, prevent PHN in patients who already have zoster, or to treat PHN. Zoster vaccine is not recommended for individuals who have received varicella vaccine, but few individuals today who are ≥60 years of age will fit into that category.

If immunosuppression is anticipated, vaccination should occur at least 14 days earlier. Persons taking antiviral medications such as acyclovir, famciclovir, and valacyclovir should discontinue those medications at least 24 hours before vaccination and remain off medication for at least 14 days. Receipt of antibody-containing blood products is not a contraindication to vaccination.

Modern Combination Vaccines

■ Background

Combination vaccines consist of two or more separate antigens combined in a single product and administered through the same syringe. Some of the first vaccines licensed in the United States were combinations. For example, the influenza vaccine (first licensed in 1945) contains antigens from three different strains of influenza virus. Likewise, the hexavalent pneumococcal polysaccharide vaccine (1947), DTwP vaccine (1948), and trivalent IPV (1955) and OPV (1963) were also combinations. The modern era of combinations, however, began in the 1990s, when combinations of routinely administered childhood vaccines (referred to herein as component vaccines) such as DTwP, DTaP, Hib, and HepB were developed.

As of 2008, the routine childhood schedule from birth through 18 years of age calls for as many as 50 shots for girls and 47 shots for boys (this includes yearly influenza vaccination). Most of these shots are concentrated in the first 2 years of life. Depending on how vaccine visits are scheduled, as many as 9 shots may be due on one day (eg, a 15-month-old may be due for HepB, DTaP, Hib, PCV7, IPV, influenza vaccine, MMR, varicella vaccine, and HepA). This causes distress for patients, parents, and health care professionals, enough so that compliance with universal vaccine programs may be threatened. Combination vaccines, which reduce the number of shots necessary without reducing the delivery of antigens, are a logical solution to this problem.

■ **Development, Evaluation, and Licensure**

Producing safe and effective combination vaccines is far more complex than simply mixing antigens together in a single vial. Adjuvants, buffers, stabilizers, and excipients can have *physical or chemical interactions* with antigens that reduce immunogenicity, and many of these interactions cannot be predicted a priori. *Antigenic competition* can occur as vaccine components vie for position in binding to major histocompatibility molecules on antigen-presenting cells at the site of injection. This may explain in part the decreased anti-PRP responses that were seen in initial attempts to combine Hib with DTaP. Another phenomenon, *carrier-induced epitopic suppression*, may cause decreased antibody responses to protein-polysaccharide conjugates (such as Hib) when there has been prior or simultaneous immunization with free (homologous) carrier protein. A similar effect is seen when different conjugates containing the same carrier protein are given at the same time. These interactions may be relevant, eg, in the situation where a child receives a tetanus toxoid-containing vaccine at the same time as a conjugate vaccine that uses tetanus toxoid as the carrier protein. When live viral vaccines are given together, *viral interference* may limit responses as the replication of one virus is inhibited by the replication of the other. This phenomenon is relevant to combinations of measles, mumps, rubella, and varicella vaccines. While these interactions are important considerations, they must be differentiated from "immune overload," a popular concept that has no scientific basis (see *Chapter 8*).

Once compatibility issues are worked out in laboratory and animal models, extensive clinical trials are required to prove that a new combination vaccine is safe and effective. FDA guidelines require that such trials compare the combination to separately but simultaneously administered component vaccines. Reactogenicity is compared with the most reactogenic of the individual components. For antigens that have an established serologic correlate of protection, it may be enough to demonstrate that the combination induces protective antibody responses. However, the FDA generally requires that *noninferiority* with component vaccines be demonstrated, defined as no more than a 10% reduction in seroprotection. While this criterion is intended to ensure that protection is not compromised for the sake of convenience, it is not clear how important it is for vaccines that induce high-quality antibody and robust anamnestic reponses. For antigens without established serologic correlates of protection, combination vaccines should demonstrate antibody responses similar to those measured in previous studies showing efficacy of individual vaccines.

■ Recommendations

In 1999, recognizing the potential advantages (**Table 9.21**), the ACIP, AAP, and AAFP issued a statement expressing a clear preference for combination vaccines over separate injections of the component vaccines. The preference for combination vaccines has been reiterated annually in the routine childhood schedule and in the *General Recommendations on Immunization* that is published every 3 to 5 years by the CDC. The only exception is MMRV, which is not preferred over separate MMR and varicella vaccines because of concerns about an increased incidence of febrile seizures after vaccination (the rate is estimated at five to nine per 10,000 first-time vaccinees, about double the rate in children who receive the separate vaccines).

Modern combination vaccines available in the United States are listed in **Table 9.22**. Contraindications and precautions for combination vaccines are the same as for the individual components. Use of combination vaccines may result in overimmunization because unnecessary doses of an antigen may be given. For example, an infant who receives the birth dose of HepB and then receives DTaP-HepB-IPV at 2, 4, and 6 months of age will receive 4 total doses of HepB, when only 3 doses are required. Such extraimmunization is not harmful and is an accepted consequence of using combination vaccines. More robust adoption of combination vaccines might occur if providers were incentivized through antigen-based reimbursement, rather than the current system of reimbursing for the administration of the injections per se (see *Chapter 4*). Providers are warned not to combine vaccines in the same syringe unless the products are specifically labeled for this purpose.

TABLE 9.21 — Potential Advantages and Disadvantages of Combination Vaccines

Potential Advantages
- Fewer injections
- Decreased pain and anxiety
- Decreased injection risk
- Fewer sharps injuries
- Fewer visits[a]
- Simplified schedule
- Decreased administration costs and overhead
- Improved billing efficiency
- Improved record-keeping and tracking
- Improved coverage rates
- Improved timeliness
- Decreased preparation time
- More efficient well-child visits
- Easier storage and inventory management
- Less vaccine wastage
- More efficient federal documentation
- Easier introduction of new vaccines

Potential Disadvantages
- Increased reactogenicity
- Difficulty attributing adverse events to specific antigens
- Confusion over antigen content and errors in record-keeping
- Extraimmunization[b]
- Fewer visits[a]
- Decreased flexibility
- Increased cost of vaccines
- Loss of revenue from administration fees[c]

[a] Fewer visits means less expense for families and may improve office efficiency. However, immunization visits serve to anchor children in the medical home, where other aspects of well-child care are delivered.

[b] An example of this is the child who receives 4 doses of HepB because a birth dose of monovalent vaccine is given followed by doses of Pediarix (DTaP-HepB-IPV) at 2, 4, and 6 months of age. There is no evidence that such extraimmunization increases reactogenicity or impairs the immune response.

[c] Providers are reimbursed per injection (see Chapter 4, *Vaccine Practice*).

■ **Effect on Quality**

The more shots that are due on a given day, the more likely it is that one or more vaccinations will be deferred to another day. In recent years, it has become clear that such deferrals may lead to reduced coverage rates and poor immunization timeliness. Several studies now suggest that use of combination vaccines, by reducing the number of shots due, can lead to improvements in coverage and timeliness. A study of administrative claims from the Georgia

TABLE 9.22 — Part 1: Modern Combination Vaccines

	Comvax	Kinrix	Pediarix	Pentacel
Trade name	Comvax	Kinrix	Pediarix	Pentacel
Abbreviation	HepB-Hib	DTaP-IPV	DTaP-HepB-IPV	DTaP-IPV/Hib
Manufacturer/distributor	Merck	GlaxoSmithKline	GlaxoSmithKline	Sanofi Pasteur
Diseases prevented[a]	Hepatitis B Invasive *Haemophilus influenzae* type b	Diphtheria Tetanus Pertussis Polio	Diphtheria Tetanus Pertussis Hepatitis B Polio	Diphtheria Tetanus Pertussis Invasive *H influenzae* type b Polio
Type of vaccine	Inactivated, engineered subunits	Inactivated, purified subunits, toxoids, and whole agent	Inactivated, purified subunits, toxoids, engineered subunit, and whole agent	Inactivated, purified subunits, toxoids, engineered subunit, and whole agent
Component vaccines[b]	Recombivax HB (HepB) PedvaxHIB (PRP-OMPC)	Infanrix (DTaP) IPV[c]	Infanrix (DTaP) Engerix-B (HepB) IPV[c]	DTaP similar to Daptacel Poliovax (IPV)[d] ActHIB (Hib)[e]
Composition	HBsAg (*adw* subtype) expressed in yeast (*Saccharomyces cerevisiae*) (5 mcg) Polyribosylribitol phosphate (7.5 mcg) conju-	Diphtheria toxoid (25 Lf units) Tetanus toxoid (10 Lf units) Inactivated pertussis toxin (25 mcg)	Diphtheria toxoid (25 Lf units) Tetanus toxoid (10 Lf units) Inactivated pertussis toxin (25 mcg)	Diphtheria toxoid (15 Lf units) Tetanus toxoid (5 Lf units) Inactivated pertussis toxin (20 mcg) Filamentous hemagglutinin (20 mcg)

gated to *Neisseria meningitidis* serogroup B (strain B11) outer membrane protein (125 mcg)	Filamentous hemagglutinin (25 mcg) Pertactin (8 mcg) Poliovirus type 1 (Mahoney), 40 D antigen units Poliovirus type 2 (MEF-1), 8 D antigen units Poliovirus type 3 (Saukett), 32 D antigen units Polioviruses propagated in Vero (African Green Monkey kidney) cells and inactivated with formaldehyde	Filamentous hemagglutinin (25 mcg) Pertactin (8 mcg) HBsAg expressed in yeast (*S cerevisiae*) (10 mcg) Poliovirus type 1 (Mahoney), 40 D antigen units Poliovirus type 2 (MEF-1), 8 D antigen units Poliovirus type 3 (Saukett), 32 D antigen units Polioviruses propagated in Vero (African Green Monkey kidney) cells and inactivated with formaldehyde	Pertactin (3 mcg) Fimbriae types 2 and 3 (5 mcg) Polyribosylribitol phosphate (10 mcg) conjugated to tetanus toxoid (24 mcg) Poliovirus type 1 (Mahoney), 40 D antigen units Poliovirus type 2 (MEF-1), 8 D antigen units Poliovirus type 3 (Saukett), 32 D antigen units Polioviruses propagated in human diploid (MRC-5) cells and inactivated with formaldehyde
Adjuvant Aluminum hydroxide (0.225 mg aluminum)	Aluminum hydroxide (≤0.6 mg aluminum)	Aluminum hydroxide Aluminum phosphate (≤0.85 mg aluminum)	Aluminum phosphate (0.33 mg aluminum)

Continued

9

TABLE 9.22 — Part 1 (*continued*)

Preservative	None	None	None	None
Trade name	Comvax	Kinrix	Pediarix	Pentacel
Excipients and contaminants	Yeast protein (≤5%) Sodium borate decahydrate (35 mcg) Sodium chloride (0.9%) Formaldehyde (≤0.0004%)	Sodium chloride (4.5 mg) Formaldehyde (≤100 mcg) Polysorbate 80 (≤100 mcg) Neomycin sulfate (≤0.05 ng) Polymyxin B (≤0.01 ng)	Sodium chloride (4.5 mg) Formaldehyde (≤100 mcg) Polysorbate 80 (≤100 mcg) Neomycin sulfate (≤0.05 ng) Polymyxin B (≤0.01 ng) Yeast protein (≤5%)	Polysorbate 80 (10 ppm) Formaldehyde (≤5 mcg) Glutaraldehyde (<50 ng) Bovine serum albumin (≤50 ng) 2-phenoxyethanol (3.3 mg) Neomycin (<4 pg) Polymyxin B sulfate (<4 pg)
Latex	Vial stopper contains dry natural rubber	Tip cap and plunger of prefilled syringe contain dry natural rubber	Tip cap and plunger of prefilled syringe contain dry natural rubber	None
Labeled ages	6 weeks to 15 months[f]	4 to 6 years	6 weeks to 6 years[f,g]	6 weeks to 4 years
Dose	0.5 mL	0.5 mL	0.5 mL	0.5 mL
Route of administration	Intramuscular	Intramuscular	Intramuscular	Intramuscular
Usual schedule	2, 4, 12 to 15 months of age[h,i]	Dose 5 of DTaP and dose 4 of IPV	2, 4, 6 months of age[h,j,k]	2, 4, 6, 15 to 18 months of age[k]

Reactogenicity (%)				
Pain	24-35	57	31-36	39-56
Redness	22-27	37	25-40	7.1-17
Swelling	27-30	26	17-28	5.0-9.7
Low-grade fever	11-14	6.5	28-39	5.8-16
High-grade fever	0.8-2.7	0.1	0.4-1.4	0-0.7
Total reduction in shots[l]	2 or 3[m]	1	5	6 or 7[m]
How supplied (number in package)	1-dose vial (10)	1-dose vial (10), Prefilled syringe (5)	1-dose vial (10), Prefilled syringe (5)	1-dose vial (5) of ActHIB, lyophilized, with 1-dose vial (5) of DTaP-IPV as diluent
Storage	Refrigerate, Do not freeze	Refrigerate, Do not freeze	Refrigerate, Do not freeze	Vaccines: refrigerate, do not freeze. Reconstituted vaccine: use immediately
Reference package insert	August 2004	June 2008	February 2007	June 2008

[a] Licensure by the FDA implies efficacy that is not inferior to the component vaccines.
[b] The combination vaccines may not be strict mixtures of the component vaccines. In some cases, the amount of antigen or the method of production may be different than the separate components.
[c] The IPV contained in Pediarix and Kinrix is not licensed or distributed separately in the United States.
[d] The IPV contained in Pentacel is licensed but not distributed separately in the United States.
[e] The liquid DTaP-IPV combination is used to reconstitute the lyophilized ActHIB.
[f] Not labeled for use in infants of HBsAg-positive or -unknown mothers, but use in these infants is considered acceptable.

Continued

9

TABLE 9.22 — Part 1 (*continued*)

g Only labeled for the primary series (not booster doses).

h With the birth dose of HepB, use of this combination vaccine will result in four total doses of HepB. This does not increase reactogenicity or compromise immunogenicity.

i Patients who receive Comvax according to this schedule do not need further doses of HepB or Hib.

j Patients who receive Pediarix according to this schedule will need DTaP boosters at 15 to 18 months and 4 to 6 years of age, as well as an IPV booster at 4 to 6 years of age.

k Patients who receive Pentacel according to this schedule do not need further doses of Hib but do need a DTaP booster at 4 to 6 years of age. Pentacel given at 2, 4, 6, and 12-18 months of age provides 4 valid doses of IPV.

l Reduction in shots across the complete routine immunization schedule if the practice uses traditional ("monovalent") vaccines and switches to the combination.

m The higher number applies if ActHIB is currently in use, because switching to Comvax reduces the total number of Hib doses needed to complete the primary series from 3 to 2.

n The lower number applies if the office uses PedvaxHIB (PRP-OMPC), because a dose of that vaccine is not given at 6 months (there is one less shot saved).

Medicaid program demonstrated higher coverage rates among children who had received a combination vaccine (either HepB-Hib or DTaP-HepB-IPV) as compared with children who had received the component vaccines, an effect that was independent of other determinants of coverage. In another analysis of the same database, 2-year-olds who had received 3 doses of DTaP-HepB-IPV had markedly fewer cumulative days undervaccinated (125 days) than did control children (334 days) for the series of 4 DTaP, 3 IPV, 1 MMR, 3 Hib, 3 HepB, and 1 varicella vaccine. Similar findings have been seen in managed-care populations.

ADDITIONAL READING

Diphtheria, Tetanus, Pertussis

Broder KR, Cortese MM, Iskander JK, et al; Advisory Committee on Immunization Practices (ACIP). Preventing tetanus, diphtheria, and pertussis among adolescents: use of tetanus toxoid, reduced diphtheria toxoid and acellular pertussis vaccines: recommendations of the Advisory Committee on Immunization Practices (ACIP). *MMWR Recomm Rep.* 2006;55(RR-3):1-34.

Cortese MM, Baughman AL, Zhang R, Srivastava PU, Wallace GS. Pertussis hospitalizations among infants in the United States, 1993 to 2004. *Pediatrics.* 2008;121:484-492.

Kretsinger K, Broder KR, Cortese MM, et al; Centers for Disease Control and Prevention; Advisory Committee on Immunization Practices; Healthcare Infection Control Practices Advisory Committee. Preventing tetanus, diphtheria, and pertussis among adults: use of tetanus toxoid, reduced diphtheria toxoid and acellular pertussis vaccine: recommendations of the Advisory Committee on Immunization Practices (ACIP) and recommendation of ACIP, supported by the Healthcare Infection Control Practices Advisory Committee (HICPAC), for use of Tdap among health-care personnel. *MMWR Recomm Rep.* 2006;55(RR-17):1-37.

Murphy TV, Slade BA, Broder KR, et al; Advisory Committee on Immunization Practices (ACIP) Centers for Disease Control and Prevention (CDC). Prevention of pertussis, tetanus, and diphtheria among pregnant and postpartum women and their infants recommendations of the Advisory Committee on Immunization Practices (ACIP). *MMWR Recomm Rep.* 2008;57(RR-4):1-51.

Pertussis vaccination: use of acellular pertussis vaccines among infants and young children. Recommendations of the Advisory Committee on Immunization Practices (ACIP) *MMWR Recomm Rep.* 1997;46(RR-7):1-25.

Tanaka M, Vitek CR, Pascual FB, Bisgard KM, Tate JE, Murphy TV. Trends in pertussis among infants in the United States, 1980-1999. *JAMA.* 2003;290:2968-2975.

Use of diphtheria toxoid-tetanus toxoid-acellular pertussis vaccine as a five-dose series. Supplemental recommendations of the Advisory Committee on Immunization Practices (ACIP). *MMWR Recomm Rep.* 2000;49(RR-13):1-8.

9

TABLE 9.22 — Part 2: Modern Combination Vaccines

Trade name	ProQuad	TriHIBit	Twinrix
Abbreviation	MMRV	DTaP/Hib	HepA-HepB
Manufacturer/distributor	Merck	Sanofi Pasteur	GlaxoSmithKline
Diseases prevented[a]	Measles Mumps Rubella Varicella	Diphtheria Tetanus Pertussis Invasive *Haemophilus influenzae* type b	Hepatitis A Hepatitis B
Type of vaccine	Live attenuated, classical	Inactivated, purified subunits, toxoids, and engineered subunit	Inactivated, whole agent, and engineered subunit
Component vaccines[b]	M-M-R II (MMR) Varivax	Tripedia (DTaP) ActHIB (PRP-T)[c]	Havrix (HepA) Engerix-B (HepB)
Composition	Measles virus, Moraten strain (derived from the Edmonston B strain), propagated in chick embryo cells, at least 1000 TCID$_{50}$ Mumps virus, Jeryl Lynn strain (actually consists of two distinct strains), propagated in chick embryo cells, at least 19,950 TCID$_{50}$	Diphtheria toxoid (6.7 Lf units) Tetanus toxoid (5 Lf units) Inactivated pertussis toxin (23.4 mcg) Filamentous hemagglutinin (23.4 mcg) Polyribosylribitol phosphate (10 mcg) conjugated to tetanus toxoid (24 mcg)	HAV, HM175 strain, propagated in human diploid (MRC-5) cells and inactivated with formalin (1440 ELISA units) HBsAg expressed in yeast (*Saccharomyces cerevisiae*) (20 mcg)

	Rubella virus, RA 27/3 strain, propagated in human diploid lung fibroblast (WI-38) cells, at least 1000 TCID$_{50}$ Varicella virus, Oka/Merck strain, propagated in human diploid (MRC-5) cells, at least 9770 plaque-forming units		
Adjuvant	None	Aluminum phosphate (≤0.17 mg aluminum)	Aluminum phosphate Aluminum hydroxide (0.45 mg aluminum)
Preservative	None	None	None
Excipients and contaminants	Sucrose (21 mg) Hydrolyzed gelatin (11 mg) Sodium chloride (2.4 mg) Sorbitol (1.8 mg) Monosodium L-glutamate (0.40 mg) Sodium phosphate dibasic (0.34 mg) Human albumin (0.31 mg) Sodium bicarbonate (0.17 mg) Potassium phosphate monobasic (72 mcg)	Gelatin Formaldehyde (≤100 mcg) Polysorbate 80 Thimerosal (≤0.3 mcg mercury) Sucrose (8.5%)	Amino acids Sodium chloride Phosphate buffer Polysorbate 20 Formalin (≤0.1 mg) Residual MRC-5 proteins (≤2.5 mcg) Neomycin sulfate (≤20 ng) Yeast protein (≤5%)

Continued

9

TABLE 9.22 — Part 2 *(continued)*

Trade name	ProQuad	TriHIBit	Twinrix
Excipients and contaminants *(continued)*	Potassium chloride (60 mcg) Potassium phosphate dibasic (36 mcg) Residual components of MRC-5 cells, including DNA and protein Neomycin (<16 mcg) Bovine calf serum (0.5 mcg) Other buffer and media ingredients		
Latex	None	Vial stopper contains dry natural rubber	Tip cap and plunger of prefilled syringe contain dry natural rubber
Labeled ages	12 months to 12 years	15 to 18 months	≥18 years
Dose	0.5 mL	0.5 mL	1 mL
Route of administration	Subcutaneous	Intramuscular	Intramuscular
Usual schedule	12 to 15 months of age Revaccination before school entry	Dose 4 of DTaP and dose 4 of Hib	0, 1, 6 months Alternative schedule: 0, 7, 21 to 30 days; booster at 12 month
Reactogenicity (%)			
Pain	22	2.3–11	35–41
Redness	14[d]	13–33	8.0–11
Swelling	8.4	8.2–28	4.0–6.0

	—	0.7-5.6	2.0-4.0
Low-grade fever	—		—
High-grade fever	21.5	—	—
Total reduction in shots[e]	2	1	2 Alternative schedule: 1
How supplied (number in package)	1-dose vial (10), lyophilized with diluent	1-dose vial (5) of ActHIB, lyophilized (5) with 1-dose vial (5) of Tripedia as diluent	1-dose vial (10) 1-dose Prefilled syringe (5)
Storage	Vaccine: freeze, can be refrigerated for up to 72 hours before reconstitution, protect from light Diluent: refrigerate or room temperature Reconstituted vaccine: use within 30 minutes	Vaccines: refrigerate, do not freeze Reconstituted vaccine: use within 30 minutes	Refrigerate Do not freeze
Reference package insert	February 2008	December 2003 December 2005	April 2007

[a] Licensure by the FDA implies efficacy that is not inferior to the component vaccines.

[b] The combination vaccines may not be strict mixtures of the component vaccines. In some cases, the amount of antigen or the method of production may be different than the separate components.

[c] The liquid Tripedia is used to reconstitute the lyophilized ActHIB.

[d] A measles-like rash occurs in about 3% of patients and a varicella-like rash in 2%.

[e] Reduction in shots across the complete routine immunization schedule if the practice uses tradional ("monovalent") vaccines and switches to the combination.

9

Ward JI, Cherry JD, Chang SJ, et al; APERT Study Group. Bordetella Pertussis infections in vaccinated and unvaccinated adolescents and adults, as assessed in a national prospective randomized Acellular Pertussis Vaccine Trial (APERT). *Clin Infect Dis*. 2006;43:151-157.

Wendelboe AM, Njamkepo E, Bourillon A, et al; Infant Pertussis Study Group. Transmission of Bordetella pertussis to young infants. *Pediatr Infect Dis J*. 2007;26:293-299.

Haemophilus influenzae type b

Centers for Disease Control and Prevention (CDC). Haemophilus influenzae invasive disease among children aged <5 years—California, 1990-1996. *MMWR Morb Mortal Wkly Rep*. 1998;47:737-740.

Centers for Disease Control and Prevention (CDC). Progress toward elimination of *Haemophilus influenzae* type b invasive disease among infants and children—United States, 1998-2000. *MMWR Morb Mortal Wkly Rep*. 2002;51:234-237.

Decker MD, Edwards KM. Haemophilus influenzae type b vaccines: history, choice and comparisons. *Pediatr Infect Dis J*. 1998;17(9 suppl):S113-S116.

Haemophilus b conjugate vaccines for prevention of Haemophilus influenzae type b disease among infants and children two months of age and older. Recommendations of the immunization practices advisory committee (ACIP). *MMWR Recomm Rep*. 1991;40(RR-1):1-7.

Hepatitis A

Advisory Committee on Immunization Practices (ACIP) Centers for Disease Control and Prevention (CDC). Update: Prevention of hepatitis A after exposure to hepatitis A virus and in international travelers. Updated recommendations of the Advisory Committee on Immunization Practices (ACIP). *MMWR Morb Mortal Wkly Rep*. 2007;56:1080-1084.

Advisory Committee on Immunization Practices (ACIP), Fiore AE, Wasley A, Bell BP. Prevention of hepatitis A through active or passive immunization: recommendations of the Advisory Committee on Immunization Practices (ACIP). *MMWR Recomm Rep*. 2006;55(RR-7):1-23.

Armstrong GL, Billah K, Rein DB, Hicks KA, Wirth KE, Bell BP. The economics of routine childhood hepatitis A immunization in the United States: the impact of herd immunity. *Pediatrics*. 2007;119:e22-e29.

Averhoff F, Shapiro CN, Bell BP, et al. Control of hepatitis A through routine vaccination of children. *JAMA*. 2001;286:2968-2973.

Fiore AE. Hepatitis A transmitted by food. *Clin Infect Dis*. 2004;38:705-715.

Innis BL, Snitbhan R, Kunasol P, et al. Protection against hepatitis A by an inactivated vaccine. *JAMA*. 1994;271:1328-1334.

Mutsch M, Spicher VM, Gut C, Steffen R. Hepatitis A virus infections in travelers, 1988-2004. *Clin Infect Dis*. 2006;42:490-497.

Rendı-Wagner P, Korinek M, Winkler B, Kundi M, Kollaritsch H, Wiedermann U. Persistence of seroprotection 10 years after primary hepatitis A vaccination in an unselected study population. *Vaccine*. 2007;25:927-931.

Shapiro CN, Coleman PJ, McQuillan GM, Alter MJ, Margolis HS. Epidemiology of hepatitis A: seroepidemiology and risk groups in the USA. *Vaccine*. 1992;10(suppl 1):S59-S62.

Victor JC, Monto AS, Surdina TY, et al. Hepatitis A vaccine versus immune globulin for postexposure prophylaxis. *N Engl J Med*. 2007;357:1685-1694.

Wasley A, Grytdal S, Gallagher K; Centers for Disease Control and Prevention (CDC). Surveillance for acute viral hepatitis—United States, 2006. *MMWR Surveill Summ*. 2008;57:1-24.

Weinbaum C, Lyerla R, Margolis HS; Centers for Disease Control and Prevention. Prevention and control of infections with hepatitis viruses in correctional settings. Centers for Disease Control and Prevention. *MMWR Recomm Rep*. 2003;52(RR-1):1-36.

Werzberger A, Mensch B, Nalin DR, Kuter BJ. Effectiveness of hepatitis A vaccine in a former frequently affected community: 9 years' follow up after the Monroe field trial of VAQTA. *Vaccine*. 2002;20:1699-1701.

9

Hepatitis B

Boxall EH, A Sira J, El-Shuhkri N, Kelly DA. Long-term persistence of immunity to hepatitis B after vaccination during infancy in a country where endemicity is low. *J Infect Dis*. 2004;190:1264-1269.

Chang MH, Chen CJ, Lai MS, et al. Universal hepatitis B vaccination in Taiwan and the incidence of hepatocellular carcinoma in children. Taiwan Childhood Hepatoma Study Group. *N Engl J Med*. 1997;336:1855-1859.

Ganem D, Prince AM. Hepatitis B virus infection—natural history and clinical consequences. *N Engl J Med*. 2004;350:1118-1129.

Mast EE, Margolis HS, Fiore AE, et al; Advisory Committee on Immunization Practices (ACIP). A comprehensive immunization strategy to eliminate transmission of hepatitis B virus infection in the United States: recommendations of the Advisory Committee on Immunization Practices (ACIP) part 1: immunization of infants, children, and adolescents. *MMWR Recomm Rep*. 2005;54(RR-16):1-31.

Mast EE, Weinbaum CM, Fiore AE, et al; Advisory Committee on Immunization Practices (ACIP) Centers for Disease Control and Prevention (CDC). A comprehensive immunization strategy to eliminate transmission of hepatitis B virus infection in the United States: recommendations of the Advisory Committee on Immunization Practices (ACIP) Part II: immunization of adults. *MMWR Recomm Rep*. 2006;55(RR-16):1-33.

Perz JF, Elm JL Jr, Fiore AE, Huggler JI, Kuhnert WL, Effler PV. Near elimination of hepatitis B virus infections among Hawaii elementary school children after universal infant hepatitis B vaccination. *Pediatrics*. 2006;118:1403-1408.

Shepard CW, Finelli L, Fiore AE, Bell BP. Epidemiology of hepatitis B and hepatitis B virus infection in United States children. *Pediatr Infect Dis J*. 2005;24:755-760.

U.S. Public Health Service. Updated U.S. Public Health Service Guidelines for the Management of Occupational Exposures to HBV, HCV, and HIV and Recommendations for Postexposure Prophylaxis. *MMWR Recomm Rep*. 2001;50(RR-11):1-52.

van der Sande MA, Waight P, Mendy M, et al. Long-term protection against carriage of hepatitis B virus after infant vaccination. *J Infect Dis*. 2006;193:1528-1535.

Weinbaum C, Lyerla R, Margolis HS; Centers for Disease Control and Prevention. Prevention and control of infections with hepatitis viruses in correctional settings. Centers for Disease Control and Prevention. *MMWR Recomm Rep*. 2003;52(RR-1):1-36.

Yusuf HR, Daniels D, Smith P, Coronado V, Rodewald L. Association between administration of hepatitis B vaccine at birth and completion of the hepatitis B and 4:3:1:3 vaccine series. *JAMA*. 2000;284:978-983.

Human Papillomavirus

Ault KA; Future II Study Group. Effect of prophylactic human papillomavirus L1 virus-like-particle vaccine on risk of cervical intraepithelial neoplasia grade 2, grade 3, and adenocarcinoma in situ: a combined analysis of four randomised clinical trials. *Lancet*. 2007;369:1861-1868.

Barr E, Tamms G. Quadrivalent human papillomavirus vaccine. *Clin Infect Dis*. 2007;45:609-617.

Block SL, Nolan T, Sattler C, et al; Protocol 016 Study Group. Comparison of the immunogenicity and reactogenicity of a prophylactic quadrivalent human papillomavirus (types 6, 11, 16, and 18) L1 virus-like particle vaccine in male and female adolescents and young adult women. *Pediatrics*. 2006;118:2135-2145.

D'Souza G, Kreimer AR, Viscidi R, et al. Case-control study of human papillomavirus and oropharyngeal cancer. *N Engl J Med*. 2007;356:1944-1956.

Dunne EF, Unger ER, Sternberg M, et al. Prevalence of HPV infection among females in the United States. *JAMA*. 2007;297:813-819.

FUTURE II Study Group. Quadrivalent vaccine against human papillomavirus to prevent high-grade cervical lesions. *N Engl J Med*. 2007;356:1915-1927.

Harper DM, Franco EL, Wheeler CM, et al; HPV Vaccine Study group. Sustained efficacy up to 4.5 years of a bivalent L1 virus-like particle vaccine against human papillomavirus types 16 and 18: follow-up from a randomised control trial. *Lancet*. 2006;367:1247-1255.

Joura EA, Leodolter S, Hernandez-Avila M, et al. Efficacy of a quadrivalent prophylactic human papillomavirus (types 6, 11, 16, and 18) L1 virus-like-particle vaccine against high-grade vulval and vaginal lesions: a combined analysis of three randomised clinical trials. *Lancet*. 2007;369:1693-1702.

Kaufman RH, Adam F., Vonka V. Human papillomavirus infection and cervical carcinoma. *Clin Obstet Gynecol.* 2000;43:363-380.

Markowitz LE, Dunne EF, Saraiya M, Lawson HW, Chesson H, Unger ER; Centers for Disease Control and Prevention (CDC); Advisory Committee on Immunization Practices (ACIP). Quadrivalent Human Papillomavirus Vaccine: Recommendations of the Advisory Committee on Immunization Practices (ACIP). *MMWR Recomm Rep.* 2007;56(RR-2):1-24.

Paavonen J, Jenkins D, Bosch FX, et al; HPV PATRICIA study group. Efficacy of a prophylactic adjuvanted bivalent L1 virus-like-particle vaccine against infection with human papillomavirus types 16 and 18 in young women: an interim analysis of a phase III double-blind, randomised controlled trial. *Lancet.* 2007;369:2161-2170.

Reisinger KS, Block SL, Lazcano-Ponce E, et al. Safety and persistent immunogenicity of a quadrivalent human papillomavirus types 6, 11, 16, 18 L1 virus-like particle vaccine in preadolescents and adolescents: a randomized controlled trial. *Pediatr Infect Dis J.* 2007;26:201-209.

Schiffman M, Castle PE, Jeronimo J, Rodriguez AC, Wacholder S. Human papillomavirus and cervical cancer. *Lancet.* 2007;370:890-907.

Villa LL, Costa RL, Petta CA, et al. High sustained efficacy of a prophylactic quadrivalent human papillomavirus types 6/11/16/18 L1 virus-like particle vaccine through 5 years of follow-up. *Br J Cancer.* 2006;95:1459-1466.

9

Influenza

Ashkenazi S, Vertruyen A, Arístegui J, et al; CAIV-T Study Group. Superior relative efficacy of live attenuated influenza vaccine compared with inactivated influenza vaccine in young children with recurrent respiratory tract infections. *Pediatr Infect Dis J.* 2006;25:870-879.

Belshe RB, Edwards KM, Vesikari T, et al; CAIV-T Comparative Efficacy Study Group. Live attenuated versus inactivated influenza vaccine in infants and young children. *N Engl J Med.* 2007;356:685-696.

Belshe RB, Mendelman PM, Treanor J, et al. The efficacy of live attenuated, cold-adapted, trivalent, intranasal influenzavirus vaccine in children. *N Engl J Med.* 1998;338:1405-1412.

Belshe RB, Nichol KL, Black SB, et al. Safety, efficacy, and effectiveness of live, attenuated, cold-adapted influenza vaccine in an indicated population aged 5-49 years. *Clin Infect Dis.* 2004;39:920-927.

Bridges CB, Thompson WW, Meltzer MI, et al. Effectiveness and cost-benefit of influenza vaccination of healthy working adults: A randomized controlled trial. *JAMA.* 2000;284:1655-1663.

Centers for Disease Control and Prevention (CDC). Interim within-season estimate of the effectiveness of trivalent inactivated influenza vaccine—Marshfield, Wisconsin, 2007-08 influenza season. *MMWR Morb Mortal Wkly Rep.* 2008;57:393-398.

Fleming DM, Crovari P, Wahn U, et al; CAIV-T Asthma Study Group. Comparison of the efficacy and safety of live attenuated cold-adapted influenza vaccine, trivalent, with trivalent inactivated influenza virus vaccine in children and adolescents with asthma. *Pediatr Infect Dis J.* 2006;25:860-869.

Hurwitz ES, Haber M, Chang A, et al. Effectiveness of influenza vaccination of day care children in reducing influenza-related morbidity among household contacts. *JAMA.* 2000;284:1677-1682.

Izurieta HS, Thompson WW, Kramarz P, et al. Influenza and the rates of hospitalization for respiratory disease among infants and young children. *N Engl J Med.* 2000;342:232-239.

Jefferson T, Smith S, Demicheli V, Harnden A, Rivetti A, Di Pietrantonj C. Assessment of the efficacy and effectiveness of influenza vaccines in healthy children: systematic review. *Lancet.* 2005;365:773-780.

Neuzil KM, Zhu Y, Griffin MR, et al. Burden of interpandemic influenza in children younger than 5 years: a 25-year prospective study. *J Infect Dis.* 2002;185:147-152.

Nichol KL, Lind A, Margolis KL, et al. The effectiveness of vaccination against influenza in healthy, working adults. *N Engl J Med.* 1995;333:889-893.

Nichol KL, Nordin JD, Nelson DB, Mullooly JP, Hak E. Effectiveness of influenza vaccine in the community-dwelling elderly. *N Engl J Med.* 2007;357:1373-1381.

Nichol KL. Cost-benefit analysis of a strategy to vaccinate healthy working adults against influenza. *Arch Intern Med.* 2001;161:749-759.

Pearson ML, Bridges CB, Harper SA; Healthcare Infection Control Practices Advisory Committee (HICPAC); Advisory Committee on Immunization Practices (ACIP). Influenza vaccination of health-care personnel: recommendations of the Healthcare Infection Control Practices Advisory Committee (HICPAC) and the Advisory Committee on Immunization Practices (ACIP). *MMWR Recomm Rep.* 2006;55(RR-2):1-16.

Poehling KA, Edwards KM, Weinberg GA, et al; New Vaccine Surveillance Network. The underrecognized burden of influenza in young children. *N Engl J Med.* 2006;355:31-40.

Recommendations of the Advisory Committee on Immunization Practices (ACIP), 2008. Prevention and control of influenza. *MMWR Recomm Rep.* 2008;57(Early Release):1-60 (Note: these recommendations are revised annually).

Reichert TA, Sugaya N, Fedson DS, Glezen WP, Simonsen L, Tashiro M. The Japanese experience with vaccinating schoolchildren against influenza. *N Engl J Med.* 2001;344:889-896.

Thompson WW, Shay DK, Weintraub E, et al. Influenza-associated hospitalizations in the United States. *JAMA.* 2004;292:1333-1340.

Thompson WW, Shay DK, Weintraub E, et al. Mortality associated with influenza and respiratory syncytial virus in the United States. *JAMA.* 2003;289:179-186.

Centers for Disease Control and Prevention (CDC). Elimination of rubella and congenital rubella syndrome—United States, 1969-2004. *MMWR Morb Mortal Wkly Rep.* 2005;54:279-282.

Centers for Disease Control and Prevention (CDC). Epidemiology of measles—United States, 2001-2003. *MMWR Morb Mortal Wkly Rep.* 2004;53:713-716.

Centers for Disease Control and Prevention (CDC). Measles—United States, January 1-April 25, 2008. *MMWR Morb Mortal Wkly Rep.* 2008;57:494-498.

Centers for Disease Control and Prevention (CDC). Mumps epidemic—Iowa, 2006. *MMWR Morb Mortal Wkly Rep.* 2006;55:366-368.

Centers for Disease Control and Prevention (CDC). Notice to readers: updated recommendations of the Advisory Committee on Immunization Practices (ACIP) for the control and elimination of mumps. *MMWR Morb Mortal Wkly Rep.* 2006;55:629-630.

Date AA, Kyaw MH, Rue AM, et al. Long-term persistence of mumps antibody after receipt of 2 measles-mumps-rubella (MMR) vaccinations and antibody response after a third MMR vaccination among a university population. *J Infect Dis.* 2008;197:1662-1668.

Dayan GH, Quinlisk MP, Parker AA, et al. Recent resurgence of mumps in the United States. *N Engl J Med.* 2008;358:1580-1589.

France EK, Glanz J, Xu S, et al; Vaccine Safety Datalink Team. Risk of immune thrombocytopenic purpura after measles-mumps-rubella immunization in children. *Pediatrics.* 2008;121:e687-e692.

Marin M, Quinlisk P, Shimabukuro T, Sawhney C, Brown C, Lebaron CW. Mumps vaccination coverage and vaccine effectiveness in a large outbreak among college students-Iowa, 2006. *Vaccine.* 2008;26:3601-3607.

Parker AA, Staggs W, Dayan GH, et al. Implications of a 2005 measles outbreak in Indiana for sustained elimination of measles in the United States. *N Engl J Med.* 2006;355:447-455.

Reef SE, Redd SB, Abernathy E, Zimmerman L, Icenogle JP. The epidemiological profile of rubella and congenital rubella syndrome in the United States, 1998-2004: the evidence for absence of endemic transmission. *Clin Infect Dis.* 2006;43(suppl 3):S126-S132.

Watson JC, Hadler SC, Dykewicz CA, Reef S, Phillips L. Measles, mumps, and rubella—vaccine use and strategies for elimination of measles, rubella, and congenital rubella syndrome and control of mumps: recommendations of the Advisory Committee on Immunization Practices (ACIP). *MMWR Recomm Rep.* 1998;47(RR-8):1-57.

Neisseria meningitidis

Advisory Committee on Immunization Practices (ACIP) Centers for Disease Control and Prevention (CDC). Report from the Advisory Committee on Immunization Practices (ACIP): decision not to recommend routine vaccination of all children aged 2-10 years with quadrivalent meningococcal conjugate vaccine (MCV4). *MMWR Morb Mortal Wkly Rep.* 2008;57:462-465.

Balmer P, Borrow R, Miller E. Impact of meningococcal C conjugate vaccine in the UK. *J Med Microbiol.* 2002;51:717-722.

Bruce MG, Rosenstein NE, Capparella JM, Shutt KA, Perkins BA, Collins M. Risk factors for meningococcal disease in college students. *JAMA.* 2001;286:688-693.

Campbell JD, Edelman R, King JC Jr, Papa T, Ryall R, Rennels MB. Safety, reactogenicity, and immunogenicity of a tetravalent meningococcal polysaccharide-diphtheria toxoid conjugate vaccine given to healthy adults. *J Infect Dis.* 2002;186:1848-1851.

Centers for Disease Control and Prevention (CDC) Advisory Committee on Immunization Practices. Revised recommendations of the Advisory Committee on Immunization Practices to Vaccinate all Persons Aged 11-18 Years with Meningococcal Conjugate Vaccine. *MMWR Morb Mortal Wkly Rep.* 2007;56:794-795.

Centers for Disease Control and Prevention. Recommendation from the Advisory Committee on Immunization Practices (ACIP) for use of quadrivalent meningococcal conjugate vaccine (MCV4) in children aged 2–10 years at increased risk for invasive meningococcal disease. *MMWR Morbib Mortal Wkly Rep.* 2007;56:1265-1266.

Kaplan SL, Schutze GE, Leake JA, et al. Multicenter surveillance of invasive meningococcal infections in children. *Pediatrics.* 2006;118:e9-79-e984.

Keyserling H, Papa T, Koranyi K, et al. Safety, immunogenicity, and immune memory of a novel meningococcal (groups A, C, Y, and W-135) polysaccharide diphtheria toxoid conjugate vaccine (MCV-4) in healthy adolescents. *Arch Pediatr Adolesc Med.* 2005;159:907-913.

Lieberman JM, Chiu SS, Wong VK, et al. Safety and immunogenicity of a serogroups A/C Neisseria meningitides oligosaccharide-protein conjugate vaccine in young children. A randomized controlled trial. *JAMA.* 1996;275:1499-1503.

Meningococcal disease and college students. Recommendations of the Advisory Committee on Immunization Practices (ACIP). *MMWR Recomm Rep.* 2000;49(RR-7):13-20.

Pichichero M, Casey J, Blatter M, et al. Comparative trial of the safety and immunogenicity of quadrivalent (A, C, Y, W-135) meningococcal polysaccharide-diphtheria conjugate vaccine versus quadrivalent polysaccharide vaccine in two- to ten-year-old children. *Pediatr Infect Dis J.* 2005;24:57-62.

Rosenstein NE, Perkins BA, Stephens DS, et al. The changing epidemiology of meningococcal disease in the United States, 1992-1996. *J Infect Dis.* 1999;180:1894-1901.

Rosenstein NE, Perkins BA, Stephens DS, Popovic T, Hughes JM. Meningococcal disease. *N Engl J Med.* 2001;344:1378-1388.

Snape MD, Pollard AJ. Meningococcal polysaccharide-protein conjugate vaccines. *Lancet Infect Dis.* 2005;5:21-30.

Polio

Centers for Disease Control and Prevention (CDC). Poliovirus infections in four unvaccinated children—Minnesota, August-October 2005. *MMWR Morb Mortal Wkly Rep*. 2005;54:1053-1055.

Centers for Disease Control and Prevention (CDC). Progress toward interruption of wild poliovirus transmission—worldwide, January 2007-April 2008. *MMWR Morb Mortal Wkly Rep*. 2008;57:489-494.

Global Polio Eradication Initiative. Annual Report 2006. http://www.polioeradication.org/content/publications/annualreport2006.asp (Accessed August 15, 2008).

Hull HF. The future of polio eradication. *Lancet Infect Dis*. 2001;1:299-303.

Poliomyelitis prevention in the United States: introduction of a sequential vaccination schedule of inactivated poliovirus vaccine followed by oral poliovirus vaccine. Recommendations of the Advisory Committee on Immunization Practices (ACIP) *MMWR Recomm Rep*. 1997;46(RR-3):1-25.

Prevots DR, Burr RK, Sutter RW, Murphy TV; Advisory Committee on Immunization Practices. Poliomyelitis prevention in the United States. Updated recommendations of the Advisory Committee on Immunization Practices (ACIP). *MMWR Recomm Rep*. 2000;49(RR-5):1-22.

9

Rotavirus

Centers for Disease Control and Prevention. ACIP provisional recommendations for the prevention of rotavirus gastroenteritis among infants and children. http://www.cdc.gov/vaccines/recs/provisional/downloads/roto-7-1-08-508.pdf (Accessed August 15, 2008).

Centers for Disease Control and Prevention (CDC). Delayed onset and diminished magnitude of rotavirus activity—United States, November 2007-May 2008. *MMWR Morb Mortal Wkly Rep*. 2008;57:697-700.

Centers for Disease Control and Prevention (CDC). Postmarketing monitoring of intussusception after RotaTeq vaccination—United States, February 1, 2006-February 15, 2007. *MMWR Morb Mortal Wkly Rep*. 2007;56:218-222.

Charles MD, Holman RC, Curns AT, Parashar UD, Glass RI, Bresee JS. Hospitalizations associated with rotavirus gastroenteritis in the United States, 1993-2002. *Pediatr Infect Dis J*. 2006;25:489-493.

Coffin SE, Elser J, Marchant C, et al. Impact of acute rotavirus gastroenteritis on pediatric outpatient practices in the United States. *Pediatr Infect Dis J*. 2006;25:584-589.

Cunliffe NA, Bresee JS, Hart CA. Rotavirus vaccines: development, current issues and future prospects. *J Infect*. 2002;45:1-9.

Dennehy PH, Cortese MM, Bégué RE, et al. A case-control study to determine risk factors for hospitalization for rotavirus gastroenteritis in U.S. children. *Pediatr Infect Dis J*. 2006;25:1123-1131.

Glass RI, Parashar UD, Bresee JS, et al. Rotavirus vaccines: current prospects and future challenges. *Lancet*. 2006;368:323-332.

Linhares AC, Velázquez FR, Pérez-Schael I, et al; Human Rotavirus Vaccine Study Group. Efficacy and safety of an oral live attenuated human rotavirus vaccine against rotavirus gastroenteritis during the first 2 years of life in Latin American infants: a randomised, double-blind, placebo-controlled phase III study. *Lancet.* 2008;371:1181-1189.

Parashar UD, Alexander JP, Glass RI; Advisory Committee on Immunization Practices (ACIP), Centers for Disease Control and Prevention (CDC). Prevention of rotavirus gastroenteritis among infants and children. Recommendations of the Advisory Committee on Immunization Practices (ACIP). *MMWR Recomm Rep.* 2006;55(RR-12):1-13.

Peter G, Myers MG; National Vaccine Advisory Committee; National Vaccine Program Office. Intussusception, rotavirus, and oral vaccines: summary of a workshop. *Pediatrics.* 2002;110:e67.

Ruiz-Palacios GM, Pérez-Schael I, Velázquez FR, et al; Human Rotavirus Vaccine Study Group. Safety and efficacy of an attenuated vaccine against severe rotavirus gastroenteritis. *N Engl J Med.* 2006;354:11-22.

Vesikari T, Matson DO, Dennehy P, et al; Rotavirus Efficacy and Safety Trial (REST) Study Team. Safety and efficacy of a pentavalent human-bovine (WC3) reassortant rotavirus vaccine. *N Engl J Med.* 2006;354:23-33.

Vesikari T, Karvonen A, Prymula R, et al. Efficacy of human rotavirus vaccine against rotavirus gastroenteritis during the first 2 years of life in European infants: randomised, double-blind controled study. *Lancet.* 2007;370:1757-1763.

Streptococcus pneumoniae

Advisory Committee on Immunization Practices. Preventing pneumococcal disease among infants and young children. Recommendations of the Advisory Committee on Immunization Practices (ACIP). *MMWR Recomm Rep.* 2000;49(RR-9):1-35.

Black S, Shinefield H, Baxter R, et al. Postlicensure surveillance for pneumococcal invasive disease after use of heptavalent pneumococcal conjugate vaccine in Northern California Kaiser Permanente. *Pediatr Infect Dis J.* 2004;23:485-489.

Butler JC, Breiman RF, Campbell JF, Lipman HB, Broome CV, Facklam RR. Pneumococcal polysaccharide vaccine efficacy. An evaluation of current recommendations. *JAMA.* 1993;270:1826-1831.

Centers for Disease Control and Prevention (CDC); Advisory Committee on immunization Practices (ACIP). Updated recommendation from the Advisory Committee on Immunization Practices (ACIP) for use of 7-valent pneumococcal conjugate vaccine (PCV7) in children aged 24-59 months who are not completely vaccinated. *MMWR Morb Mortal Wkly Rep.* 2008;57:343-344.

Centers for Disease Control and Prevention (CDC). Direct and indirect effects of routine vaccination of children with 7-valent pneumococcal conjugate vaccine on incidence of invasive pneumococcal disease—United States, 1998-2003. *MMWR Morb Mortal Wkly Rep.* 2005;54:893-897.

Centers for Disease Control and Prevention (CDC). Invasive pneumococcal disease in children 5 years after conjugate vaccine introduction—eight states, 1998-2005. *MMWR Morb Mortal Wkly Rep.* 2008;57:144-148.

Grijalva CG, Nuorti JP, Arbogast PG, Martin SW, Edwards KM, Griffin MR. Decline in pneumonia admissions after routine childhood immunisation with pneumococcal conjugate vaccine in the USA: a time-series analysis. *Lancet.* 2007;369:1179-1186.

Grijalva CG, Poehling KA, Nuorti JP, et al. National impact of universal childhood immunization with pneumococcal conjugate vaccine on outpatient medical care visits in the United States. *Pediatrics.* 2006;118:865-873.

Kyaw MH, Lynfield R, Schaffner W, et al; Active Bacterial Core Surveillance of the Emerging Infections Program Network. Effect of introduction of the pneumococcal conjugate vaccine on drug-resistant Streptococcus pneumoniae. *N Engl J Med.* 2006;354:1455-1463.

Lexau CA, Lynfield R, Danila R, et al; Active Bacterial Core Surveillance Team. Changing epidemiology of invasive pneumococcal disease among older adults in the era of pediatric pneumococcal conjugate vaccine. *JAMA.* 2005;294:2043-2051.

O'Brien KL, Millar EV, Zell ER, et al. Effect of pneumococcal conjugate vaccine on nasopharyngeal colonization among immunized and unimmunized children in a community-randomized trial. *J Infect Dis.* 2007;196:1211-1220.

Poehling KA, Lafleur BJ, Szilagyi PG, et al. Population-based impact of pneumococcal conjugate vaccine in young children. *Pediatrics.* 2004;114:755-761.

Poehling KA, Talbot TR, Griffin MR, et al. Invasive pneumococcal disease among infants before and after introduction of pneumococcal conjugate vaccine. *JAMA.* 2006;295:1668-1674.

Prevention of pneumococcal disease: recommendations of the Advisory Committee on Immunization Practices (ACIP). *MMWR Recomm Rep.* 1997;46(RR-8):1-24.

Robinson KA, Baughman W, Rothrock G, et al; Active Bacterial Core Surveillance (ABCs)/Emerging Infections Program Network. Epidemiology of invasive Streptococcus pneumoniae infections in the United States, 1995-1998: Opportunities for prevention in the conjugate vaccine era. *JAMA.* 2001;285:1729-1735.

Tsai CJ, Griffin MR, Nuorti JP, Grijalva CG. Changing epidemiology of pneumococcal meningitis after the introduction of pneumococcal conjugate vaccine in the United States. *Clin Infect Dis.* 2008;46:1664-1672.

Whitney CG, Pilishvili T, Farley MM, et al. Effectiveness of seven-valent pneumococcal conjugate vaccine against invasive pneumococcal disease: a matched case-control study. *Lancet.* 2006;368:1495-1502.

Varicella

Centers for Disease Control and Prevention (CDC). A new product (VariZIG) for postexposure prophylaxis of varicella available under an investigational new drug application expanded access protocol. *MMWR Morb Mortal Wkly Rep*. 2006;55:209-210.

Chaves SS, Gargiullo P, Zhang JX, et al. Loss of vaccine-induced immunity to varicella over time. *N Engl J Med*. 2007;356:1121-1129.

Galea SA, Sweet A, Beninger P, et al. The safety profile of varicella vaccine: a 10-year review. *J Infect Dis*. 2008;197(suppl 2):S165-S169.

Izurieta HS, Strebel PM, Blake PA. Postlicensure effectiveness of varicella vaccine during an outbreak in a child care center. *JAMA*. 1997;278:1495-1499.

Marin M, Güris D, Chaves SS, Schmid S, Seward JF; Advisory Committee on Immunization Practices, Centers for Disease Control and Prevention (CDC). Prevention of varicella: recommendations of the Advisory Committee on Immunization Practices (ACIP). *MMWR Recomm Rep*. 2007;56(RR-4):1-40.

Meyer PA, Seward JF, Jumaan AO, Wharton M. Varicella mortality: trends before vaccine licensure in the United States, 1970-1994. *J Infect Dis*. 2000;182:383-390.

Prevention of varicella. Update recommendations of the Advisory Committee on Immunization Practices (ACIP). *MMWR Recomm Rep*. 1999;48(RR-6):1-5.

Reynolds MA, Watson BM, Plott-Adams KK, et al. Epidemiology of varicella hospitalizations in the United States, 1995-2005. *J Infect Dis*. 2008;197(suppl 2):S120-S126.

Seward JF, Watson BM, Peterson CL, et al. Varicella disease after introduction of varicella vaccine in the United States, 1995-2000. *JAMA*. 2002;287:606-611.

Vázquez M, LaRussa PS, Gershon AA, et al. Effectiveness over time of varicella vaccine. *JAMA*. 2004;291:851-855.

Vázquez M, LaRussa PS, Gershon AA, Steinberg SP, Freudigman K, Shapiro ED. The effectiveness of the varicella vaccine in clinical practice. *N Engl J Med*. 2001;344:955-960.

Zhou F, Harpaz R, Jumaan AO, Winston CA, Shefer A. Impact of varicella vaccination on health care utilization. *JAMA*. 2005;294:797-802.

Zhou F, Ortega-Sanchez IR, Guris D, Shefer A, Lieu T, Seward JF. An economic analysis of the universal varicella vaccination program in the United States. *J Infect Dis*. 2008;197(suppl 2):S156-S164.

Zoster

Dworkin RH, Johnson RW, Breuer J, et al. Recommendations for the management of herpes zoster. *Clin Infect Dis*. 2007;44(suppl 1):S1-S26.

Gnann JW Jr, Whitley RJ. Clinical practice. Herpes zoster. *N Engl J Med*. 2002;347:340-346.

Harpaz R, Ortega-Sanchez IR, Seward JF; Advisory Committee on Immunization Practices (ACIP) Centers for Disease Control and Prevention (CDC). Prevention of herpes zoster: recommendations of the Advisory Committee on Immunization Practices (ACIP). *MMWR Recomm Rep*. 2008;57(RR-5):1-30.

Kimberlin DW, Whitley RJ. Varicella-zoster vaccine for the prevention of herpes zoster. *N Engl J Med*. 2007;356:1338-1343.

Oxman MN, Levin MJ, Johnson GR, et al; Shingles Prevention Study Group. A vaccine to prevent herpes zoster and postherpetic neuralgia in older adults. *N Engl J Med*. 2005;352:2271-2284.

Reynolds MA, Chaves SS, Harpaz R, Lopez AS, Seward JF. The impact of the varicella vaccination program on herpes zoster epidemiology in the United States: a review. *J Infect Dis*. 2008;197(suppl 2):S224-S227.

Thomas SL, Hall AJ. What does epidemiology tell us about risk factors for herpes zoster? *Lancet Infect Dis*. 2004;4:26-33.

Wood M. Understanding pain in herpes zoster: an essential for optimizing treatment. *J Infect Dis*. 2002;186(suppl 1):S78-S82.

Modern Combination Vaccines

Centers for Disease Control and Prevention. Licensure of a diphtheria and tetanus toxoids and acellular pertussis adsorbed, inactivated poliovirus, and *Haemophilus* b conjugate vaccine and guidance for use in infants and children. *MMWR* 2008;57:1079-1080.

Centers for Disease Control and Prevention. Licensure of a diphtheria and tetanus toxoids and acellular pertussis adsorbed and inactivated poliovirus vaccine and guidance for use as a booster dose. *MMWR* 2008;57:1078-1079.

Combination vaccines for childhood immunization: recommendations of the Advisory Committee on Immunization Practices (ACIP), the American Academy of Pediatrics (AAP), and the American Academy of Family Physicians (AAFP). *Pediatrics*. 1999;103:1064-1077.

Freed GL, Cowan AE, Clark SJ, Santoli J, Bradley J. Use of a new combined vaccine in pediatric practices. *Pediatrics*. 2006;118:e251-e257.

Happe LE, Lunacsek OE, Kruzikas DT, Marshall GS. Impact of a pentavalent combination vaccine on immunization timeliness in a state Medicaid population. *Pediatr Infect Dis J*. 2008. In press.

Happe LE, Lunacsek OE, Marshall GS, Lewis T, Spencer S. Combination vaccine use and vaccination quality in a managed care population. *Am J Manag Care*. 2007;13:506-512.

Marshall GS, Happe LE, Lunacsek OE, et al. Use of combination vaccines is associated with improved coverage rates. *Pediatr Infect Dis J*. 2007;26:496-500.

Proceedings of the International Symposium on Combination Vaccines. 2-4 February 2000. *Clin Infect Dis*. 2001;33(suppl 4):S261-S375.

Specialized Vaccines

Anthrax

■ Pathogen

Bacillus anthracis is a large, aerobic, spore-forming, toxin-producing gram-positive rod with a "jointed bamboo-rod" appearance and "Medusa's head" colony morphology. Pathogenicity is mediated by two secreted virulence factors: lethal toxin and edema toxin.

■ Clinical Features

Anthrax is of most interest as a potential agent of bioterrorism (see Chapter 2, *Vaccine Infrastructure in the United States*). *Inhalational anthrax* is characterized by a flu-like illness, dyspnea, and hemorrhagic thoracic lymphadenitis and mediastinitis. *Cutaneous anthrax* is characterized by a painless ulcer with extensive surrounding edema, eschar formation, and regional adenopathy. Both of these forms of disease would be seen after a bioterrorism attack and either can lead to meningitis. The *gastrointestinal* (bloody diarrhea, hemorrhagic mesenteric adenitis) and *oropharyngeal* (oral or esophageal ulcers and regional adenopathy) forms of anthrax result from ingestion of large numbers of vegetative bacilli (usually in poorly cooked meat) and would therefore be unlikely to result from an attack. After the spores are ingested by phagocytes, they are transported to regional lymph nodes, where they germinate into vegetative cells after variable (and potentially extended) periods of time. Replicating cells then elaborate toxins that lead to massive hemorrhage, edema, necrosis, and cytokine release. Early antibiotic therapy for symptomatic disease is essential, but the effects of local tissue damage and systemic toxinosis may be irreversible.

■ Epidemiology and Transmission

Anthrax spores are found in soil worldwide and may remain viable for years. Infection occurs in grazing animals who ingest the spores, and natural human infection occurs almost exclusively after contact with infected animals and animal products (one classic example is *woolsorter's disease*, inhalational anthrax linked to the processing of hides and wool in enclosed spaces). Up to 20,000 annual cases of anthrax are estimated to occur worldwide, but this disease in the United States was rare until October 2001. Only 18 cases of inhalational anthrax were reported between 1900 and 1976, and no cases of that particular form of the disease were reported after 1976. Between 1944 and 1994, only 224 cases of cutaneous anthrax were reported, with one case occurring in 2000.

Anthrax is an attractive agent of bioterrorism because the infection can be lethal, natural immunity does not exist, the organism can be engineered into antibiotic resistance, and the infectious dose of spores is very low. It is easily grown in the laboratory, and the spores can be weaponized into a highly concentrated powder with uniform small particle size and low electrostatic charge, features that reduce clumping and facilitate aerosol dispersal. Such aerosols are odorless and invisible, can spread over large areas, and would probably not be detected until cases occurred. The lethality of aerosolized weapons-grade anthrax was demonstrated after the accidental release of anthrax spores (possibly as little as 1 g) on April 2, 1979, from a Soviet bioweapons facility in Sverdlovsk (now called Ekaterinburg). As many as 250 cases and 100 deaths occurred downwind (away from the city of over 1 million people) of the release, mostly from inhalational disease. Most cases occurred within 10 days, although some occurred 6 weeks later. While the majority of victims were exposed in a narrow 4-km band extending from the military facility to the southern city limit, cases did occur many miles away and livestock in several towns downwind of the release were affected.

In September and October 2001, at least five letters containing high-grade Ames strain anthrax spores were mailed through the United States postal service from Trenton, NJ, to sites in Florida, New York City, and Washington, DC. One letter was known to contain 2 g of powder and between 100 billion and 1 trillion spores. A total of 22 anthrax cases occurred in seven eastern states between September 22 and November 16; 11 were inhalational (five deaths) and 11 cutaneous (no deaths). Twelve victims were mail handlers, demonstrating the propensity for weaponized spores to disperse from relatively sealed containers. Cross-contamination was evidenced by the isolation of anthrax from over 100 environmental samples along the path of the letters.

In 1970, the WHO estimated that a release of 50 kg of spores over an urban population of 5 million would result in 250,000 cases and 100,000 deaths. The experience in the United States in 2001 indicates that this might have been an underestimate. Unlike smallpox, all cases occurring after an attack would result from primary exposure, because the infection is not transmitted from person to person. However, secondary aerosolization of particles that settle after a primary release could continue to cause disease for some time.

■ Background on Immunization Program

Antibiotic therapy after exposure can prevent inhaled spores from germinating and causing disease. In fact, there were no cases of anthrax among over 10,000 people who took antibiotics (primarily ciprofloxacin or doxycycline) for at least 60 days following the October 2001 attacks. In May 2002, the Working Group on Civilian Biodefense concluded that antibiotic therapy in conjunction with vaccination would be optimal for exposed persons, and current recommendations incorporate that concept.

Pre-exposure vaccination is based on a quantifiable risk for exposure and is not recommended for the general public. Although a vaccine has been licensed since 1970, it was in limited use until 1991 when the United States military immunized 150,000 service members deployed for the Gulf War. The Anthrax Vaccine Immunization Program was started in March 1998 with the routine immunization of personnel deployed to high-risk areas. In June 2002, the Department of Defense reintroduced the program (which had slowed because of dwindling vaccine supplies) because of intelligence assessments indicating possible risk of exposure to military personnel.

■ Available Vaccines

Characteristics of the anthrax vaccine licensed in the United States are given in **Table 10.1**.

■ Efficacy and/or Immunogenicity

Protection has been demonstrated in a macaque model of inhalational anthrax. Although correlates of protective immunity are not defined, 95% of adults receiving at least 3 doses of the vaccine develop a 4-fold rise in antibodies to protective antigen. One controlled trial of a similar vaccine among 1249 mill workers (379 were immunized) demonstrated 92.5% efficacy. No inhalational cases occurred among vaccinees, but three cutaneous cases occurred in incompletely vaccinated individuals. Case surveillance data from 1962 to 1974 suggest that anthrax in mill workers or those living near mills occurred exclusively in unvaccinated or incompletely vaccinated individuals.

■ Safety

In an open-label safety study, 15,907 doses of BioThrax were administered to 7000 at-risk individuals using the 6-dose schedule. Mild local reactions (erythema only or induration <30 mm) occurred in 8.6% of vaccinees, moderate reactions (edema or induration between 30 mm and 120 mm) in 0.9%, and severe reactions (edema or induration >120 mm accompanied by limitation of motion or axillary lymph node tenderness) in 0.15%. There were only four reports of systemic reactions such as fever, chills, nausea, and general body aches. In a study of 28 volunteers, injection-site tenderness was reported in 71% after dose 1, 61% after dose 2, and 58% after dose 3. The respective rates of erythema were 43%, 32%, and 12%, occurrence of a subcutaneous nodule 36%, 39%, and 4%, and induration 21%, 18%, and 8%. Fewer than 10% of volunteers had notable systemic reactions, and all of these were transient.

In a study involving >4300 service personnel in Korea, 2% of individuals reported limitation in work performance after dose 1 or dose 2 but <1% lost ≥1 day of work. Surveillance for adverse events in the Department of Defense program between 1998 and 2000 involving >400,000 recipients of >1.5 million doses

TABLE 10.1 — Anthrax Vaccine

Trade Name	BioThrax
Abbreviation	—
Manufacturer/distributor	BioPort
Type of vaccine	Inactivated, purified subunits
Composition	Cell-free filtrate of microaerophilic cultures of the avirulent, noncapsulated *Bacillus anthracis* strain V770-NP1-R
	Includes 83kDa protective antigen
Adjuvant	Aluminum hydroxide (0.6 mg aluminum)
Preservative	Benzethonium chloride (25 mcg/mL) Formaldehyde (100 mcg/mL)
Excipients and contaminants	Sodium chloride (0.85%)
Latex	Vial stopper contains dry natural rubber
Labeled indications	Pre-exposure prophylaxis
Labeled ages	18 to 65 years
Dose	0.5 mL
Route of administration	Subcutaneous
Labeled schedule	0, 2, 4 weeks, 6, 12, 18 months Booster doses every year
How supplied (number in package)	10-dose vial (1)
Storage	Refrigerate Do not freeze
Reference package insert	January 2002

revealed no unexpected patterns of reactogenicity but did note higher rates of local reactions in women than in men. In another series of >10,000 doses in US Army Medical Research Institute of Infectious Diseases (USAMRIID) employees, local reactions were noted in 4% and systemic reactions in 1%, and there were no long-term sequelae. An IOM study concluded that the anthrax vaccine is safe, and epidemiologic studies provide no evidence linking the vaccine to Gulf War Syndrome.

- *Contraindications*:
  - Allergic reaction to previous dose of vaccine or any vaccine component
- *Precautions*:
  - Moderate or severe acute illness
  - Pregnancy
  - History of Guillain-Barré syndrome

- Previous anthrax disease
- Latex allergy

■ Recommendations

Recommendations for civilian use of anthrax vaccine were published in 2000 and include the following:

- Routine vaccination of persons working with production quantities of *B anthracis* cultures and in activities with the potential for aerosol dispersal
- Vaccination of persons working with imported animal hides, furs, bone meal, wool, animal hair, or bristles only if existing standards and restrictions would be insufficient to prevent exposure to spores
- Routine vaccination is *not* recommended for workers in routine clinical laboratories or veterinarians
- Routine vaccination is *not* recommended for emergency first responders, federal responders, medical practitioners, or private citizens

These recommendations were supplemented in 2002 in the wake of the anthrax attacks, to include the following:

- *Pre-exposure vaccination:*
  - Workers making repeated entries into known contaminated areas (with concomitant prophylactic antibiotic use during the period of risk and for 60 days thereafter, unless the entire 6-dose series is completed and annual boosters are updated)
  - Laboratory workers handling environmental specimens and performing confirmatory testing for *B anthracis* (excluding workers using standard Biosafety Level 2 practices in routine processing of clinical samples or environmental swabs)
- *Postexposure vaccination:*
  - A 3-dose regimen (0, 2, 4 weeks) under an investigational new-drug protocol, with concomitant antibiotics until 7 to 14 days after the third dose
  - Partially or fully vaccinated individuals should receive at least 30 days of antibiotics and should continue with the licensed vaccine regimen
  - Fully vaccinated persons working in Biosafety Level 3 laboratories under recommended conditions and those wearing appropriate personal protective equipment need not receive antibiotics

Use of anthrax vaccine in the military is summarized below:

- Vaccination is mandatory for Department of Defense service members, emergency-essential designated civilians, and contractor personnel performing mission-essential services assigned to Central Command area of responsibility for ≥15 consecutive days, Korean Peninsula for ≥15 consecutive days, special units with biowarfare or bioterrorism related missions, and specialty units with approved exception to policy

10

- Vaccination occurs up to 120 days prior to deployment or arrival in higher threat areas
- Vaccination is voluntary for Department of Defense service members and government civilian employees of the Department of Defense who are not in the mandatory groups and have received at least one dose of anthrax vaccine during or after 1998
- Vaccination is voluntary for Department of Defense civilians and adult family members, as well as contractors and their accompanying United States–citizen family members
- Vaccine manufacturing and research personnel and others, as designated by the Assistant Secretary of Defense for Health Affairs, are vaccinated

Influenza A (H5N1)

■ The Pathogen

See Chapter 9, *Routine Vaccines*, for a general discussion of influenza viruses. Influenza A (H5N1) is known to be widespread in poultry and wild birds and probably remains restricted to those hosts because of preferential binding of the H5 molecule to alpha 2,3-linked sialic acid receptors on avian cells. The influenza A (H5N1) strain that emerged in humans in Southeast Asia in 2005 (bird flu) is entirely of avian origin (ie, not the product of reassortment). Its ability to spread to humans appears to be due to the ability of its HA molecule to bind to alpha 2,6-linked sialic acid receptors, which are present on human cells. Its increased virulence compared with human strains (which are virulent enough) may be explained by the presence of multiple basic amino acids in the region of the connecting peptide that links the two HA subunits—this allows for cleavage by ubiquitous intracellular proteases, thus enhancing infectivity and expanding tissue tropism. Other virulence factors also may be involved.

■ Clinical Features

Bird flu typically manifests as febrile pneumonia that progresses rapidly to respiratory failure. Additional clinical and laboratory features include dyspnea, sore throat, headache, elevated transaminases, leukopenia, and thrombocytopenia. Mortality rates are extremely high, ranging from 39% to 88% in various studies, and young adults are disproportionately represented. Death usually occurs during the second week of illness.

■ Epidemiology and Transmission

Between May 2005 and December 2007, bird flu was reported in 340 humans, most of whom lived in Southeast Asia, Eurasia, and Africa. The median age of affected individuals was around 18 years, and the vast majority of patients were <40 years old; this is strikingly different from seasonal influenza, which disproportionately affects the young and the old, but it is reminiscent of the

1918 pandemic influenza A (H1N1) Spanish flu strain. Humans are infected directly from birds; risk factors include handling of sick or dead poultry; slaughtering, defeathering, or preparing sick poultry for consumption; eating undercooked poultry products; and other close contact with birds, such as ducks. Some cases may have been acquired through contaminated fomites, and whereas there is no evidence of sustained human-to-human transmission, limited transmission might have occurred from very close contact with severely affected individuals.

■ Background on Immunization Program

There is no population-level immunity to influenza A (H5N1). Therefore, transmission of the virus to bird populations in close proximity to humans could result in increased human disease. If the virus adapted to growth in humans and learned how to spread from person to person, a pandemic could result. The vaccine might provide limited protection in the few months that it would take to manufacture a vaccine specifically tailored to a particular emergent strain of H5N1.

■ Available Vaccines

Characteristics of the influenza A (H5N1) vaccine licensed in the United States are given in **Table 10.2**. The vaccine is based on a laboratory strain of influenza A (commonly used to produce seasonal influenza vaccines) that was modified to carry the genes encoding the HA and NA of the human isolate A/Vietnam/1203/2004 (H5N1, clade 1). The HA gene was mutated to prevent cleavage of the mature protein, reducing pathogenicity and allowing the vaccine to grow efficiently in embryonated chicken eggs. The vaccine virus is inactivated with formaldehyde, chemically disrupted, and purified, in much the same way as the trivalent split-virus inactivated vaccine. Influenza A (H5N1) vaccine is not commercially available but will be purchased by the federal government for inclusion in the National Stockpile for distribution by public health officials, if necessary.

■ Efficacy and/or Immunogenicity

Licensure was based on immunogenicity rather than efficacy. Among 99 subjects receiving 2 doses of the 90-mcg formulation of the vaccine, 43% achieved a 4-fold or greater rise in hemagglutination inhibition antibody titer and a minimum titer of 1:40.

■ Safety

No serious adverse events related to the vaccine were reported among 103 subjects in a randomized, placebo-controlled, double-blind, multicenter trial. Local reactions included pain (74%), tenderness (70%), erythema (20%), and induration (15%). Headache was reported in 36% of vaccinees, malaise in 22%, myalgia in 16%, nausea in 10%, and fever in 7%.

• *Contraindications*:
 – None

TABLE 10.2 — Influenza A (H5N1) Vaccine

Trade name	Influenza Virus Vaccine, H5N1
Abbreviation	—
Manufacturer/distributor	Sanofi Pasteur
Type of vaccine	Inactivated, purified subunits (split virus)
Composition	Influenza A/Vietnam/1203/2004 (H5N1, clade 1) Propagated in embryonated eggs Inactivated with formaldehyde Hemagglutinin (90 mcg)
Adjuvant	None
Preservative	Thimerosal (50 mcg mercury)
Excipients and contaminants	Sodium phosphate–buffered isotonic sodium chloride Porcine gelatin (500 mcg) Formaldehyde ($\leq$200 mcg) Polyethylene glycol p-isooctylphenyl ether ($\leq$0.05%) Sucrose ($\leq$2.0%)
Latex	None
Labeled indications	Persons at risk of increased exposure to influenza A (H5N1)
Labeled ages	18 to 64 years
Dose	1 mL
Route of administration	Intramuscular
Labeled schedule	0, 1 month
How supplied (number in package)	5-dose vial (1)
Storage	Refrigerate Do not freeze Protect from light
Reference package insert	April 2007

- *Precautions*:
  - Severe allergic reaction to influenza vaccine or any vaccine component
  - Egg allergy: Being able to eat eggs (even in baked goods) without adverse effects is a reasonable indication of a very low risk of anaphylaxis. Mild or local manifestations of allergy to eggs or feathers are not a contraindication. Skin testing can be done and desensitization may be possible.
  - Guillain-Barré syndrome within 6 weeks of a prior dose of influenza vaccine

■ **Recommendations**
General recommendations have not been issued.

Japanese Encephalitis

■ **The Pathogen**

Japanese encephalitis virus (JEV) is a mosquito-borne flavivirus with a single-stranded RNA genome surrounded by a protein nucleocapsid and a lipid envelope. It is antigenically related to West Nile virus and St. Louis encephalitis virus.

■ **Clinical Features**

Only 1 in 250 to 1 in 1000 infections with JEV results in symptomatic illness, but up to 25% of those who do develop encephalitis may progress to coma and death. Others may have less severe disease characterized by aseptic meningitis. Illness begins abruptly with fever, lethargy, headache, abdominal pain, nausea, and vomiting. Mental status changes, including disorientation, personality change, agitation, delirium, and abnormal movements (including tremor, ataxia, choreoathetosis, rigidity, and extrapyramidal signs) are common, with progression to confusion, delirium, and coma. Mutism is a presenting sign in some cases. Up to 75% of patients present with or develop seizures. One third of patients develop cranial nerve palsies and some develop generalized or asymmetric muscular weakness, flaccid or spastic paralysis, and clonus.

Analysis of the CSF shows moderate lymphocytic pleocytosis and normal or moderately elevated protein. Imaging of the brain may show diffuse white matter edema, abnormal signal in the thalamus, and hemorrhage. Hyponatremia due to inappropriate secretion of antidiuretic hormone is a frequent complication. After a week of illness there may be gradual improvement, but some patients experience a rapidly fatal course. Complete recovery may require months to years, but one third of patients will have chronic neurologic sequelae, such as memory loss, motor and cranial nerve paresis, movement disorders, chronic seizures, cortical blindness, or behavioral disorders. JEV may cause intrauterine infection and miscarriage when it is acquired in the first or second trimester of pregnancy.

■ **Epidemiology and Transmission**

JEV is endemic throughout China, Southeast Asia, the Indian subcontinent, Indonesia, the Philippines, and Australia. In temperate areas, transmission generally occurs from May through September with periodic seasonal epidemics. In subtropical Asia, transmission is hyperendemic and the season is longer, from March through October. In tropical Asia, transmission occurs year-round without noticeable seasonable epidemics. In areas where the virus is endemic, almost all individuals will have been infected by early adulthood.

The virus is spread by *Culex* mosquitoes, which breed in ground pools (eg, rice paddies and ditches) in rural areas. These mosquitoes feed on aquatic birds and other animals that remain asymptomatic despite infection. Domestic pigs in particular have sustained viremia and serve as host to many feeding mosquitoes. Humans, horses, and domestic animals are incidental hosts. The risk of transmission is highest in rural areas, and the incidence of disease correlates with abundance of mosquitoes, proximity of pigs and birds, rainy season, and irrigation of agricultural fields. Most cases occur in children 2 to 10 years of age. Persons who travel extensively in or move to endemic areas acquire symptomatic infection at a rate of 1 per 50,000 persons per month. The risk of disease in short-term travelers to developed or urban areas is <1 per million; the risk for travelers to rural areas during the season of risk is somewhere between 1 in 5000 to 1 in 20,000 travelers per week. The risk of infection increases with travel during the transmission season, exposure to rural areas, extended period of travel or residence, and outdoor activities, especially in the evenings when mosquitoes are active.

■ Background on Immunization Program

Residing in air-conditioned or screened-in areas, avoiding outdoor activities, and using permethrin-treated mosquito nets, insect repellents, and protective clothing can reduce the risk of infection. Societal changes, such as urbanization, less agriculture, use of pesticides, centralized pig rearing, and improved standards of living, may also contribute to lower disease rates. However, there are still 175,000 annual cases worldwide among children <15 years of age, resulting in 45,000 deaths and 78,000 survivors with chronic disabilities. Since 1996, childhood immunization programs in China, Taiwan, Japan, and Korea have resulted in marked decreases in the number of reported cases.

■ Available Vaccines

Characteristics of the Japanese encephalitis (JE) vaccine licensed in the United States are given in **Table 10.3**.

■ Efficacy and/or Immunogenicity

Children 1 to 14 years of age were given a monovalent Nakayama-NIH strain vaccine ($N = 21,628$), a bivalent vaccine that also contained the Beijing strain ($N = 22,080$), or tetanus toxoid as placebo ($N = 21,516$) in a clinical trial in Thailand. Subjects received 2 doses of vaccine 7 days apart. Efficacy of each vaccine was 91%. Based on this study, a 2-dose primary series is used in many parts of Asia. However, <80% of vaccinees in US trials developed protective antibody levels after 2 doses, and responses were short-lived. In contrast, >99% of subjects demonstrated adequate responses to regimens consisting of 3 doses over a 30-day period. The duration of protection after primary immunization is not well defined. In the Thai field trial, efficacy was maintained through 2 years of surveillance, but further follow-up data were not available. All 21 US Army personnel followed for 2 years after vaccination retained seroprotective antibody levels.

TABLE 10.3 — Japanese Encephalitis Vaccine

Trade name	JE-Vax
Abbreviation	JE vaccine
Manufacturer/distributor	Biken/Sanofi Pasteur
Type of vaccine	Inactivated, whole agent
Composition	Nakayama-NIH strain
	Propagated in mouse brain
	Inactivated with formaldehyde
Adjuvant	None
Preservative	Thimerosal (0.007%)
Excipients and contaminants	Gelatin (500 mcg)
	Formaldehyde (<100 mcg)
	Polysorbate 80 (<0.0007%)
	Mouse serum protein (<50 ng)
Latex	None
Labeled indications	Immunization against JE
Labeled ages	≥1 years
Dose:	
Age 1 to 2 years	0.5 mL
Age ≥3 years	1 mL
Route of administration	Subcutaneous
Labeled schedule:	
Primary series	0, 7, 30 days
Abbreviated primary series	0, 7, 14 days
Booster dose in 2 years	
How supplied (number in package)	1-dose vial (3), lyophilized, with diluent
	10-dose vial, lyophilized, with diluent
Storage:	
Vaccine	Refrigerate
Diluent	Refrigerate, do not freeze
Reconstituted vaccine	Use within 8 hours
Reference package insert	February 1997

In a Japanese study, individuals maintained seroprotective levels for 3 years after the primary series.

■ Safety

Injection site tenderness, redness, and swelling have been reported in about 20% of vaccinees. Systemic side effects, such as fever, headache, malaise, rash, chills, dizziness, myalgia, nausea, vomiting, and abdominal pain, have been reported in approximately 10%. Most reactions occur within 3 days of the first dose and within 2 weeks of the second dose. In one study, <5% of travelers immunized with a 3-dose regimen reported systemic complaints, 0.2% reported hives, and 0.1% facial swelling. Vaccinees may rarely experience generalized urticaria and angioedema. For this reason, patients should be observed for 30 minutes after vaccination and warned about the possibility of delayed urticaria and angioedema of the extremities, face and oropharynx, airway, and especially the lips. Most such reactions occur within 10 days of vaccination, so travelers should remain in areas where they have access to medical care for that period of time. Persons with a history of idiopathic urticaria or urticaria after hymenopteran envenomation, drugs, or other provocations appear to be at increased risk.

Vaccinees should avoid alcohol intake during the 48 hours following vaccination because of a study showing increased risk of hypersensitivity reactions in persons who had unusual alcohol consumption during this time period. The same study showed an increased risk for hypersensitivity reactions in persons who received other vaccines within the 7 days before receipt of a JE vaccine. Therefore, other vaccines that need to be given should be given concurrently rather than before JE vaccine.

- *Contraindications:*
  - Allergic reaction to previous dose of vaccine or any vaccine component (this includes proteins of rodent or neural origin that were present in experimental hantavirus vaccines produced in Korea and China and a French neurotropic yellow fever vaccine strain that was discontinued in 1982)
- *Precautions:*
  - Moderate or severe acute illness
  - Pregnant women can be immunized when the risks of immunization are outweighed by the risk of infection to the mother and developing fetus

■ Recommendations

JE vaccine is not recommended for all persons traveling to or residing in Asia. Factors that should be considered in the decision to administer vaccine include the incidence of JE in the location of intended stay, the conditions of housing, nature of activities, duration of stay, and the possibility of unexpected travel to high-risk areas. In general, vaccination *should be considered* for use in persons spending a month or longer in epidemic or endemic areas during the transmission season, especially if travel will include rural areas. Depending on the epidemic circumstances, vaccination *should be considered* for persons spending <30 days who are at particularly high risk, such as those engaging in extensive outdoor activities in rural areas. Travelers are advised to take personal precautions to reduce exposure to mosquito bites. Current CDC advisories should be consulted with regard to disease activity in specific locales. The decision to use JE vaccine should balance the risk of exposure, the risk of disease, the availability and acceptability of repellents and other protective measures, and the side effects of vaccination.

Laboratory workers with potential exposure to infectious JEV *should be vaccinated.*

The recent occurrence of disseminated encephalomyelitis in some Japanese children after receipt of the mouse brain-derived vaccine led to suspension of its use in the Japanese immunization program. Production has been discontinued and existing supplies will be exhausted in a few years. Live attenuated vaccines are available in some countries, and a live attenuated chimeric vaccine is under development. The most likely candidate vaccine to be licensed in the United States in the near future is an inactivated whole agent vaccine derived from JEV strain SA_{14}-14-2 grown in Vero cell culture and adjuvanted with aluminum hydroxide.

Rabies

■ The Pathogen

Rabies virus is an enveloped, bullet-shaped, single-stranded RNA virus in the Rhabdoviridae family, genus *Lyssavirus*. The virion surface is covered with glycoprotein (G-protein) spikes, which mediate attachment to the heavily sialated gangliosides on neuronal cells. Attachment also may occur at nicotinic acetylcholine receptors in muscle, facilitating entry into peripheral nerves. The virus moves by retrograde axoplasmic flow from the site of inoculation to neuronal cell bodies, where it replicates and spreads to the brain; from there it may spread further to other organs, such as salivary and lacrimal glands. Gross pathologic changes in the brain include vascular congestion and edema, and the characteristic cellular abnormality is eosinophilic cytoplasmic neuronal inclusions called *Negri bodies*. The clinical severity of the disease is disproportionate to the degree of histopathologic derangement.

■ Clinical Features

Rabies presents in four sequential stages: the incubation period, prodrome, acute neurologic phase, and coma/death. Two thirds of patients present with a *furious form*, characterized by fluctuating consciousness, phobic spasms, dilated pupils, and hypersalivation. The other one third present with a *paralytic form*, which is differentiated from Guillain-Barré syndrome by the presence of fever, intact sensation, and urinary incontinence. The incubation period is typically a few weeks to 2 months but may be many years. Animal bites to the head usually result in shorter incubation periods than bites to the extremities.

There are no symptoms during the *incubation phase*, but the *prodrome*, which lasts 2 to 10 days, is characterized by fever, headache, malaise, fatigue, anorexia, anxiety, agitation, irritability, insomnia, or depression, and pain, pruritus, or paresthesia at the site of the bite. The *neurologic phase*, which lasts 2 to 12 days, is characterized by hyperactivity, disorientation, hallucinations, bizarre behavior, aggressiveness, seizures, paralysis, hydrophobia, aerophobia, hyperventilation, and cholinergic mani-

417

festations, including hypersalivation, lacrimation, mydriasis, and hyperpyrexia. Paralysis occurs in 20% of cases. Agitation may be precipitated by tactile, auditory, visual, or other stimuli, and hydrophobia, characterized by painful spasms of the pharynx and larynx, may be precipitated by eating or drinking or even the sight of liquids. At the end of the neurologic phase, the patient may become comatose. Death from respiratory or cardiac arrest usually occurs within 7 days, although with supportive care, coma may last for months. There are only a handful of reported survivors, most of whom have neurologic sequelae. Successful treatment of a 15-year-old girl from Wisconsin was reported in 2005; the strategy included therapeutic coma, using gamma-aminobutyric acid-receptor agonists along with N-methyl-D-aspartate–receptor antagonists.

■ Epidemiology and Transmission

All mammals can be infected with rabies, but only carnivorous mammals and bats are considered true reservoirs. Transmission from animals to humans occurs by exposure to saliva, usually through an animal bite, scratch, or contact with mucous membranes. Infection by aerosol has been reported in laboratories that handle the virus and in caves inhabited by bats (here, direct infection of the olfactory apparatus is implicated). Rabies can also be transmitted by allografts. In nature, dogs, wolves, foxes, coyotes, jackals, raccoons, skunks, weasels, bats, and mongooses are most commonly infected. However, in some areas of the world, dogs and cats account for the majority of animal rabies and the greatest number of exposures to humans. In the United States, where domestic animal rabies is well-controlled through vaccination of animals, most human exposures come from contact with wild animals, such as skunks, raccoons, and bats. Silver-haired bats have become a particular problem because the strains they carry may infect human skin more easily and their bites may be too small to see. Small rodents (eg, squirrels, rats, and mice) and lagomorphs (eg, rabbits and hares) rarely carry rabies.

Most animal exposures in the United States involve dogs, cats, and rodents; the vast majority of these exposures carry a very low risk for rabies transmission, even though postexposure prophylaxis is commonly given. Insectivorous bats are now the most common source of human infection in the United States. In at least half of cases, there is no known bite—in some cases, the bite may simply have been imperceptible or might have occurred during sleep; in others, transmission could have occurred through a scratch or bat saliva coming into contact with a mucous membrane or break in the skin.

■ Background on Immunization Program

There are an estimated 50,000 human rabies cases each year worldwide; only one or two of these occur in the United States. The long incubation period makes rabies uniquely suited to postexposure prophylaxis through both vaccination and passive immunization with human rabies immune globulin (HRIG); in this respect, rabies is similar to hepatitis B. The common occurrence of animal contacts combined with the near certainty of death if rabies occurs leads to frequent consideration of postexposure prophylaxis. However, postexposure prophylaxis is considered *urgent*, not *emergent*—in other words, the time frame in which to administer prophylaxis is hours, not minutes, and in some cases may be days (eg, if signs of rabies develop in an animal during quarantine).

Postexposure prophylaxis is cost saving (from the societal perspective) when given to individuals bitten by test-positive rabid animals or untested reservoir or vector animals. For other risk situations, the cost-effectiveness of postexposure prophylaxis varies widely. For example, it costs $2.9 million per life saved by administering prophylaxis after a bite from an untested cat, $403 million per life saved after a bite from an untested dog, and $4 billion per life saved after a lick from an untested dog.

Pre-exposure vaccination for individuals likely to encounter the virus can simplify postexposure treatment by eliminating the need for HRIG and reducing the number of vaccine doses needed. It also protects people who may have unapparent exposures or whose postexposure therapy might be delayed. Pre-exposure vaccination is particularly important for individuals who are at high risk of exposure, but who may be in situations where modern prophylaxis is not available.

■ Available Vaccines

Characteristics of the rabies vaccines licensed in the United States are given in **Table 10.4**.

HRIG is used in conjunction with vaccination for postexposure prophylaxis. Two preparations are available in the United States. They consist of IgG derived from pooled plasma of human donors who have been hyperimmunized with rabies vaccine; they are therefore polyclonal (contain a variety of antibodies, including antibodies to other organisms). Both products are initially purified by cold ethanol fractionation and then formulated for IM administration as follows:

- *HyperRAB S/D* (Talecris Biotherapeutics) is treated with a solvent (tri-n-butyl phosphate), a detergent (sodium cholate), and heat (30ºC) for 6 hours in order to inactivate potential blood borne viruses. The immune globulin is then purified by precipitation and ultrafiltration. The final product is 15% to 18% protein at a pH of 6.4-7.2 with 0.21-0.32 M glycine and no preservative; the average potency is 150 IU/mL. It is supplied in 2 mL- (300 IU) and 10 mL- (1,500 IU) vials that should be stored in the refrigerator (do not freeze).
- *Imogam Rabies—HT* (Sanofi Pasteur) is stabilized with 0.3 M glycine then heat treated (58-60ºC) for 10 hours in order to inactivate potential bloodborne viruses. The final product

TABLE 10.4 — Rabies Vaccines[a]

Trade name	Imovax Rabies	RabAvert
Abbreviation	HDCV	PCECV
Manufacturer/distributor	Sanofi Pasteur	Novartis
Type of vaccine	Inactivated, whole agent	Inactivated, whole agent
Composition	PM-1503-3M strain	Flury LEP strain
	Propagated in human diploid (MRC-5) cells	Propagated in chick embryo fibroblasts
	Inactivated with beta-propiolactone	Inactivated with beta-propiolactone
	$\geq$2.5 IU rabies antigen	$\geq$2.5 IU rabies antigen
Adjuvant	None	None
Preservative	None	None
Excipients and contaminants	Albumin (<100 mg)	Polygeline (processed bovine gelatin) (<12 mg)
	Neomycin sulfate (<150 mcg)	Human serum albumin (<0.3 mg)
	Phenol red (20 mcg)	Potassium glutamate (1 mg)
		Sodium EDTA (0.3 mg)
		Ovalbumin (<3 ng)
		Neomycin (<1 mcg)
		Chlorotetracycline (<20 ng)
		Amphotericin B (<2 ng)
Latex	None	None
Labeled indications	Pre-exposure (primary series and booster dose) and postexposure prophylaxis	Pre-exposure (primary series and booster dose) and postexposure prophylaxis

Labeled ages	All ages	All ages
Dose	1 mL	1 mL
Route of administration	Intramuscular	Intramuscular
Labeled schedule:		
Pre-exposure	0, 7, 21, or 28 days; periodic booster doses	0, 7, 21, or 28 days; periodic booster doses
Postexposure (unvaccinated)[b]	0, 3, 7, 14, 28 days	0, 3, 7, 14, 28 days
Postexposure (previously vaccinated)	0, 3 days	0, 3 days
How supplied (number in package)	1-dose vial (1), lyophilized, with diluent	1-dose vial (1), lyophilized, with diluent
Storage:		
Vaccine	Refrigerate	Refrigerate
Diluent	Refrigerate, do not freeze	Refrigerate, protect from light
Reconstituted vaccine	Use immediately	Use immediately
Reference package insert	December 2005	April 2004

[a] Two vaccines are no longer available in the United States: Rabies Vaccine Adsorbed (BioPort) and Imovax Rabies I.D. (Sanofi Pasteur).
[b] HRIG should also be given to exposed, previously unvaccinated individuals (see **Table 10.7**).

is 10% to 18% protein at a pH of 6.8 and has no preservative; the minimum potency is 150 IU/mL. It is supplied in 2 mL-(300 IU) and 10-mL (1,500 IU) vials that should be stored in the refrigerator (do not freeze).

■ Efficacy and/or Immunogenicity

Essentially all persons given pre- or postexposure prophylaxis achieve seroprotective concentrations of antibody. Multiple studies have demonstrated that postexposure prophylaxis with cell culture–derived vaccine and HRIG provide absolute protection against rabies—in fact, there has never been a failure of properly administered postexposure prophylaxis in the United States.

■ Safety

Local reactions to human diploid cell vaccine (HDCV) occur in 60% to 90% of vaccinees, with local pain occurring in 21% to 77%. Mild systemic symptoms, such as fever, headache, dizziness, and gastrointestinal complaints, occur in 7% to 56%. Systemic hypersensitivity, including urticaria, pruritic rash, and angioedema, may be seen in up to 6% of individuals receiving booster doses. This is thought to be mediated by IgE antibodies to human albumin that is chemically altered by betapropiolactone.

Local reactions to purified chick embryo cell vaccine (PCECV) occur in 11% to 57% of vaccinees, with local pain occurring in 2% to 23%. Mild systemic symptoms are seen in 0% to 31%. From 1997 to 2005, the reporting rate to VAERS for adverse events was 30 per 100,000 doses distributed, and for serious adverse events it was 3 per 100,000 doses distributed.

Local reactions to HRIG include pain, tenderness, erythema, and induration. Systemic reactions are reported in 75% to 81% of recipients.

- *Contraindications*:
  - In the event of exposure to rabies, there are no contraindications to vaccination or use of HRIG.
- *Precautions*:
  - Allergic reaction to previous dose of vaccine or any vaccine component
  - *Immunosuppression*: Immunosuppressive agents should not be administered during postexposure prophylaxis unless absolutely essential. When an immunosuppressed person is given pre- or postexposure prophylaxis, antibody titers should be checked (a rapid fluorescent focus inhibition test that demonstrates complete virus neutralization at a serum dilution of 1:5 is considered to be indicative of protection).
  - Patients with selective IgA deficiency may be at increased risk for anaphylactic reactions to HRIG because it may contain minute amounts of IgA.

■ Recommendations

Table 10.5 gives recommendations for pre-exposure prophylaxis. **Table 10.6** lists the situations where postexposure prophylaxis should be considered, and **Table 10.7** gives the postexposure regimens. Cell culture–derived rabies vaccines are considered interchangeable, although situations where one would need to complete a series with one vaccine that was initiated with a different vaccine should be very rare.

Oral vaccination of wildlife has proven effective in preventing spread of enzootic disease. Traditional approaches have utilized bait seeded with live attenuated rabies strains. A recent approach uses a vaccinia recombinant expressing the G protein of rabies virus.

Smallpox

■ The Pathogen

Variola virus is a very large, brick-shaped, enveloped DNA virus in the genus *Orthopoxvirus* that replicates in the cytoplasm and is closely related to vaccinia, cowpox, and monkeypox. Direct organ damage by viral infection is unusual, as is secondary bacterial infection. Instead, death results from toxemia associated with circulating immune complexes and viral antigens. Encephalitis can occur and is similar to the acute perivascular demyelination syndromes that may complicate measles and varicella infection, or smallpox vaccination.

■ Clinical Features

Initial infection takes place at mucosal surfaces of the oropharynx or respiratory tract. Three to 4 days later, viremia leads to visceral dissemination, but the patient remains asymptomatic. Secondary viremia leads to a marked prodromal illness, which begins 12 to 14 days after infection and is characterized by high fever, malaise, headache, backache, prostration, chills, vomiting, delirium, and/or abdominal pain. Rash begins 1 to 4 days into the prodrome and is coincident with a decrease in fever; maculopapular lesions initially appear in the mouth and on the face and forearms, spreading to the trunk and legs. The lesions evolve slowly into vesicles and pustules, which are characteristically deep-seated, round, firm, and discrete, although some may coalesce. Eventually, the lesions develop an umbilicated appearance with a central dimple. Fever usually continues until scabs form, about 2 weeks into the illness. Scars are evident after the scabs separate.

Variola major refers to the typical smallpox syndrome, which is easily recognized and accounts for the vast majority of cases; mortality rates approximate 30%. *Hemorrhagic smallpox* follows a shorter incubation period and is characterized by an extreme prodrome, the development of dusky erythema, and the eruption of petechiae and hemorrhage into skin and mucous membranes. Pregnant women are disproportionately affected and the syndrome is uniformly fatal. In *malignant (flat) smallpox*, the onset is equally abrupt, but the initial confluent lesions never evolve into pustules, instead remaining flat, soft, and velvety. Mortality

TABLE 10.5 — Indications for Pre-exposure Rabies Prophylaxis

Intensity of Exposure	Nature of Exposure	Examples	Vaccination
Continuous	Continuous Possible high concentration of virus May go unrecognized Bite, nonbite, aerosol[a]	Rabies research laboratory workers[b] Rabies biologics production workers	3-dose primary series Serology every 6 months Booster dose if titer[c] falls <1:5
Frequent	Episodic with recognized source May go unrecognized Bite, nonbite, aerosol[a]	Rabies diagnostic laboratory workers[b] Spelunkers Veterinarians and staff Animal-control and wildlife workers in enzootic areas All persons who frequently handle bats	3-dose primary series Serology every 2 years Booster dose if titer[c] falls <1:5
Infrequent	Episodic with recognized source Bite or nonbite[a]	Veterinarians, animal-control, and wildlife workers in nonenzootic areas Veterinary students Travelers to enzootic areas where immediate access to medical care is limited	3-dose vaccine series

Rare | Episodic with recognized source | General US population (including epizootic areas) | Not necessary
Bite or nonbite[a]

[a] See **Table 10.6** for explanation of types of exposure.

[b] Judgment of relative risk and monitoring of immunization status is the responsibility of the laboratory supervisor. See *Biosafety in Microbiological and Biomedical Laboratories*. 4th ed. Washington, DC: US Government Printing Office; 1999. Centers for Disease Control and Prevention Web site. Available at http://www.cdc.gov/OD/ohs/biosfty/bmbl4/bmbl4toc.htm. Accessed August 15, 2008.

[c] Rapid fluorescent focus inhibition test.

Centers for Disease Control and Prevention. *MMWR*. 2008;57(RF-3):1-28.

10

TABLE 10.6 — Indications for Postexposure Rabies Prophylaxis[a]

Animal	Animal Evaluation and Disposition	Recommendations
Dog, cat, ferret	Healthy and quarantined for 10-day observation period[b]	Do not begin prophylaxis routinely Institute prophylaxis at first sign of rabies in the animal[c]
	Rabid or suspected rabid	Institute prophylaxis immediately[c]
	Unknown or not available for observation	Consult public health officials[d]
Skunk, raccoon, fox, other carnivore (eg, coyote, bobcat, wild-animal hybrid), bat	Regard as rabid[e]	Consider immediate prophylaxis[c]
Livestock, small rodent (eg, squirrel, chipmunk, rat, mouse, hamster, guinea pig, gerbil), large rodent (eg, woodchuck or groundhog, beaver), lagomorph (eg, rabbit, hare), other mammal[f]	Consider individually	Consult public health officials[d]

[a] *Bite* exposures occur when there has been any penetration of the skin by teeth. *Nonbite* exposures include scratches, abrasions, open wounds, or mucous membranes contaminated with saliva or other potentially infectious material (eg, brain or neural tissue). Contact between intact skin and saliva does not constitute an exposure; neither does casual petting or handling or contact with blood, urine, or feces. However, any potential contact with a bat deserves evaluation because bat bites are small and can go unrecognized. Exposure is assumed to have occurred if a person in the same room as a bat might have been unaware that a bite or direct contact had occurred. Examples include a sleeping person who awakens to find a bat in the room or finding a bat in the room with an unattended child, mentally disabled person, or intoxicated person. *Aerosol* exposure is rare but has been reported in laboratories that handle the virus and in caves infested with millions of bats. *Human-to-human* transmission occurs almost exclusively through tissue or organ transplantation.

[b] The animal should be quarantined and observed for 10 days. This usually takes place under the supervision of the local health department, which specifies approved facilities (private or government) and monitors the animal's behavior. If signs of rabies develop (eg, aggressive or combative behavior, irritability, hyperreaction to stimuli, or paralysis), the animal should be euthanized and the brain sent for detection of rabies virus antigens by direct fluorescent antibody test (this is usually done at the state lab).

[c] **Table 10.7** gives the recommended prophylaxis regimens. If prophylaxis is initiated but the animal is found not to have rabies by direct fluorescent antibody testing of the brain, prophylaxis may be discontinued.

[d] The epidemiology of rabies is complex and varies from region to region. Local and state public health officials should be consulted to determine the likelihood of exposure in specific situations.

[e] These animals should be regarded as rabid unless proved negative by immunofluorescence testing of the brain (this is usually done at the state lab). Prophylaxis should be initiated unless the brain is known to be negative or expeditious testing is under way. Prophylaxis should be considered more urgent if the exposure was from an animal species in the area known to carry rabies; if the animal exhibited abnormal behavior or signs of illness, had an unexplained wound, attacked without provocation (bites that result from attempts to feed or handle an apparently healthy animal should generally be regarded as *provoked*); or if the person's wounds were severe or involved the head and neck. Every effort should be made by properly trained officials to obtain the animal for euthanization and testing; quarantine for observation is *not* recommended.

[f] Bites of small rodents and lagomorphs almost never require prophylaxis. Previous recommendations pointed out that large rodents, such as woodchucks, could survive an attack by a rabid animal and go on to develop rabies. This should be considered in areas where raccoon rabies is prevalent.

Clinician outreach and communication activity clinical briefing: human rabies prevention, March 22, 2005. Centers for Disease Control and Prevention Web site. http://emergency.cdc.gov/coca/summaries/pdf/rabies_032205.pdf. Accessed August 15, 2008; Centers for Disease Control and Prevention. *MMWR.* 2008;57(RR-3):1-28.

TABLE 10.7 — Postexposure Prophylaxis Regimens[a]

Vaccination Status	Treatment	Regimen
Not previously vaccinated	Wound cleansing	Immediately cleanse all wounds thoroughly with soap and water
		Use a virucidal agent like povidone-iodine solution if available
	HRIG	Administer 20 IU/kg (0.133 mL/kg)[b]
		Infiltrate the full dose around the wound and give any remaining volume intramuscularly at another site[c]
		Do not exceed the recommended dose[d]
		Use separate syringes for HRIG and vaccine
	Rabies vaccine	Administer 1 mL intramuscularly on days 0, 3, 7, 14, and 28[e]
Previously vaccinated[f]	Wound cleansing	Immediately cleanse all wounds thoroughly with soap and water
		Use a virucidal agent like povidone-iodine solution if available
	HRIG	Not recommended
	Rabies vaccine	Administer 1 mL intramuscularly on days 0 and 3[e]

[a] Postexposure prophylaxis should be initiated regardless of the time that has elapsed since the exposure. State or local health departments should be contacted for patients whose postexposure prophylaxis was initiated outside of the United States, because the regimens and products used may be suboptimal. For bites, the need for tetanus immunization and prophylactic antibiotics should be assessed. Wound closure should be avoided if possible.

[b] HRIG should be given at the same time the vaccine series is initiated. If not given on the day of the first dose of vaccine (day 0), it may be given up to and including day 7. Beyond this it is not indicated because the vaccine is presumed to have induced antibodies at that point.

[c] The intramuscular site, if used, should be different from the site where the first dose of vaccine is given. Subsequent doses of the vaccine may be given in the same muscle where the HRIG was given, if that is a preferred site for vaccination.

[d] Exceeding the dose of HRIG may suppress the antibody response to vaccination.

e The deltoid area is the only acceptable site for adults and older children. The anterolateral thigh can be used for young children (see **Table 4.5**). The gluteal area should never be used. The series does not need to be reinitiated because of minor interruptions of the vaccine schedule—just pick up where you left off, maintaining the intervals between doses specified in the schedule. If major deviations occur, test for antibody after completing the series (a rapid fluorescent focus inhibition test that demonstrates complete virus neutralization at a serum dilution of 1:5 is considered to be indicative of protection).

f This includes: 1) individuals who received a full pre- or postexposure series of one of the currently licensed cell culture–derived vaccines or of Rabies Vaccine Adsorbed (which is no longer available in the United States); and 2) individuals who received another type of rabies vaccine and had a documented antibody response. Serologic testing at the time of exposure is not recommended.

Centers for Disease Control and Prevention. *MMWR*. 2008;57(RR-3):1-28.

10

in this form approaches 100% as well. *Modified smallpox* occurs in previously vaccinated individuals, and although the prodrome may be severe, the lesions are fewer in number, more superficial, and evolve more rapidly; death is rare. *Variola minor (alastrim)*, caused by a less-pathogenic strain of the virus, is differentiated by fewer constitutional symptoms, sparse rash, and excellent prognosis. *Variola sine eruptione* is asymptomatic or self-limited with fever and flulike symptoms; it occurs in previously vaccinated individuals or infants with maternal antibodies. There is no clinical experience with antiviral treatment, but cidofovir may have some activity.

Failure to diagnose the first wave of cases during a smallpox attack would have grave consequences. For this reason, and given the fact that most practicing physicians today have never seen a case, attention has focused on recognizing the clinical signs and symptoms and differentiating smallpox from other conditions that bear similarities, most notably chickenpox. **Table 10.8** provides clues to accurate and timely diagnosis. Suspected cases should immediately be reported to state or local health departments. The CDC also maintains a 24/7 Emergency Operations Center that is available to health care providers at 770-488-7100.

■ **Epidemiology and Transmission**

Natural smallpox has been *eradicated* from the face of the earth, but the variola virus itself is not extinct, existing as it is in US and Russian government laboratory freezers (see Chapter 1, *Introduction to Vaccinology*). The possibility exists that the virus could get into the wrong hands and be used as a weapon of bioterrorism.

Certain features of smallpox make it attractive as a weapon, including the small infectious dose, high mortality rate, absence of natural and vaccine-induced immunity at the population level, lack of established therapy, historical fear and panic related to the disease, and person-to-person spread, which would amplify the effect of a primary release by generating secondary and tertiary cases. Epidemic disease in developed countries today would have the potential for great devastation because of the high point prevalence of atopic skin disease and relative immunoincompetency resulting from immunosuppressive therapy, chronic conditions, HIV infection, and aging.

Fortunately, variola virus is labile, and <90% remains viable for 24 hours after aerosol release in the presence of ultraviolet light. Transmission occurs through direct contact with body fluids and inhalation of aerosols and droplet nuclei expelled from the oropharynx of infected persons. Close contact is usually required, and secondary attack rates vary from about 40% to 90% under these circumstances. Distant airborne transmission is rare, but fomites such as bedding or clothing can transmit the virus. Transmission does not occur through insects or animals. Patients are most infectious 7 to 10 days after the rash develops;

since this occurs after a debilitating prodromal illness, patients are likely to be easily recognized and bedridden at the time they are most contagious. Transmission from subclinical cases is of little epidemiologic importance.

■ **Background on Immunization Program**

Universal pre-event vaccination would constitute an absolute deterrent to a smallpox attack and could be conducted under controlled conditions. However, this approach is not favored by scientists because the overall risk of an attack is considered to be low, the population at risk cannot be determined, and the risks of vaccination are substantial. The strategy of *surveillance and containment*, or *ring vaccination*, involves the isolation of suspected and confirmed cases and the identification, vaccination, and monitoring of their contacts. Vaccination can be extended to household contacts of contacts as well, or other people with indirect exposure, and the strategy can be supplemented by local quarantine and travel restrictions. This strategy, which was highly successful during the global eradication campaign, is workable because vaccination is effective if given soon after exposure. Ring vaccination, however, might not work as well in a largely nonimmune, highly mobile population experiencing a multisite intentional aerosol release of virus. In addition, the logistical complexity of this approach is daunting, especially in the face of the potential for public panic. The CDC has developed large-scale vaccination clinic guidelines, available at http://www.bt.cdc.gov/agent/smallpox/response-plan/files/annex-3.pdf (Accessed August 15, 2008), to assist state and local health departments in expanding vaccination rings if this becomes necessary. *Universal postevent vaccination* would be logistically difficult and would provide little additional benefit to ring vaccination, although the CDC National Pharmaceutical Stockpile has protocols for simultaneous delivery of vaccine to every state and territory within 24 hours of an event. The current US vaccination plan combines limited pre-event vaccination with ring vaccination.

■ **Available Vaccines**

The origin of vaccinia virus is not clear, but it appears to be a hybrid between cowpox and smallpox that is not found in nature. In October 2002, the FDA relicensed Dryvax (Smallpox Vaccine, Dried, Calf Lymph Type), a product manufactured by Wyeth until 1982, but in storage at the CDC since then, for active immunization against smallpox. Relicensure was intended to facilitate administration of the vaccine outside of investigational protocols. Dryvax was a lyophilized preparation of the New York City Board of Health strain of vaccinia harvested from lymph contained in skin lesions that develop after scarification of calves. As of December 2002, two lots of Dryvax with a total of 2.7 million doses were approved for release under licensure. In 2002, approximately 85 million doses of a similar vaccine (in liquid

TABLE 10.8 — Diagnosis of Smallpox[a]

Clinical Finding	Smallpox[b]	Chickenpox[c]
Major Criteria		
Prodrome	Fever ≥101°F (38.3°C) beginning 1 to 4 days before rash and at least one of the following: prostration, headache, backache, chills, vomiting, severe abdominal pain	None or mild
Lesion morphology	Deep-seated, firm, round, well-circumscribed vesicles or pustules, may be umbilicated or confluent	Superficial vesicles (resembling dewdrops on a rose petal)
Lesion development	Same stage of development on any one part of the body	Appear in crops and are at different stages of development on any one part of the body
Minor Criteria		
Distribution	Centrifugal (concentrated on face and distal extremities)	Centripetal (concentrated on trunk)
Initial lesions	Oral mucosa, palate, face, forearms	Face or trunk
General appearance	Toxic or moribund	Well-appearing
Evolution	Slow (from macules to papules to pustules over days)	Rapid (from macules to papules to vesicles to pustules to crusts in <24 hours)
Palms and soles	Involved	Spared

[a] If the patient has all three major criteria, the risk of smallpox is high and authorities should be notified immediately. If the patient has a febrile prodrome and one other major criterion or ≥4 minor criteria, the risk is moderate and urgent evaluation is indicated.

[b] Other conditions to be considered in the differential diagnosis include disseminated herpes zoster or herpes simplex, impetigo, drug eruptions, erythema multiforme, Stevens-Johnson syndrome, enterovirus infection, scabies, secondary syphilis, bullous pemphigoid, and molluscum contagiosum. Cowpox

and monkeypox resemble smallpox but can only be acquired directly from the respective animals. The differential diagnosis of hemorrhagic smallpox includes meningococcemia, hemorrhagic varicella, Rocky Mountain spotted fever, ehrlichiosis, and gram-negative sepsis.

[c] Other clues to the diagnosis of chickenpox include absence of a personal history of varicella or varicella vaccination and exposure to chickenpox or shingles. Most cases will occur in children because most adults are immune. The lesions are usually intensely pruritic and scarring is unusual.

Evaluating patients for smallpox. Centers for Disease Control and Prevention Web site. http://www.bt.cdc.gov/agent/smallpox/diagnosis/evalposter .asp. Accessed August 15, 2008: Smallpox: images. Centers for Disease Control and Prevention Web site. http://www.bt.cdc.gov/agent/smallpox/ smallpox-images. Accessed August 15, 2008.

10

433

formulation) that had been in cold storage since the 1950s were discovered by Sanofi Pasteur and donated to the CDC for further study. Since studies indicated that Dryvax could be diluted up to 1:5 without diminution in the response rate in naïve subjects, it was estimated that sufficient doses were on hand in the event of an emergency.

A new, second-generation smallpox vaccine called ACAM2000 was licensed in August 2007 and will replace Dryvax in the Strategic National Stockpile. Characteristics of this vaccine are given in **Table 10.9**.

Handling and administration of smallpox vaccine is different from all other vaccines, as summarized.

- *Reconstitution*
  - Wear gloves, use aseptic technique, and avoid contact of the vaccine with skin, eyes, and mucous membranes.
  - Bring the vaccine up to room temperature.
  - Lift up the cap seals on the vaccine and diluent vials.
  - Wipe off the rubber stopper with alcohol and allow it to dry.
  - Draw up 0.3 mL of diluent in the 1-mL tuberculin syringe fitted with a 25-gauge 5/8-inch needle that is provided with the vaccine.
  - Transfer the contents of the syringe to the vaccine vial.
  - Gently swirl without letting the liquid get on the rubber stopper. The reconstituted vaccine is clear to slightly hazy, colorless to straw-colored, and free from particulates.
- *Administration*
  - Providers must be properly educated on administration technique and must provide vaccinees with an FDA-approved Medication Guide.
  - Wear gloves, use aseptic technique, and avoid contact of the vaccine with skin, eyes, and mucous membranes.
  - Preparation of the skin with alcohol is not required (this may inactivate the virus). Use soap and water if the site is grossly contaminated. If alcohol is used, the skin must be allowed to dry thoroughly before inoculation.
  - Remove the vaccine vial cap (maintain sterile conditions for later recapping).
  - Remove the bifurcated needle from its individual wrapping. Dip the bifurcated needle into the reconstituted vaccine and withdraw. A sufficient amount of liquid (approximately 0.0025 mL) is retained between the prongs by capillary action.
  - Hold the needle between the thumb and first finger, perpendicular to the vaccinee's skin. Lay your wrist on the vaccinee's arm below the deltoid region. Use your other hand to pull the skin taught from underneath.
  - Deposit the drop of vaccine on the skin. Using firm strokes from the wrist, make 15 rhythmic perpendicular insertions through the drop into the skin within a 5-mm area. A trace of blood should be visible after each puncture. *Do not*

reinsert the needle into the vial between punctures or after the whole procedure.

– Discard the bifurcated needle immediately in a leak-proof, puncture-proof biohazard waste container. When ready for disposal, the vaccine vial, stopper, diluent syringe, and vented needle should be placed in a similar container. The container can be disposed of in the usual way.

– Absorb excess vaccine and blood with sterile gauze and discard in a biohazard container.

– Close the vaccine vial by reinserting the cap and return it to the refrigerator.

– Cover the site with gauze and adhesive tape. If the vaccinee will have direct patient contact, cover the gauze with a semipermeable dressing such as OpSite (Smith & Nephew) or Tegaderm (3M) (some of these products are supplied with attached gauze pads). Semipermeable dressings should not be used alone because they macerate the skin.

• *Postvaccination Care*
– Vaccinees should make sure a layer of clothing covers the dressing and should exercise meticulous hand hygiene after touching the site or dressings.

– Change the dressing every 3 to 5 days or more often if exudates accumulate (dressings can be discarded in the household trash if sealed in a plastic bag).

– Avoid rubbing and scratching.

– Do not put salves or ointments on the site.

– Keep the site dry. Showering or bathing can continue. If the site is uncovered it should not be touched. The site should be blotted dry with gauze, which should then be discarded in a sealed plastic bag in the household trash. If a towel is used for drying the site, it should not be used on the rest of the body.

– Separately wash clothing or other material that comes into contact with the site, using hot water with detergent and/or bleach.

• *Assessing Response*
– The subject should return for examination in 7 days.

– A red, pruritic papule should form 2 to 5 days after vaccination. This becomes vesicular then pustular and reaches a maximum size by 8 to 10 days. The pustule dries and forms a scab, which separates by 14 to 21 days, leaving a pitted scar.

– Failure to develop a skin lesion as described indicates failure of vaccination, and revaccination should be considered, unless the vaccinee had been previously vaccinated (pre-existing immunity can modify the cutaneous reaction). Images of appropriate primary and revaccination responses are shown in the package insert, and images of normal and adverse reactions can be viewed at www.bt.cdc.gov/training/smallpoxvaccine/reactions (Accessed August 15, 2008).

TABLE 10.9 — Smallpox Vaccine[a]

Trade name	ACAM2000[b]
Abbreviation	—
Manufacturer/distributor	Acambis
Type of vaccine	Live attenuated, classical
Composition	Vaccinia, New York Board of Health strain
	Propagated in African green monkey kidney cells
	2.5 to 12.5×10^5 PFU/dose
Adjuvant	None
Preservative	None
Excipients and contaminants	HEPES (pH 6.5 to 7.5) (6 to 8 mM)
	Human serum albumin (2%)
	Sodium chloride (0.5% to 0.7%)
	Mannitol USP (5%)
	Neomycin (trace)
	Polymyxin B (trace)
	Glycerin USP (50% v/v)
	Phenol USP (0.25% v/v)
Latex	None
Labeled indications	Active immunization against smallpox disease
Labeled ages	All ages
Dose	15 punctures *(see text)*
Route of administration	Percutaneous (scarification)
Labeled schedule[c]	1 dose
	Booster doses every 3 years (for individuals with occupational exposures)
How supplied (number in package)	100-dose vial, lyophilized, with diluent, bifurcated needles, and tuberculin syringe for reconstitution
Storage:	
Vaccine	Freeze
Diluent	Room temperature
Reconstituted vaccine	May be used at room temperature for 6 to 8 hours; may be refrigerated for up to 30 days
Reference package insert	August 2007

[a] Dryvax (Smallpox Vaccine, Dried, Calf Lymph Type; Wyeth) is no longer available in the United States. Any remaining lots of Dryvax should have been destroyed by March 31, 2008.

Continued

436

b ACAM2000 is not commercially available but rather will be purchased by the federal government for inclusion in the Strategic National Stockpile.
c Until 1972, smallpox vaccine was given in the United States 1 time to children at 1 year of age. For those who receive pre-event vaccination today, a single dose is recommended with a booster every 10 years. Revaccination every 3 years should be considered for workers with occupational exposure to orthopox viruses. The vaccine will completely prevent or significantly modify smallpox if given 3 to 4 days postexposure; vaccination 4 to 7 days postexposure probably modifies the severity of the disease.

■ Efficacy and/or Immunogenicity

Studies with Dryvax suggest that protection persists for at least 5 years after primary vaccination. Antibody levels steadily decline 5 to 10 years following vaccination, and although detectable cellular responses may persist, it must be assumed that immunity to smallpox wanes. Revaccination even one time results in boosted antibody levels that may persist for 30 years.

Two randomized, multicenter studies were conducted comparing ACAM2000 to Dryvax. One study looked at 1647 individuals who had been vaccinated over 10 years earlier; 1242 received ACAM2000 and 405 received Dryvax. Successful revaccination was slightly less common in the ACAM2000 group, but antibody titers were not inferior. The second study looked at 1037 vaccinia-naïve subjects; 780 received ACAM2000 and 257 received Dryvax. In this case, vaccination success rates were not inferior, although antibody titers were lower. Overall, ACAM2000 was noninferior to Dryvax where it counts most—major cutaneous reaction in vaccinia-naïve subjects and strength of antibody response in vaccinia-experienced subjects (whose pre-existing immunity might have modified the cutaneous reaction).

■ Safety

Smallpox vaccine is the most reactogenic and dangerous of all licensed vaccines. By definition, successfully vaccinated individuals develop a pustule at the inoculation site that lasts several weeks. Many experience additional local reactions and associated systemic complaints. In about one third of patients, these symptoms may lead to missed work, school, or recreational activities, or to trouble sleeping. Common side effects for ACAM2000 include itching, soreness, fever, headache, rash, and fatigue. As with Dryvax, transmission to individuals who are pregnant, immunocompromised, or have chronic skin problems can lead to serious complications. In order to prevent serious adverse events, a Risk Minimization Action Plan has been implemented for ACAM2000. This includes provision of an FDA-approved Medication Guide to recipients, education of health care providers, expedited adverse-event reporting, and a strategy for risk-management evaluation.

Potential complications of vaccination include inadvertent inoculation, generalized vaccinia, erythema multiforme, eczema vaccinatum, post-vaccinal encephalitis or encephalomyelitis, progressive vaccinia, contact vaccinia, and fetal infection. In March 2003, the CDC reported 10 cases of myopericarditis occurring shortly after vaccination among 240,000 primary military vaccinees, as well as two similar cases in civilians. The incidence of myopericarditis was substantially higher than in unvaccinated historical cohorts, raising suspicion of a causal relationship. Cardiac ischemic events were also reported in five civilians. In a study of military personnel in early 2003, 18 cases of probable myopericarditis were seen among 230,734 primary vaccinees, whereas no cases were seen among 95,622 vaccinees who had been previously vaccinated. A causal relationship was supported by temporal clustering (7 to 19 days following vaccination), wide geographic distribution, a lack of evidence for alternative etiologies, and a 3.6-fold increase in incidence above expected rates. Interestingly, no increase in cardiac deaths was seen in New York City after a mass vaccination campaign in 1947 where the same vaccine strain was used. The risk of myocarditis and/or pericarditis after vaccination with ACAM2000 is estimated to be 1 in 175 previously unvaccinated adults.

- *Contraindications (postexposure vaccination)*:
  - In the event of exposure to smallpox, there are no contraindications to vaccination.
- *Contraindications (pre-exposure vaccination, potential vaccinees and their household or sexual contacts)*:
  - *Eczema, atopic dermatitis, other acute, chronic, or exfoliative skin conditions*: burns, impetigo, chickenpox, contact dermatitis, shingles, herpes, severe acne, psoriasis, Darier's disease (keratosis follicularis), even if currently inactive. Two screening questions have been suggested by the CDC:
    - Have you or a member of your household ever been diagnosed with eczema or atopic dermatitis?
    - Have you or a family member ever had an itchy, red, scaly rash that lasts for >2 weeks and often comes and goes?
  - *Immunodeficiency or immunosuppression*: solid organ or bone marrow transplantation, generalized malignancy, leukemia, lymphoma, agammaglobulinemia, autoimmune disease, treatment with radiation, antimetabolites, alkylating agents, corticosteroids (in similar doses to those outlined in Chapter 7, *Vaccination in Special Circumstances*), chemotherapy agents or organ transplant medications, and HIV infection (routine testing is not recommended, but should be done in individuals with risk factors, those who are unsure of their status and those who are concerned that they could have HIV infection)
  - *Pregnancy*: currently pregnant or planning to become pregnant in the next 4 weeks (vaccinated women should be counseled not to become pregnant for 4 weeks)

- For reassurance, women can perform a urine pregnancy test on the first morning void on the day of vaccination.
- Routine pregnancy testing is not recommended.
- Inadvertent vaccination during pregnancy is not ordinarily a reason to terminate the pregnancy, although the mother should be aware of the extremely rare occurrence of fetal vaccinia.
- *Contraindications (pre-exposure vaccination, potential vaccinees only)*:
  – Allergic reaction to previous dose of vaccine or any vaccine component
  – Moderate or severe acute illness
  – Infants <12 months of age (ACIP advises against vaccination of individuals <18 years of age)
  – Breast-feeding
  – Cardiac risk
    - Known underlying heart disease, with or without symptoms
    - Persons with three or more risk factors, including hypertension, diabetes, hypercholesterolemia, first-degree relative under age 50 years with heart disease, and smoking
    - Verbal screening for risk factors is recommended
    - Special follow-up for persons with risk factors who have already been vaccinated is not recommended

10

Vaccinia immune globulin (VIG), a polyclonal immune globulin product made from blood of recently vaccinated blood donors, can be used to treat complications of vaccination. As of 2008, there are 2700 treatment doses of VIG available at the CDC, enough to treat expected complications from >27 million vaccinations. The usual dose is 0.6 mL/kg intramuscularly, and indications include progressive vaccinia, eczema vaccinatum, severe generalized vaccinia, and inadvertent inoculation resulting in a large number of lesions, toxicity, or significant pain. Cidofovir may help limit viral replication. Both VIG and cidofovir are available through CDC under an investigational new-drug protocol. Civilian providers seeking access should first contact their state health department, which may refer them to the CDC (800-232-4636).

Section 304 of the Homeland Security Act of 2002 (P.L. 107-296) provides liability protection (with certain caveats) in the case of injury to a vaccinee or a contact for smallpox vaccine manufacturers, health care institutions, licensed health care professionals, and public health agencies that administer vaccine programs. The Smallpox Emergency Personnel Protection Act of 2003 (Public Law 108-20) authorized the establishment of the Smallpox Vaccine Injury Compensation Program, which provides benefits and lost employment income to public health and medical response team members and others who are injured by smallpox vaccine (the final rules for this program were published in the Federal Register in May 2006). Individuals and parties eligible for compensation include vaccine recipients, unvaccinated individuals injured after acquiring the vaccine virus from others through physical contact, and estates and survivors in the event of death. More information can be found at http://www.hrsa.gov/smallpoxinjury (Accessed August 15, 2008).

■ Recommendations

In June 2001, the ACIP recommended against pre-event vaccination of any group other than laboratory and health care workers involved in orthopox research. Certain groups were targeted for vaccination post-event, including people with primary exposure, close contacts of cases (face-to-face, household, or <2 meters distance), medical personnel with potential patient contact, clinical laboratory personnel, and ancillary personnel with potential exposure to infectious waste. The earliest vaccinations were to be targeted to persons who had been vaccinated in the past. These recommendations were reviewed in the wake of the anthrax attacks of October 2001, and supplemental recommendations made were in June 2002 to vaccinate the following groups:

- *Smallpox Response Teams*: At least one team would be maintained in each state and territory, to include a medical team leader, public health advisor, epidemiologists, disease investigators, diagnostic laboratory scientists, nurses, medical personnel, vaccinators, and security and law enforcement officials.
- *Smallpox Health Care Teams*: These are individuals who would care for initial cases at predesignated isolation and care facilities.

Recognizing the fact that smallpox patients would likely present to any hospital, the ACIP issued revised recommendations in October 2002, and supplemental recommendations from ACIP and the Healthcare Infection Control Practices Advisory Committee (HICPAC) were issued in final form in April 2003. It was recommended that all acute care hospitals establish Smallpox Health Care Teams. These teams should provide hospital-based in-room evaluation and management for the first 7 to 10 days, using 8- to 12-hour shifts. Team members should include the following:

- Emergency department and intensive care unit staff, including physicians and nurses
- General medical and primary care staff
- House staff
- Medical subspecialists, including infectious disease specialists, experienced physicians, dermatologists, ophthalmologists, pathologists, surgeons, and anesthesiologists
- Infection control professionals
- Respiratory therapists
- Radiology technicians
- Security personnel
- Housekeeping staff

The following comments were offered:

- Clinical laboratory workers were not included because clinical specimens were expected to contain low levels of virus and standard precautions were considered to be protective.
- Although emergency medical technicians (EMTs) would not routinely be vaccinated, hospital-based EMTs could be vaccinated if included on the teams.
- Designated vaccinated staff should examine all vaccinated health care workers each day, assess vaccine take, and change the dressings if indicated.
- Persons handling the vaccine should also be vaccinated.
- Routine leave for vaccinated health care workers was not recommended. However, leave would be indicated for systemic illness, extensive lesions that cannot be covered, or inability to adhere to infection control precautions.
- Institutions should take a phased in, staggered approach to vaccination, beginning with groups of previously vaccinated individuals.
- Rigorous screening for contraindications was recommended, but routine pregnancy and HIV testing was not.

The federal plan announced in December 2002 called for voluntary vaccination of up to 500,000 health and safety workers constituting local Smallpox Response Teams. By mid-2003 it was clear that the federal plan to vaccinate civilians was proceeding much slower than anticipated; in all, only 40,000 civilians had been vaccinated, and the CDC had effectively ceased efforts to vaccinate additional people. The concomitant DOD plan called for stepwise, compulsory vaccination, first involving up to 5000 members of smallpox epidemic response teams, then 10,000 to 25,000 medical team members, then up to 500,000 mission-critical forces. As of January 2005, >700,000 service members had been vaccinated.

Smallpox vaccination is recommended for laboratory workers who directly handle cultures or animals infected with nonhighly attenuated vaccinia viruses or vaccinia recombinants, as well as other orthopoxviruses that infect humans (eg, monkeypox and cowpox). Vaccination should also be considered for health care workers who may contact materials contaminated with such viruses.

Smallpox vaccine may be administered simultaneously with all inactivated vaccines and live vaccines except for varicella, in which case ≥4 weeks should separate the 2 inoculations. Tuberculin skin tests should be deferred at least 1 month following smallpox vaccination to minimize the risk of false-negatives. Blood donation by vaccinees (as well as individuals with contact vaccinia) should be deferred until the scab spontaneously separates or 21 days postvaccination, whichever is later.

Under all circumstances, *pre-event* vaccination of civilians is voluntary. A complete information packet for potential vaccinees is available at http://www.bt.cdc.gov/agent/smallpox/vaccination/infopacket.asp (Accessed August 15, 2008).

Typhoid Fever

■ The Pathogen

Salmonella typhi (also known as *Salmonella enterica* subspecies *enterica* serotype Typhi) is a motile, nonlactose-fermenting, gram-negative bacillus. Infection begins in the gut, where the organism invades Peyer's patches, multiplies in macrophages, and disseminates to the mesenteric lymph nodes, reticuloendothelial organs, and ultimately the bloodstream. The Vi capsular antigen interferes with complement binding and enhances virulence. *S typhi* produces a cholera-like toxin that causes efflux of electrolytes and water into the intestinal lumen.

■ Clinical Features

Typhoid fever refers to enteric fever caused by *S typhi*, although other salmonella species can cause a less-severe form of enteric fever. The incubation period is 5 to 21 days depending on inoculum size and health of the host. The onset is insidious, with fever and abdominal pain accompanied by malaise and anorexia. Fever climbs to higher peaks each day, reaching 104°F (40°C) by the end of the first week; interestingly, adults display relative bradycardia for the level of fever. Early on, up to 50% of patients have constipation and 30% diarrhea. Diarrhea is more common in infants and is typically small-volume and pea souplike, containing red blood cells and leukocytes, but not gross blood. During the first week of illness, children complain of headache and often are irritable, drowsy, or delirious. Adults may display psychosis or delirium, and arthralgia and back pain are common. Patients may appear toxic, have meningismus, a coated tongue with musty odor, and a tender doughy abdomen with slight guarding. During the second week of illness, a rash may appear on the abdomen or chest consisting of crops of 10 to 15 salmon-colored, blanching, slightly raised lesions measuring 2 to 4 mm, referred to as *rose spots*. The spleen may be palpable and tender and respiratory symptoms may develop. Untreated, the illness lasts 4 to 6 weeks.

Complications generally occur during the third or fourth week and include intestinal hemorrhage or perforation, which occurs in approximately 3% of patients. The patient's mental status may progress to coma. Additional complications include hepatitis, cholecystitis, arthritis, osteomyelitis, parotitis, endocarditis, myocarditis, pericarditis, pneumonia, meningitis, pyelonephritis, pancreatitis, and orchitis. Laboratory abnormalities include anemia, leukopenia or leukocytosis, thrombocytopenia, and elevated hepatic and muscle enzymes. Relapses occur in 5% to 20% of cases even after appropriate therapy, although they are usually milder than the initial illness. Infants are more likely than adults to develop massive hepatosplenomegaly and thrombocytopenia, and they have a higher mortality rate. However, young children may have *S typhi* bacteremia with mild disease manifestations. Typhoid fever during pregnancy increases the risk of premature labor and spontaneous abortion. Up to 4% of patients who recover from typhoid fever become chronic carriers of *S typhi* and are potential sources of infection for others.

S typhi can also cause nontyphoidal gastroenteritis, bacteremia, and extraintestinal focal infection.

■ Epidemiology and Transmission

There are an estimated 12 to 33 million cases of typhoid fever each year in the world, with the highest incidence in Asia (especially the Indian subcontinent), Central and South America, and Africa. In endemic areas, the annual incidence is as high as 500 to 900 cases per 100,000 people, and the peak is in school-aged children. In developed countries, the incidence is only 0.2 to 3.7 cases per 100,000. Four-hundred cases are reported in the United States each year, with the highest risk among international travelers.

Humans are the only reservoir of *S typhi* and transmission is by the fecal-oral route; the infectious dose is about 10^7 organisms. Patients with cholecystitis or gallstones are especially vulnerable to chronic carriage and may excrete up to 10^9 organisms per gram of stool. Direct person-to-person transmission is unusual; rather, disease spreads through feces-contaminated food or water. For this reason, countries with inadequate sanitation systems, overcrowded living conditions, and limited potable water have the highest rates of disease. Laboratory workers have acquired infection through accidents and health care workers have acquired infection from patients because of poor hand-washing. Occasionally, transplacental transmission occurs from a bacteremic mother to the fetus, and infants may be infected at the time of birth through exposure to bacteria shed in the mother's stool.

■ Background on Immunization Program

Worldwide, approximately 500,000 people die each year of typhoid fever. In endemic areas, aside from the human costs, the direct medical and indirect societal costs are high. Interest in vaccination is highest in areas where antibiotic treatment is not readily available and where antibiotic-resistant strains have increased in prevalence. Outbreaks of multidrug-resistant *S typhi* infection have occurred in the Indian subcontinent, Southeast Asia, and Africa and have been associated with high rates of complications and death. Vaccination might be beneficial for persons at high risk for disease, including children, international travelers, and military personnel. Persons who travel from low-risk to high-risk areas are particularly susceptible because they have not developed immunity through repeated exposure to low doses of *S typhi* over time.

■ **Available Vaccines**

Characteristics of the typhoid fever vaccines licensed in the United States are given in **Table 10.10**.

■ **Efficacy and/or Immunogenicity**

In a clinical trial of TViPSV conducted in Nepal, 3454 subjects received a liquid formulation of the vaccine and 3454 controls received a pneumococcal polysaccharide vaccine. Most subjects were 5 to 44 years of age; 165 children 2 to 4 years of age were included. Efficacy against blood culture–confirmed typhoid fever was 74% during the 20-month follow-up period. In a second trial conducted in South Africa, a lyophilized formulation was evaluated in school children 5 to 15 years of age who received the vaccine ($N = 5692$) or a meningococcal (serogroups A and C) polysaccharide vaccine as placebo ($N = 5692$). Efficacy was 55% against blood culture–confirmed typhoid fever during a 3-year follow-up period. Four-fold or greater increases in antibody to the Vi polysaccharide were seen in 88% to 96% of US adults who received one dose of the vaccine.

The efficacy of Ty21a was first evaluated in Egypt, where 16,486 children aged 6 to 7 years were given 3 doses of a liquid formulation on alternate days; 15,902 children were given placebo. Efficacy was 95% during a 3-year surveillance period. A series of field trials were then performed in Santiago, Chile. The first one, which compared 1 or 2 doses given 1 week apart, involved 82,543 school-aged children. Efficacy at 24 months was 29% and 59%, respectively. Another trial, which compared three doses on alternate days to three doses given 21 days apart, involved 109,594 school-aged children. Efficacy was best in the group that received the shorter schedule, reaching 69% over 4 years and with persistent efficacy demonstrated at 5 years. Subsequent studies established that efficacy was best using a 4-dose, alternate-day regimen.

■ **Safety**

TViPSV causes local tenderness in 97% to 98% of vaccinees; pain is seen in 27% to 41%, induration in 5% to 15%, and erythema in 4% to 5%. Systemic signs and symptoms include malaise (4% to 24%), headache (16% to 20%), myalgia (3% to 7%), and nausea (2% to 8%). Fever $\geq 100°F$ occurs in <2% of vaccinees. Reactogenicity is similar after reimmunization but is less pronounced in children. Postmarketing surveillance in countries where >14 million doses were distributed demonstrated some systemic reactions but very few serious adverse events. From 1995 to 2002, the reporting rate to VAERS for adverse events was 4.5 per 100,000 doses distributed, and for serious adverse events, it was 0.34 per 100,000 doses distributed.

Ty21a is less reactogenic than TViPSV. Symptoms reported during clinical studies included abdominal pain (6%), nausea (6%), headache (5%), fever (3%), diarrhea (3%), vomiting (2%), and rash (1%), but only nausea occurred more frequently than in placebo groups. In field trials involving >500,000 school children, this vaccine did not cause serious adverse reactions. Postmarketing surveillance in the early 1990s, during which time 60 million doses were distributed, revealed only a handful of adverse events and only one serious allergic reaction. From 1991 to 2002, the reporting rate to VAERS for adverse events was 9.7 per 100,000 doses distributed, and for serious adverse events, was 0.59 per 100,000 doses distributed.

- *Contraindications*:
  - Both vaccines: allergic reaction to previous dose of vaccine or any vaccine component
  - Ty21a: immune impairment
- *Precautions*:
  - Both vaccines: moderate or severe acute illness
  - Ty21a: concomitant antibiotics or proguanil therapy (these may inactivate the vaccine)

■ Recommendations

Routine immunization is *not* recommended in the United States. This includes sewage sanitation workers, persons attending rural summer camps, and people living in areas in which natural disasters such as floods have occurred. Further, there is no evidence that typhoid vaccine is useful in controlling common-source outbreaks.

Vaccination *is*, however, recommended for the following groups:
- Travelers to endemic areas (especially developing countries in Latin America, Asia, and Africa) who will have prolonged exposure to potentially contaminated food and water (individuals should be cautioned that vaccination is not a substitute for careful avoidance of contaminated food and drink); typhoid vaccine is not *required* for international travel, but is *recommended*.
- Persons with intimate exposure (eg, household contact) to a documented carrier of *S typhi* (the vaccine cannot be used to *treat* chronic carriers)
- Microbiology laboratory workers who are in frequent contact with *S typhi*
- Persons living in endemic areas outside the United States

There are no data on interchangeability of typhoid vaccines. However, if a booster series is necessary in a person who previously received the inactivated whole-cell vaccine, it is reasonable to give 4 doses of Ty21a or 1 dose of TViPSV. There is no evidence that concomitant administration of either vaccine with other live oral or live or inactivated parenteral vaccines impairs immune responses.

TABLE 10.10 — Typhoid Vaccines[a]

Trade name	Typhim Vi	Vivotif
Abbreviation	TViPSV	Ty21a
Manufacturer/distributor	Sanofi Pasteur	Berna
Type of vaccine	Inactivated, purified subunit	Live attenuated, engineered
Composition	Capsular polysaccharide Vi extracted from strain *Salmonella enterica serovar typhi*, *S typhi* Ty2 Vi polysaccharide (25 mcg)	Strain *Salmonella typhi* Ty21a mutagenized and selected for attenuation 2 to 6.8×10^9 colony-forming units
Adjuvant	None	None
Preservative	Phenol (0.25%)	None
Excipients and contaminants	Polydimethylsiloxane (residual) Fatty-acid ester-based antifoam (residual) Sodium chloride (4.15 mg) Disodium phosphate (0.065 mg) Monosodium phosphate (0.023 mg)	Sucrose (26 to 130 mg) Ascorbic acid (1 to 5 mg) Amino acid mixture (1.4 to 7 mg) Lactose (100 to 180 mg) Magnesium stearate (3.6 to 4.4 mg)
Latex	None	None
Labeled indications	Active immunization against typhoid fever	Immunization against disease caused by *S typhi*
Labeled ages	≥ 2 years	>6 years
Dose	0.5 mL	1 capsule
Route of administration	Intramuscular	Oral (swallow 1 hour before meal with a cold or lukewarm drink)

Labeled schedule	1 dose Booster doses every 2 years (for individuals with continued exposure)	0, 2, 4, 6 days[b] Booster series of 4 doses every 5 years (for individuals with continued exposure)
How supplied (number in package)	20-dose vial (1)	4 capsules in a single foil blister package
Storage	Refrigerate Do not freeze	Refrigerate
Reference package insert	August 2004	August 2006

[a] Typhoid Vaccine USP (Wyeth), a phenol-inactivated, whole-cell vaccine for parenteral administration, is no longer produced.
[b] Some experts recommend repeating the series if all 4 doses are not given within 3 weeks.

10

447

Yellow Fever

■ The Pathogen

Yellow fever virus (YFV) is a flavivirus with a single-stranded RNA genome surrounded by a protein nucleocapsid and a lipid envelope. After inoculation by the bite of an infected mosquito, the virus spreads through lymphatics to the viscera, and viremia ensues. The liver is particularly affected, with the appearance of necrotic masses (Councilman's bodies) in hepatocytes.

■ Clinical Features

YFV infection may be asymptomatic or present as a viral syndrome of varying severity. The classic yellow fever (YF) triad of jaundice, hemorrhage, and albuminuria occurs in 10% to 20% of patients, and the associated case fatality rate is 20% to 50%. The onset of symptoms is abrupt with fever, headache, backache, malaise, myalgia, nausea, vomiting, prostration, photophobia, restlessness, irritability, and dizziness; epistaxis and bleeding from the gums may also occur. Children may experience febrile seizures. Examination reveals congestion of the skin, conjunctivae, and mucous membranes. Leukopenia, albuminuria, and elevated serum transaminase levels may be present. After about 3 days of illness, most patients experience a remission of symptoms, but this may be brief and relapse may occur with prostration, marked venous congestion, extreme bradycardia, severe nausea, vomiting, epigastric pain, jaundice, marked albuminuria and anuria, hematemesis (referred to as *vomito negro*), and melena. The hemorrhagic manifestations may be so severe as to cause hypotension, shock, acidosis, myocardial dysfunction, arrhythmias, and death, usually after 7 to 10 days. CNS signs include delirium, agitation, seizures, stupor, and coma, and complications include pneumonia, parotitis, skin infections, and renal abscesses.

■ Epidemiology and Transmission

Transmission of the *jungle* form of YF involves tree hole–breeding mosquitoes and nonhuman primates in the rain forests of Africa and South America. Humans exposed to the mosquitoes in this environment, such as forestry workers, soldiers, and settlers, may acquire the infection and travel to urban areas where *Aedes aegypti* mosquitoes become infected after feeding on them. These mosquitoes may in turn infect other persons, leading to epidemics of *urban* YF (jungle and urban YF are clinically indistinguishable). *A aegypti* breeds in and around houses and thereby sustains interhuman transmission. YFV is also transmitted vertically from infected female mosquitoes to their offspring. This mode of transmission is important to survival of the virus during prolonged dry periods.

YF occurs throughout sub-Saharan Africa and tropical South America. Epidemics are common in Africa, where approximately 20,000 cases and 5000 deaths were reported between 1986 and

1991. After accounting for underreporting, the true annual number of cases is thought to be about 200,000. Epidemics of YF have reappeared in the urban centers of West Africa and may reappear in tropical urban centers in the Americas in the near future. In South America, approximately 100 cases are reported in forested areas annually. Mass vaccination campaigns and mosquito-control programs have been instituted in South America in an attempt to prevent urban outbreaks. Interestingly, YF has never been reported in Asia.

■ Background on Immunization Program

As with JE, control of mosquitoes and mosquito exposures can reduce the risk of infection, but this is not always possible. From 1986 to 1995, a total of 23,543 cases and 6421 deaths were reported to the WHO, a dramatic increase compared with previous intervals. The case-fatality rate during this same period was 24% in Africa and 64% in South America. Perhaps the most important rationale for vaccination is the risk of reemergence of YF carried by *A aegypti* mosquitoes in urban areas of the Americas. This is a possibility because *A aegypti* infests many areas that are currently free of YF, including coastal regions of South America, the Caribbean, North America, the Middle East, coastal eastern Africa, the Indian subcontinent, Asia, and Australia. Travelers to and expatriates living in tropical Africa and America are candidates for vaccination as well.

■ Available Vaccines

Characteristics of the YF vaccine licensed in the United States are given in **Table 10.11**.

■ Efficacy and/or Immunogenicity

While the efficacy of YF vaccine has never been tested in a controlled clinical trial, numerous observations suggest efficacy. For example, neutralizing antibodies can be demonstrated in 90% of vaccinees in 10 days and in 99% by 30 days. Infection of laboratory workers disappeared after vaccination became routine, and in Brazil and other South American countries, YF only occurs in people who have not been immunized. Immunization during outbreaks results in rapid disappearance of new cases, and high rates of coverage in endemic areas are followed by marked reduction in disease incidence. During an epidemic in Nigeria in 1986, vaccine efficacy was estimated at 85%, although there were important methodologic problems with the assessment. Immunity following vaccination persists for at least 30 to 35 years and probably for life.

■ Safety

Reactions to YF vaccine are typically mild. Studies between 1953 and 1994 showed that <5% of vaccinees experience erythema and pain at the infection site, headaches, and fever, typically 5 to 7 days after immunization. A study in 2001 in 715

TABLE 10.11 — Yellow Fever Vaccine

Trade name	YF-Vax
Abbreviation	YF vaccine
Manufacturer/distributor	Sanofi Pasteur
Type of vaccine	Live attenuated, classical
Composition	YFV strain 17D-204
	Propagated in chick embryos
	$\geq 4.74 \log_{10}$ plaque-forming units
Adjuvant	None
Preservative	None
Excipients and contaminants	Sorbitol
	Gelatin
	Sodium chloride
Latex	Vial stopper contains dry natural latex rubber
Labeled indications	Immunization of persons living in or traveling to endemic areas as well as laboratory personnel
Labeled ages	≥ 9 months
Dose	0.5 mL
Route of administration	Subcutaneous
Labeled schedule	1 dose
	Booster doses every 10 years (for individuals with continued exposure)
How supplied (number in package)	1-dose vial (5), lyophilized, with diluent
	5-dose vial (5), lyophilized, with diluent
Storage	Refrigerate
	Do not freeze
Reference package insert	April 2005

adults demonstrated mild systemic reactions such as headache, myalgia, malaise, and asthenia in 10% to 30% of subjects. The rate of systemic adverse events appears to be higher in older vaccinees.

Two important serious adverse events should be mentioned:

- *Vaccine-associated neurotropic disease*: Formerly known as *postvaccination encephalitis*, this has been reported in 21 persons who received a 17D vaccine strain between 1952 and 2004; 16 cases were in infants ≤ 9 months of age. A study from Senegal estimated the incidence of vaccine-associated neurotropic disease in children 6 months to 2 years of age to be 3 per 100,000, and a study from Kenya estimated the overall incidence to be 5.3 per 1,000,000 vaccinees.

- *Vaccine-associated viscerotropic disease*: Formerly known as *febrile multiple organ-system failure*, this typically begins 2 to 5 days after vaccination and is characterized by fever, myalgia, and headache that progresses to hypotension, respiratory failure, elevated hepatic transaminases, hyperbilirubinemia, lymphocytopenia, thrombocytopenia, and renal failure. There is probably a spectrum of disease ranging from moderate illness with focal organ dysfunction (up to 4% of vaccinees experience mild, transient elevation of hepatic transaminases) to severe disease with multiple organ failure and death. The liver pathology resembles that seen with wild-type YF, but the disease appears to be related to host factors rather than reversion to virulence of the vaccine virus. The risk in the US civilian population has been estimated at 1 per 400,000 doses.

- *Contraindications*:
  - Allergic reaction to previous dose of vaccine or any vaccine component
  - Egg allergy: Being able to eat eggs (even in baked goods) without adverse effects is a reasonable indication of a very low risk of anaphylaxis. Mild or local manifestations of allergy to eggs or feathers are not a contraindication. Skin testing can be done and desensitization may be possible (the procedure is described in the package insert).
  - Age <9 months
  - Immune impairment
- *Precautions*:
  - Moderate or severe acute illness
  - Pregnancy
  - Latex allergy

■ Recommendations

Vaccination is *recommended* for the following individuals:
- Those traveling to or living in areas of South America and Africa where YF is officially reported
- Those traveling outside of urban areas in countries that do not officially report the disease but that lie in YF endemic zones
- Travelers to countries that require a certificate of vaccination against YF
- Laboratory personnel who might be exposed to virulent YFV or to concentrated preparations of the 17D vaccine strain

YF vaccine can only be administered at a site approved by the WHO (the CDC's Division of Global Migration and Quarantine and state and territorial health departments can designate nonfederal vaccination centers). Vaccinees must receive an *International Certificate of Vaccination or Prophylaxis* that has been completed, signed, and validated with the center's stamp. New certificates have been produced since December 15, 2007, in response to a 2005 revision of the International Health Regulations; persons vaccinated before that date may use the old certificate until it expires. Certain countries in Africa require evidence of vaccination from all entering travelers. Some countries waive the requirements for travelers from areas where no evidence of substantial risk exists who will be staying <2 weeks. Certain countries require persons, even if only in transit, to have a valid certificate if they have been in countries either known or thought to have YF, or even where YF does not exist but where *A aegypti* mosquitoes are found. The best advice is to check the web sites listed below before travel.

Because of the risk of vaccine-associated encephalitis, infants <6 months of age should not be vaccinated under any circumstances. Physicians considering immunization of infants between 6 and 9 months of age should contact the Division of Vector-Borne Diseases (970-221-6400) or the Division of Global Migration and Quarantine (404-498-1600) at the CDC. Vaccination of pregnant women may also be considered if travel cannot be postponed and if exposure is very likely, even though this is a live virus vaccine (data from two studies showed that only 1 of 81 infants born to mothers vaccinated during pregnancy had evidence of fetal infection and none had congenital anomalies). However, seroconversion may be markedly reduced, and the CDC should be contacted in these cases as well.

In general, immunosuppressed individuals should not be vaccinated, including those with congenital or acquired immunodeficiency, symptomatic HIV infection, leukemia, lymphoma, generalized malignancy, or those taking corticosteroids, alkylating medications, or antimetabolites, or those undergoing radiation. Patients with HIV infection who are not immunosuppressed can be offered the vaccine. Low-dose (≤20 mg prednisone or equivalent) or short-term (<2 weeks) corticosteroid therapy or intraarticular, bursal, or tendon injections with corticosteroids should not be immunosuppressive. In any circumstance, if international travel requirements are the *only* reason for vaccination of an individual at high risk for vaccine complications, consideration should be given to writing a waiver letter.

There is no evidence that concomitant administration of YF vaccine with vaccines other than cholera impairs immune responses, although all permutations have not been tested. In general, if other live vaccines are not given simultaneously, ≥4 weeks should elapse between them, unless time constraints do not allow. Neither immune globulin nor chloroquine therapy adversely affects antibody responses.

Up-to-date information regarding the risk of YF in various regions and vaccination requirements for travelers can be found at the following sources:
- WHO Yellow Fever home page: http://www.who.int/topics/ yellow_fever/en/index.html (Accessed August 15, 2008)
- CDC Yellow Fever home page: http://www.cdc.gov/ncidod/ dvbid/yellowfever/index.htm (Accessed August 15, 2008)

Diseases for Which Vaccines Are No Longer Available in the United States

Table 10.12 lists vaccines that are no longer available in the United States.

ADDITIONAL READING

Anthrax

Advisory Committee on Immunization Practices. Use of anthrax vaccine in the United States. *MMWR Recomm Rep*. 2000;49(RR-15): 1-20.

Centers for Disease Control and Prevention (CDC). Occupational health guidelines for remediation workers at Bacillus anthracis-contaminated sites—United States, 2001-2002. *MMWR Morb Mortal Wkly Rep*. 2002;51(35):786-789.

Centers for Disease Control and Prevention (CDC). Use of anthrax vaccine in response to terrorism: supplemental recommendations of the Advisory Committee on Immunization Practices. *MMWR Morb Mortal Wkly Rep*. 2002;51(45):1024-1026.

Dixon TC, Meselson M, Guillemin J, Hanna PC. Anthrax. *N Engl J Med*. 1999;341(11):815-826.

Grabenstein JD. Vaccines: countering anthrax: vaccines and immuno-globulins. *Clin Infect Dis*. 2008;46(1):129-136.

Inglesby TV, O'Toole T, Henderson DA, et al; Working Group on Civilian Biodefense. Anthrax as a biological weapon, 2002: updated recommendations for management. *JAMA*. 2002;287(17):2236-2252.

Military Vaccine Agency, Office of the Army Surgeon General. Anthrax vaccine immunization program (AVIP): questions and answers. http://www.anthrax.osd.mil/documents/Anthrax_QA.pdf. Accessed August 15, 2008.

Swartz MN. Recognition and management of anthrax–an update. *N Engl J Med*. 2001;345(22):1621-1626.

Influenza (H5N1)

Writing Committee of the Second World Health Organization Consulta-tion on Clinical Aspects of Human Infection with Avian Influenza A (H5N1) Virus, Abdel-Ghafar AN, Chotpitayasunondh T, Gao Z, et al. Update on avian influenza A (H5N1) virus infection in humans. *N Engl J Med*. 2008;358(3):261-273.

Japanese Encephalitis

Hoke CH, Nisalak A, Sangawhipa N, et al. Protection against Japanese en-cephalitis by inactivated vaccines. *N Engl J Med*. 1988;319(10):608-614.

Inactivated Japanese encephalitis virus vaccine. Recommendations of the Advisory Committee on Immunization Practices (ACIP). *MMWR Recomm Rep*. 1993;42(RR-1):1-15.

TABLE 10.12 — Vaccines That are No Longer Available in the United States

Pathogen	Disease(s)	Vaccine	Comments
Adenovirus types 4 and 7	Epidemic acute respiratory disease and pharyngoconjunctival fever	Live viruses administered orally in an enteric-coated capsule	Produced from 1971 to 1996 Exclusively used in the military
Vibrio cholerae	Cholera	Dukoral (SBL Vaccin AB): oral, inactivated vaccine consisting of recombinant cholera toxin B subunit and heat- and formalin-inactivated V cholerae strains	Immunization is not recommended for any travelers to or from endemic or epidemic areas Parenterally-administered, phenol-inactivated whole cell vaccine is no longer produced
		Orochol (Berna Biotech): oral, live attenuated vaccine consisting of V cholerae strain CVD 103-HgR	
Borrelia burgdorferi	Lyme disease	LYMErix (GlaxoSmithKline): recombinant OspA that induces antibodies that kill the bacteria in the tick after a blood meal	Introduced in 1998 but withdrawn in 2002 because of decreased demand Considered for high-risk individuals
Yersinia pestis	Plague	Formaldehyde-inactivated whole-cell vaccine (Cutter, Greer Laboratories)	Available until 1999
Mycobacterium tuberculosis	Tuberculosis	Bacille Calmette-Guérin	Protective against meningitis and miliary disease

Ruff TA, Eisen D, Fuller A, Kass R. Adverse reactions to Japanese encephalitis vaccine. *Lancet*. 1991;338(8771):881-882.

Shlim DR, Solomon T. Japanese encephalitis vaccine for travelers: exploring the limits of risk. *Clin Infect Dis*. 2002;35(2):183-188.

Tauber E, Kollaritsch H, Korinek M, et al. Safety and immunogenicity of a Vero-cell-derived, inactivated Japanese encephalitis vaccine: a non-inferiority, phase III, randomised controlled trial. *Lancet*. 2007;370(9602):1847-1853.

Thongcharoen P. Japanese encephalitis virus encephalitis: an overview. *Southeast Asian J Trop Med Public Health*. 1989;20(4):559-573.

Rabies

De Serres G, Dallaire F, Côte M, Skowronski DM. Bat rabies in the United States and Canada from 1950 through 2007: human cases with and without bat contact. *Clin Infect Dis*. 2008;46(9):1329-1337.

Manning SE, Rupprecht CE, Fishbein D, et al; Advisory Committee on Immunization Practices Centers for Disease Control and Prevention (CDC). Human rabies prevention–United States, 2008: recommendations of the Advisory Committee on Immunization Practices. *MMWR Recomm Rep*. 2008;57(3):1-28.

Messenger SL, Smith JS, Rupprecht CE. Emerging epidemiology of bat-associated cryptic cases of rabies in humans in the United States. *Clin Infect Dis*. 2002;35(6):738-747.

Moran GJ, Talan DA, Mower W, et al. Appropriateness of rabies postexposure prophylaxis treatment for animal exposures. Emergency ID Net Study Group. *JAMA*. 2000;284(8):1001-1007.

Plotkin SA. Rabies. *Clin Infect Dis*. 2000;30(1):4-12.

Rupprecht CE, Gibbons RV. Clinical practice. Prophylaxis against rabies. *N Engl J Med*. 2004;351(25):2626-2635.

Willoughby RE Jr, Tieves KS, Hoffman GM, et al. Survival after treatment of rabies with induction of coma. *N Engl J Med*. 2005;352(24):2508-2514.

Smallpox

Bozzette SA, Boer R, Bhatnagar V, et al. A model for a smallpox-vaccination policy. *N Engl J Med*. 2003;348(5):416-425.

Casey CG, Iskander JK, Roper MH, et al. Adverse events associated with smallpox vaccination in the United States, January-October 2003. *JAMA*. 2005;294(21):2734-2743.

Frey SE, Couch RB, Tacket CO, et al; National Institute of Allergy and Infectious Diseases Smallpox Vaccine Study Group. Clinical responses to undiluted and diluted smallpox vaccine. *N Engl J Med*. 2002;346(17):1265-1274.

Frey SE, Newman FK, Cruz J, et al. Dose-related effects of smallpox vaccine. *N Engl J Med*. 2002;346(17):1275-1280.

Henderson DA, Inglesby TV, Bartlett JG, et al. Smallpox as a biological weapon: medical and public health management. Working Group on Civilian Biodefense. *JAMA*. 1999;281(22):2127-2137.

Halloran ME, Longini IM Jr, Nizam A, Yang Y. Containing bioterrorist smallpox. *Science*. 2002;298(5597):1428-1432.

Rotz LD, Dotson DA, Damon IK, Becher JA; Advisory Committee on Immunization Practices. Vaccinia (smallpox) vaccine: recommendations of the Advisory Committee on Immunization Practices (ACIP), 2001. *MMWR Recomm Rep*. 2001;50(RR-10):1-25.

Wharton M, Strikas RA, Harpaz R, et al; Advisory Committee on Immunization Practices; Healthcare Infection Control Practices Advisory Committee. Recommendations for using smallpox vaccine in a pre-event vaccination program. Supplemental recommendations of the Advisory Committee on Immunization Practices (ACIP) and the Healthcare Infection Control Practices Advisory Committee (HICPAC). *MMWR Recomm Rep*. 2003;52(RR-7):1-16.

Typhoid Fever

Acharya IL, Lowe CU, Thapa R, et al. Prevention of typhoid fever in Nepal with the Vi capsular polysaccharide of Salmonella typhi. A preliminary report. *N Engl J Med*. 1987;317(18):1101-1104.

Begier EM, Burwen DR, Haber P, Ball R; Vaccine Adverse Event Reporting System Working Group. Postmarketing safety surveillance for typhoid fever vaccines from the Vaccine Adverse Event Reporting System, July 1990 through June 2002. *Clin Infect Dis*. 2004;38(6):771-779.

Ferreccio C, Levine MM, Rodriguez H, Contreras R. Comparative efficacy of two, three, or four doses of TY21a live oral typhoid vaccine in enteric-coated capsules: a field trial in an endemic area. *J Infect Dis*. 1989;159(4):766-769.

Levine MM, Ferreccio C, Black RE, Germanier R. Large-scale field trial of Ty21a live oral typhoid vaccine in enteric-coated capsule formulation. *Lancet*. 1987;1(8541):1049-1052.

Lin FY, Ho VA, Khiem HB, et al. The efficacy of a Salmonella typhi Vi conjugate vaccine in two-to-five-year-old children. *N Engl J Med*. 2001;344(17):1263-1269.

Mahle WT, Levine MM. Salmonella typhi infection in children younger than five years of age. *Pediatr Infect Dis J*. 1993;12(8):627-631.

Parry CM, Hien TT, Dougan G, White NJ, Farrar JJ. Typhoid fever. *N Engl J Med*. 2002;347(22):1770-1782.

Taylor DN, Pollard RA, Blake PA. Typhoid in the United States and the risk to the international traveler. *J Infect Dis*. 1983;148(3):599-602.

Typhoid immunization. Recommendations of the Immunization Practices Advisory Committee (ACIP). *MMWR Recomm Rep*. 1990;39(RR-10):1-5.

Yellow Fever

Barnett ED. Yellow fever: epidemiology and prevention. *Clin Infect Dis*. 2007;44(6):850-856.

Centers for Disease Control and Prevention (CDC). Adverse events associated with 17D-derived yellow fever vaccination—United States, 2001-2002. *MMWR Morb Mortal Wkly Rep.* 2002;51(44):989-993.

Centers for Disease Control and Prevention (CDC). Fever, jaundice, and multiple organ system failure associated with 17D-derived yellow fever vaccination, 1996-2001. *MMWR Morb Mortal Wkly Rep.* 2001;50(30):643-645.

Cetron MS, Marfin AA, Julian KG, et al. Yellow fever vaccine. Recommendations of the Advisory Committee on Immunization Practices (ACIP), 2002. *MMWR Recomm Rep.* 2002;51(RR-17):1-11.

Centers for Disease Control (CDC). Requirements for use of a new International Certificate of Vaccination or Prophylaxis for yellow fever vaccine. *MMWR* 2008;56:1345-1346.

Kitchener S. Viscerotropic and neurotropic disease following vaccination with the 17D yellow fever vaccine, ARILVAX. *Vaccine.* 2004;22(17-18):2103-2105.

Monath TP, Nichols R, Archambault WT, et al. Comparative safety and immunogenicity of two yellow fever 17D vaccines (ARILVAX and YF-VAX) in a phase III multicenter, double-blind clinical trial. *Am J Trop Med Hyg.* 2002;66(5):533-541.

Poland JD, Calisher CH, Monath TP, Downs WG, Murphy K. Persistence of neutralizing antibody 30-35 years after immunization with 17D yellow fever vaccine. *Bull World Health Organ.* 1981;59(6):895-900.

10

Vaccine Resources

(All web sites accessed August 15, 2008)

Governmental Agencies

Centers for Medicare & Medicaid Services (CMS)
http://www.cms.hhs.gov

Department of Defense (DOD)
http://www.defenselink.mil

Department of Health and Human Services
- National Institutes of Health (NIH):
  - National Institute of Allergy and Infectious Diseases (NIAID)
    http://www3.niaid.nih.gov
  - Division of Microbiology and Infectious Diseases (DMID)
    http://www3.niaid.nih.gov/about/organization/dmid
  - Vaccine Research Center (VRC)
    http://www.niaid.nih.gov/vrc/default.htm
  - Vaccine and Treatment Evaluation Units (VTEU)
    http://www.niaid.nih.gov/factsheets/vteu.htm
- Food and Drug Administration (FDA):
  - Center for Biologics Evaluation and Research (CBER)
    http://www.fda.gov/CBER
  - Vaccines and Related Biological Products Advisory Committee (VRBPAC)
    http://www.fda.gov/CBER/advisory/vrbp/vrbpmain.htm
  - Vaccine Adverse Events Reporting System (VAERS, cosponsored by CDC)
    http://vaers.hhs.gov
- Centers for Disease Control and Prevention (CDC):
  - National Center for Immunization and Respiratory Diseases (NCIRD)
    http://www.cdc.gov/vaccines
  - Advisory Committee on Immunization Practices (ACIP)
    http://www.cdc.gov/vaccines/recs/ACIP/default.htm
  - Vaccines for Children Program (VFC)
    http://www.cdc.gov/vaccines/programs/vfc/default.htm
- Health Resources and Services Administration (HRSA):
  - National Vaccine Injury Compensation Program (VICP)
    http://www.hrsa.gov/vaccinecompensation
  - Advisory Commission on Childhood Vaccines (ACCV)
    http://www.hrsa.gov/vaccinecompensation/accv.htm
- National Vaccine Program Office (NVPO)
  http://www.hhs.gov/nvpo
  - National Vaccine Advisory Committee (NVAC)—http://www.hhs.gov/nvpo/nvac

Office of General Counsel (OGC)
http://www.ogc.doc.gov

US Agency for International Development (USAID)
http://www.usaid.gov

International Agencies

Pan American Health Organization (PAHO)
http://www.paho.org/english/ad/fch/im/Vaccines.htm

World Health Organization (WHO)
http://www.who.int/immunization/en

Professional Associations

American Academy of Family Physicians (AAFP)
http://www.aafp.org

American Academy of Pediatrics (AAP)
http://www.cispimmunize.org

American College Health Association (ACHA)
www.acha.org

American Nurses Association (ANA)
http://nursingworld.org

American Pharmacists Association (APhA)
http://www.pharmacist.com

American Public Health Association (APHA)
http://www.apha.org

**Association for Prevention Teaching and Research (APTR)
(formerly the Association of Teachers of Preventive Medicine)**
http://www.atpm.org

Infectious Diseases Society of America (IDSA)
http://www.idsociety.org

Pediatric Infectious Diseases Society (PIDS)
http://www.pids.org

Advocacy, Implementation, and Safety

All Kids Count
http://www.allkidscount.org

Allied Vaccine Group
http://www.vaccine.org

Brighton Collaboration
http://www.brightoncollaboration.org

Children's Hospital of Philadelphia Vaccine Education Center
http://www.vaccine.chop.edu

Children's Vaccine Program at PATH
http://www.childrensvaccine.org

Clinical Immunization Safety Assessment Network (CISA)
http://www.vaccinesafety.org

Every Child by Two (ECBT)
http://www.ecbt.org

Vaccinate Your Baby
http://www.vaccinateyourbaby.org

Global Alliance for Vaccines and Immunization (GAVI)
http://www.gavialliance.org

Immunization Action Coalition (IAC)
http://www.immunize.org

Institute for Vaccine Safety, Johns Hopkins Bloomberg School of Public Health
http://www.vaccinesafety.edu

National Foundation for Infectious Diseases (NFID)
http://www.nfid.org

National Network for Immunization Information (NNii)
http://www.immunizationinfo.org

Parents of Kids With Infectious Diseases (PKID)
http://www.pkids.org

Sabin Vaccine Institute (SVI)
http://www.sabin.org

Voices for Vaccines
http://www.voicesforvaccines.org

Coverage and Assessment

Behavioral Risk Factor Surveillance System (BRFSS)
http://www.cdc.gov/brfss

Comprehensive Clinic Assessment Software Application (CoCASA)
http://www.cdc.gov/vaccines/programs/cocasa

Healthcare Effectiveness Data and Information Set (HEDIS)
http://web.ncqa.org/tabid/59/Default.aspx

National Health Interview Survey (NHIS)
http://www.cdc.gov/nchs/nhis.htm

National Immunization Survey (NIS)
http://www.cdc.gov/nis

National Notifiable Diseases Surveillance System (NNDSS)
http://www.cdc.gov/ncphi/disss/nndss/nndsshis.htm

Books

Allen A. *Vaccine: The Controversial Story of Medicine's Greatest Lifesaver*. New York: WW Norton; 2008.

Arguin PM, Kozarsky PE, Reed C. *CDC Health Information for International Travel 2008*. St Louis, MO: Elsevier; 2007.

Atkinson W, Hamborsky J, McIntyre L, Wolfe C. *Epidemiology and Prevention of Vaccine-Preventable Diseases.* 10th ed. Washington, DC: Public Health Foundation; 2007.

Colgrove J. *State of Immunity: The Politics of Vaccination in Twentieth-Century America*. Berkeley, CA: University of California Press; 2006.

Gold R. *Your Child's Best Shot: A Parent's Guide to Vaccination*. Ottawa, Ontario; Canadian Paediatric Society; 2006.

Myers MG, Pineda D. *Do Vaccines Cause That?! A Guide for Evaluating Vaccine Safety Concerns*. Galveston, TX: Immunizations for Public Health; 2008.

Offit P. *The Cutter Incident: How America's First Polio Vaccine Led to the Growing Vaccine Crisis*. New Haven, CT: Yale University Press; 2007.

Offit PA. *Vaccinated: One Man's Quest to Defeat the World's Deadliest Diseases*. New York: HarperCollins Publishers; 2007.

Offit PA, Bell LM. *Vaccines: What You Should Know*. Hoboken, NJ: John Wiley & Sons, Inc; 2003.

Oshinsky DM. *Polio: An American Story*. New York; Oxford University Press; 2006.

Pickering, LK, ed. *Red Book: 2006 Report of the Committee on Infectious Diseases*. 27th ed. Elk Grove Village, IL: American Academy of Pediatrics; 2006.

Plotkin SA, Orenstein WA, Offit PA. *Vaccines*. 5th ed. St Louis, MO: Elsevier; 2008.

Manufacturers

Acambis
http://www.acambis.com

Berna Biotech
http://www.bernabiotech.ch

Bioport
http://www.bioport.com

CSL Biotherapies
http://www.cslbiotherapies-us.com

GlaxoSmithKline
http://www.gsk.com

MedImmune
http://www.medimmune.com

Merck
http://www.merck.com

Novartis
http://www.novartis.com

Sanofi Pasteur
http://www.sanofipasteur.com

Wyeth
http://www.wyeth.com

State Health Department Immunization Programs

State health department web sites can be accessed through the following URL: http://www.cdc.gov/mmwr/international/relres .html.

11

12   Abbreviations/Nomenclature

AAFP	American Academy of Family Physicians
AAP	American Academy of Pediatrics
ACCV	Advisory Commission on Childhood Vaccines
ACHA	American College Health Association
ACIP	Advisory Committee on Immunization Practices
AIDS	acquired immune deficiency syndrome
AOM	acute otitis media
ANA	American Nurses Association
APC	antigen-presenting cell
APhA	American Pharmaceutical Association
APHA	American Public Health Association
ASD	autistic-spectrum disorder
ATPM	Association of Teachers of Preventive Medicine
AVG	Allied Vaccine Group
BCG	Bacille Calmette-Guérin (tuberculosis vaccine)
BIG	botulism immune globulin
BLA	Biologics License Application
BRFSS	Behavioral Risk Factor Surveillance System
cAMP	cyclic adenosine monophosphate
CASA	Clinical Assessment Software Application
CBER	Center for Biologics Evaluation and Research
CDC	Centers for Disease Control and Prevention
CHD	congenital heart disease
CI	confidence interval
CISA	Clinical Immunization Safety Assessment (Network)
CLD	chronic lung disease (bronchopulmonary dysplasia)
CMS	Centers for Medicare and Medicaid Services, formerly known as the Health Care Financing Administration (HCFA)
CMV	cytomegalovirus
CMV-IGIV	cytomegalovirus immune globulin, intravenous
CNS	central nervous system
CPT	Current Procedural Terminology
CRM_{197}	cross-reactive material (a mutant diphtheria toxin)
CSF	cerebrospinal fluid
CTL	cytotoxic T lymphocyte
DHHS	Department of Health and Human Services
DMEM	Dulbecco's Modified Eagle Medium
DMID	Division of Microbiology and Infectious Diseases
DNA	deoxyribonucleic acid
DOD	Department of Defense
DT	diphtheria, tetanus vaccine (infant/child formulation)
DTaP	diphtheria, tetanus, acellular pertussis vaccine (infant/child formulation)

DTwP...................diphtheria, tetanus, whole-cell pertussis vaccine
EBV.................Epstein Barr virus
EDTA ....ethylene diamine tetraacetic acid
EMLA ....eutectic mixture of local anesthetic
EMTs...................emergency medical technicians
EPA.....................Environmental Protection Agency
ETEC...................enterotoxigenic *Escherichia coli*
FDA.....................(US) Food and Drug Administration
FHA.....................filamentous hemagglutinin
FIM ....fimbriae (also known as agglutinogens)
FQHC..................federally qualified health center
GAS.....................group A streptococcus
GCP.....................Good Clinical Practices
GI ....gastrointestinal
GLP ....Good Laboratory Practices
GMP...................Good Manufacturing Practices
GVHD.................graft-versus-host disease
HA......................hemagglutin
HAV ....hepatitis A virus
HBIG..................hepatitis B immune globulin
HbOC ....polyribosylribotol phosphate (the capsular polysaccharide
                         of *Haemophilus influenzae* type b) conjugated to mutant
                         diphtheria protein CRM_{197}
HBsAb.................antibody to hepatitis B surface antigen
HBsAg.................hepatitis B surface antigen
HBV ....hepatitis B virus
HCFA ....Health Care Financing Administration, now known as the
                         Centers for Medicare and Medicaid Services (CMS)
HCP.....................health care personnel
HDCV ....human diploid cell vaccine
HEDIS.................Health Plan Employer Data and Information Set
HepA ....hepatitis A vaccine
HepB ....hepatitis B vaccine
HEPES ....N-2-hydroxyethylpiperazine-N'2-ethanesulfonic acid
HHS.....................(Department of) Health and Human Services
Hib.......................*Haemophilus influenzae* type b vaccine
HICPAC ....Healthcare Infection Control Practices Advisory Committee
HIPAA.................Health Insurance Portability and Accountability Act
HIV......................human immunodeficiency virus
HKML.................heat-killed *Mycobacterium leprae*
HPV.....................human papillomavirus virus
HPV2...................human papillomavirus vaccine, 2-valent
HPV4...................human papillomavirus vaccine, 4-valent
HRIG...................human rabies immune globulin
HRV ....(live-attenuated) human rotavirus vaccine
HSCT ....hematopoietic stem cell transplant
IAC......................Immunization Action Coalition
IBD......................inflammatory bowel disease

ICD-9-CM	International Classification of Diseases, 9th Revision, Clinical Modification
IDSA	Infectious Diseases Society of America
IG	immune globulin
IgE	immunoglobulin E
IgG	immunoglobulin G
IGIM	(polyclonal) immune globulin, intramuscular
IGIV	(polyclonal) immune globulin, intravenous
IgM	immunoglobulin M
IIS	Immunization Information Systems (also known as registries)
IM	intramuscular
IN	intranasal
IOM	Institute of Medicine
IPV	inactivated poliovirus vaccine
ISRC	Immunization Safety Review Committee
ITP	immune thrombocytopenic purpura
IU	international unit
IV	intravenous
JEV	Japanese encephalitis virus
KNOW	Kids Need Options With Vaccines
LAIV	live-attenuated influenza virus vaccine
LEP	low egg passage
LRI	lower respiratory infection
MCD	mad cow disease
MCV4	meningococcal conjugate vaccine, 4-valent
MHC	major histocompatibility complex
MMR	measles, mumps, rubella vaccine
MMRV	measles, mumps, rubella, varicella vaccine
MPSV4	meningococcal polysaccharide vaccine, 4-valent
MR	measles, rubella vaccine
MRI	magnetic resonance imaging
MS	multiple sclerosis
NCES	National Childhood Encephalopathy Study
NCIRD	National Center for Immunization and Respiratory Diseases
NCQA	National Committee on Quality Assurance
NCVIA	National Childhood Vaccine Injury Act
NDC	National Drug Code
NHIS	National Health Interview Survey
NIAID	National Institute of Allergy and Infectious Diseases
NIH	National Institutes of Health
NIP	National Immunization Program
NIS	National Immunization Survey
NNDSS	National Notifiable Disease Surveillance System
NNii	National Network for Immunization Information
NVAC	National Vaccine Advisory Committee
NVPO	National Vaccine Program Office
NVSN	New Vaccine Surveillance Network

12

OGC ....Office of General Counsel
OPV...................oral polio vaccine
OSHA................Occupational Safety and Health Administration
PAHO ....Pan American Health Organization
PAVE ....People Advocating Vaccine Education
PCECV................purified chick embryo cell vaccine
PCV7 ....pneumococcal conjugate vaccine, 7-valent
PDD...................pervasive developmental disorder
PDD...................pervasive developmental disorder
PDUFA...............Prescription Drug User Fee Act
PFU ....plague-forming units
PHN.................postherpetic neuralgia
PHS ....(US) Public Health Service
PI.......................package insert (also known as product information)
PIV3 ....(bovine) parainfluenza virus type 3
PO ....per os (orally by mouth)
PPSV23 ....pneumococcal polysaccharide vaccine, 23-valent
PRN...................pertactin
PROVE ....Parents Requesting Open Vaccine Education
PRP....................polyribosylribitol phosphate
PRP-D ....polyribosylribitol phosphate (the capsular polysaccharide of *Haemophilus influenzae* type b) conjugated to diphtheria toxoid
PRP-OMPC.........polyribosylribitol phosphate (*Haemophilus influenzae* type b)–meningococcal outer membrane protein conjugate vaccine
PRP-T................polyribosylribitol phosphate (*Haemophilus influenzae* type b)–tetatus protein conjugate vaccine
PRV ....pentavalent (bovine) rotavirus vaccine
PS ....(capsular) polysaccharide
PT ....pertussis toxin
QALY.................quality-adjusted life year
RBC....................red blood cell
RET ....Reportable Events Table
RHC ....rural health clinic
RhoGAM.............Rho(D) immune globulin
RIG.....................rabies immune globulin
RNA ....ribose nucleic acid
RR ....relative risk
RRV-TV ....rhesus-human reassortant rotavirus vaccine-tetravalent
RSV....................respiratory syncytial virus
RSV-IGIV ....respiratory syncytial virus immune globulin, intravenous
RSVmAB ....respiratory syncytial virus monoclonal antibody
RVU ....relative value unit
SC.......................subcutaneous
SCHIP ....State Children's Health Insurance Program
SIDS...................sudden infant death syndrome
SIV ....simian immunodeficiency virus
sp ....species

TB	tuberculosis
Tc	cytotoxic T cells
$TCID_{50}$	median tissue culture infective dose
TCR	T-cell receptor
Td	tetanus, diphtheria vaccine (adolescent/adult formulation)
Tdap	tetanus, diphtheria, acellular pertussis vaccine (adolescent/adult formulation)
TFSCV	Task Force on Safer Childhood Vaccines
TIG	tetanus immune globulin
TIV	trivalent inactivated influenza virus vaccine
tRNA	transfer ribonucleic acid
TST	tuberculin skin test, formerly referred to as PPD (purified protein derivative)
TT	tetanus toxoid
TViPSV	typhoid Vi polysaccharide vaccine
Ty21a	(oral) typhoid vaccine
URI	upper respiratory infection
US$	United States currency
USAID	US Agency for International Development
USAMRIID	US Army Medical Research Institute of Infectious Diseases
USP	United States Pharmacopoeial Convention
v/v	percent by volume in volume (mL per 100 mL of solution)
VAERS	Vaccine Adverse Event Reporting System
VAR	varicella
VariZIG	varicella-zoster immune globulin
VFC	Vaccines for Children (Program)
VICP	(National) Vaccine Injury Compensation Program
VIG	vaccinia immune globulin
VIS	Vaccine Information Statement
VIT	Vaccine Injury Table
VLP	virus-like particle
VRAN	Vaccination Risk Awareness Network
VRBPAC	Vaccines and Related Biological Products Advisory Committee
VRC	(Dale and Betty Bumpers) Vaccine Research Center
VSD	Vaccine Safety DataLink
VTEU	Vaccine and Treatment Evaluation Unit
VZV	varicella-zoster virus
WBC	white blood cell
WHO	World Health Organization
WI-38	human lung fibroblast (cell)
WIC	(US Department of Agriculture's Special Supplemental Nutrition Program for) Women, Infants and Children
YFV	yellow fever virus

12

TABLE 12.1 — Vaccine and Infectious Agent Nomenclature

	Infectious Agents		
Disease	**Name**	**Abbreviation**	**Vaccine Designation(s)**
Anthrax	*Bacillus anthracis*	*B anthracis*	Anthrax vaccine
Diphtheria, tetanus (lockjaw), pertussis (whooping cough)	*Corynebacterium diphtheriae* *Clostridium tetani* *Bordetella pertussis*	*C diphtheriae* *C tetani* *B pertussis*	DTwP, DTaP, Tdap, DT, Td, TT
Haemophilus influenzae type b (invasive)	*H influenzae* type b	*H influenzae* type b	Hib (PRP-OMPC, PRP-T)
Hepatitis A	Hepatitis A virus	HAV	HepA
Hepatitis B	Hepatitis B virus	HBV	HepB
Human papillomavirus–induced cervical cancer and genital warts	Human papillomavirus	HPV	HPV2, HPV4[a]
Influenza	Influenza virus	—	TIV, LAIV
Japanese encephalitis	Japanese encephalitis virus	JEV	JE vaccine
Measles, mumps, rubella	Measles virus Mumps virus Rubella virus	—	MMR
Meningococcal meningitis and sepsis	*Neisseria meningitidis*	*N meningitidis*	MCV4, MPSV4[a]
Pneumococcal pneumonia, meningitis, and sepsis	*Streptococcus pneumoniae*	*S pneumoniae*	PCV7, PPSV23[a]
Polio	Poliovirus	—	IPV, OPV

470

Disease	Organism		Vaccine
Rabies	Rabies virus	—	Rabies vaccine
Rotavirus gastroenteritis	Rotavirus	—	PRV, HRV
Smallpox	Variola virus	—	Smallpox vaccine (vaccinia)
Tuberculosis	*Mycobacterium tuberculosis*	*M tuberculosis*	BCG
Typhoid fever	*Salmonella typhi*	*S typhi*	TViPSV, Ty21a
Varicella (chickenpox)	Varicella zoster virus	VZV	Varicella vaccine
Yellow fever	Yellow fever virus	YFV	YF vaccine
Zoster (shingles)	Varicella zoster virus	VZV	Zoster vaccine
Modern combination vaccines[b]			HepB-Hib
			DTaP/Hib
			DTaP-IPV/Hib
			DTaP-IPV
			DTaP-HepB-IPV
			MMRV
			HepA-HepB

[a] Numbers indicate the valency of the vaccine. For example, HPV2 contains two serotypes (16 and 18), whereas HPV4 contains four serotypes (6, 11, 16, 18).

[b] Dashes indicate that the components are premixed (eg, DTaP-HepB-IPV); slash marks indicate that the components must be combined prior to administration (eg, DTaP/Hib, where liquid DTaP/Hib is used to reconstitute the lyophilized Hib).

12

Note: Page numbers in *italics* indicate figures.
Page numbers followed by a "t" indicate tables.

13

13

13

13

13

13

13

13

13

13

13

13

13

13

13

13

13

13

13